# RABIES

# RABIES

Proceedings of Working Conference on Rabies sponsored
by the Japan-United States Cooperative Medical Science Program

edited by
YASUITI NAGANO
and
FRED M. DAVENPORT



UNIVERSITY PARK PRESS
Baltimore • London • Tokyo

UTP 3047-67581-5149
Printed in Japan



Originally published in 1971 by
University of Tokyo Press

UNIVERSITY PARK PRESS
Baltimore • London • Tokyo

**Library of Congress Cataloging in Publication Data**

Working Conference on Rabies, Tokyo, 1970
Rabies: proceedings.
Sponsored by the Japan-United States Cooperative Medical Science Program.
Includes bibliographical references.
1. Rabies—Congresses. I. Nagano, Yasuiti, 1906– ed. II. Davenport, Fred M., 1914– ed. III. United States-Japan Cooperative Medical Science Program. IV. Title.
RC148.W68 1970 616.9'53 72-37006
ISBN 0-8391-0624-6

# LIST OF CONTRIBUTORS

ANUSKIEWICZ, W.
Microbiology Research Section, Cutter Laboratories, Berkeley, California, U.S.A.
BERAN, George W.
Silliman University, Dumaguete City, Negros Oriental, Philippines
CABASSO, V. J.
Microbiology Research Section, Cutter Laboratories, Berkeley, California, U.S.A.
CONSTANTINE, Denny G.
Cell Culture Laboratory, Naval Biomedical Research Laboratory, Oakland, California, U.S.A.
EMMONS, Richard W.
Viral and Rickettsial Disease Laboratory, California State Department of Public Health, Berkeley, California, U.S.A.
FENJE, Paul
Connaught Medical Research Laboratories, Toronto, Canada
HADDOCK, Robert L.
Department of Public Health and Social Services, Government of Guam, Agana, Guam
HUMPHREY, George L.
Veterinary Section, California State Department of Public Health, Berkeley, California, U.S.A.
ISHII, Keizo
Central Virus Diagnostic Laboratory, National Institute of Health, Murayama, Tokyo, Japan
JOHNSON, Harald N.
Viral and Rickettsial Disease Laboratory, California State Department of Public Health, Berkeley, California, U.S.A.
JOHNSON, Richard T.
Department of Neurology, The Johns Hopkins Hospital, Baltimore, Maryland, U.S.A.
KITAMOTO, Osamu
The Institute of Medical Science, University of Tokyo, Tokyo, Japan
KOPROWSKI, Hilary
The Wistar Institute of Anatomy & Biology, Philadelphia, Pennsylvania, U.S.A.
LENNETTE, Edwin H.
Viral and Rickettsial Disease Laboratory, California State Department of Public Health, Berkeley, California, U.S.A.
LOOFBOUROW, J. C.
Office of Occupational Medicine, Cowell Student Health Center, University of California, Davis, Davis, California, U.S.A.
NAGANO, Yasuiti
Virus Laboratory, The Kitasato Institute, Tokyo, Japan
NAKAMURA, Junji
Nippon Institute for Biological Science, Tachikawa, Tokyo, Japan
NOBUTO, Kenzo
Animal Health Division, Bureau of Animal Industry, Ministry of Agriculture and Forestry, Tokyo, Japan
NOMURA, Yoshitoshi
Nippon Institute for Biological Science, Tachikawa, Tokyo, Japan

Otani, S.
The Institute of Medical Science, University of Tokyo, Tokyo, Japan
Póstic, Bosko
University of Pittsburgh, Pittsburgh, Pennsylvania, U.S.A.
Roby, R. E.
Microbiology Research Section, Cutter Laboratories, Berkeley, California, U.S.A.
Shibuki, M.
The Institute of Medical Science, University of Tokyo, Tokyo, Japan
Shimada, Koji
Yakult Institute for Microbiological Research, Kunitachi, Tokyo, Japan
Shiraki, Hirotsugu
Department of Neuropathology, Institute of Brain Research, Faculty of Medicine, University of Tokyo, Tokyo, Japan
Shope, Robert E.
The Yale Arbovirus Research Unit, Department of Epidemiology and Public Health, Yale University School of Medicine, New Haven, Connecticut, U.S.A.
Sikes, Keith R.
Viral Zoonoses Section, National Communicable Diseases Center, Lawrenceville, Georgia, U.S.A.
Tierkel, Ernest S.
Office of the Assistant Secretary for Health and Scientific Affairs, Department of Health & Education, Washington, D.C., U.S.A.
Tignor, Gregory H.
The Yale Arbovirus Research Unit, Department of Epidemiology and Public Health, Yale University School of Medicine, New Haven, Connecticut, U.S.A.
Wiktor, T. J.
The Wistar Institute of Anatomy & Biology, Philadelphia, Pennsylvania, U.S.A.

# PREFACE

Today, with the ption exceof Oceania and the Antarctic, the whole world is harassed by the threat of rabies. Although the exact number is not known, several thousand people die of rabies each year. The number of persons receiving prophylactic vaccine, that is, the number of persons in danger of rabies infection, is over one million a year. The number of domestic dogs, cats and other pets and wild animals, such as foxes, found to be rabid has been increasing yearly.

Rabies thus poses a major threat to mankind, and its total eradication greatly desired. Yet, although the disease has been known to mankind since ancient times, there are still many aspects of rabies which are not understood.

For example, we do not know how rabies epizootics occur among wild animals nor do we know a sure way to eradicate such epizootics. Only recently did we learn of the airborne transmission of rabies from bats to humans.

In postwar Japan, a major rabies outbreak lasted until 1956, however, for the past 15 years there have been no outbreaks among humans or animals. Since there is no wild life reservoir of rabies in Japan, our only concern is the control of rabies in the dog population. The vaccination of dogs has been vigorously enforced and in 1956, the last year of the outbreak, more than half of the 1,600,000 registered dogs in Japan were vaccinated. However, the major source of infection was unregistered dogs, estimated to number between 1 and 1.5 million at the time. It is hard to believe that the vaccination of a little over half the registered dogs checked the spread of rabies in the total dog population, but there is no other credible explanation.

The advisability of injecting immune serum together with postbite vaccine inoculation is still a source of controversy.

To prevent rabies infection, the replication of the virus in the central nervous system must be stopped. The best method would be to prevent the virus from ever reaching the central nervous system. However, we do not know whether the rabies virus is transmitted to the central nervous system through the peripheral nerves or through the blood circulation.

There are numerous other matters which need to be investigated and clarified before rabies can be eradicated. The Japan-U.S. Cooperative Medical Science Program, Panel on Viral Diseases held a working conference in Tokyo on October 12, 13 and 14, 1970, to promote research on rabies. This volume comprises the proceedings of that conference.

I would like to express my gratitude to Prof. M. Matumoto of the University of Tokyo, Dr. K. O. Phifer of the National Institutes of Health, U.S.A. and Miss H. Komatsu of The Kitasato Institute for their editorial assistance.

October, 1971 Yasuiti NAGANO

# CONTENTS

# RABIES

# Historical Review of Rabies in Asia

Ernest S. Tierkel

*Office of the Assistant Secretary for Health and Scientific Affairs, Department of Health and Education, Washington, D.C. 20201*

Perhaps the earliest reference to rabies in Asia is one that occurs in the pre-Mosaic Eshnunna Code which predates the better known code of Hammurabi of ancient Babylon in the twenty-third century B.C. In this code the following excerpt is found: "If a dog is mad the authorities have brought the fact to the knowledge of its owner; if he does not keep it in, it bites a man and causes his death, then the owner shall pay two-thirds of a mina (40 shekels) of silver. If it bites a slave and causes his death he shall pay 15 shekels of silver."

Activity in the study of rabies in Asia began in the post-Pasteurian period about the turn of this century. Institutes were established in a number of Asian countries, the most notable of which were in India (Kasauli, Coonoor), Indochina (Saigon, Hanoi), Iran (Teheran), and Java (Bandung). Most of these served as centers for the production of rabies vaccine and also for administration of the vaccine to exposed people. As methods for the preservation and distribution of rabies vaccine improved over the years, many of the Asian countries began to decentralize rabies treatment centers making it no longer necessary for exposed persons to undertake long voyages for anti-rabies vaccination regimens.

At least two notable original contributions to the prevention and control of rabies have emanated out of this historical backdrop of rabies research in Asian institutes. The first was from India in 1919 when David Semple, at Kasauli, introduced the first vaccine produced from fixed rabies virus inactivated by treatment of heat and phenol. The Semple vaccine eventually became the biologic of choice in many countries of both the eastern and western hemispheres. The other contribution was the development and utilization of the first practical vaccine for dogs in 1921 by the Japanese workers, S. Umeno and Y. Doi. The success of this canine vaccine, a phenolized rabbit brain product, stimulated interest in trials of dog vaccination in the United States which led ultimately to the eminently effective use of single-dose canine vaccination for the control of dog rabies.

Definitive information on the status of rabies in Asian countries was first made possible by the annual World Rabies Survey begun in 1959 by the Veterinary Public Health Unit of the World Health Organization. The data collected in these annual surveys are based upon replies to a questionnaire (Annex) sent to each member country. The questionnaire requests data relating to the incidence of rabies in animals and man, the incriminating animal vector species, the number of human post-exposure immunizations administered (with and without serum), the number and types of reactions to biological prophylaxis, rabies mortality in treated and untreated individuals and the types and quantity of rabies vaccine produced for use in man and animals.

It is interesting to note that in the decade covered by annual WHO surveys (1958 through 1968), the same five areas continued to report that they were free of rabies. These are Taiwan, Hong Kong, Japan, Malaysia, and Singapore. Taiwan reported that the last case in man was identified on 28 December 1958 and the last case in a dog on 8 March 1959. The last case reported in Hong Kong was in a dog in November 1955; in Malaysia, in January 1958; in Singapore, in a dog in 1953; and in Japan the last human case was diagnosed 16 April 1954 and the last canine case, August 26, 1956. Malaysia has continued to be reported as a rabies-free area, but has reported occasional animal cases and human exposures in its northernmost province.

Included in the responses to the annual questionnaires are comments from the rabies endemic countries which point out that the morbidity and mortality statistics indicated in their reports by no means reflect the actual experience in rabies in their countries. The meager data available to the respondants for the most part cover only those cases in man and animals which occur in areas near institutes engaged in rabies work.

Of those countries in Asia where rabies has continued to be a major communicable disease problem, the two which stand out are India and the Philippines, especially in terms of human mortality. Other countries recognizing it as a sizable problem are Thailand, Burma, Pakistan, Ceylon, Indonesia, and Vietnam. The eighth WHO report (1966) points out the variance in Thailand between the nineteen officially reported human cases and the unofficial observation of several hundred during the year. This discrepancy between official and unofficial data is common in most countries and is, of course, a reflection of the poorly developed surveillance network in communicable diseases. Burma declared, at the WHO regional seminar on zoonoses in Southeast Asia last year, that the SEARO of WHO should review its communicable disease activities, citing that rabies control programs should be given higher priority in the assignment of projects. Sporadic outbreaks and incidents have been reported in Laos, Cambodia, and Korea.

The following highlights have been recorded regarding the spread of rabies in each of the reporting countries: Cambodia feels that the disease is endemic throughout the country even though most cases have been diagnosed in and around Phnom Penh because of the availability of nearby diagnostic services. In India the disease has been distributed rather ubiquitously throughout the country and indeed seems to be on the increase in some areas. The Philippines reports that the disease is endemic and that cases occur in all provinces. Korea reports moderate incidence throughout the country. In Laos the disease has been identified in the urban regions of Vientiane and Luang Prabang. Mongolia reports an increase of the spread of rabies in the Central Region, particularly in wildlife. In Pakistan the disease has been occurring endemically in both eastern and western wings of the country with no special trend of its spread. Ceylon reports highest incidence of rabies in the Western Province, with the city of Colombo and the Central Province next in incidence rank. Vietnam has reported that the rabies problem has grown in the urban centers of the country.

In all of the Asian countries, dogs have been identified as the principal vector animal in transmission to man and other animals. Among the wild fauna most often implicated as both vectors and natural reservoirs are wolves in Iran; wolves and jackals in Afghanistan; jackals in Pakistan and Nepal; jackals and mongooses in India; khorsacs (a small steppe fox) in Mongolia.

The great majority of Asian countries reported Semple vaccine as the type of vaccine produced for use in post-exposure immunization of man, with little or no change in the ten year period from 1958 to 1968. The areas listing production of Semple vaccine in the first report (1958) were Burma, Cambodia, Taiwan, Hong Kong, India, Indonesia, Iran, Malaya, Philippines and Thailand. Japan reported producing ultraviolet irradiated as well as Semple type vaccine. In the tenth report (1968), the survey revealed that Fermi type vaccine was produced in East Pakistan, Japan, and presumably in Afghanistan, whereas Semple vaccine was produced in West Pakistan. Taiwan and Japan reported producing U-V vaccine. Sheep and goats have served as the animal of choice for the production of these brain tissue vaccines in all of the Asian countries except Indonesia which has used monkeys as the source of vaccine production. In Japan, Thailand, and Taiwan rabbit brain is also used for human rabies vaccine. The production of anti-rabies serum for passive immunization in severe exposures seems to have been limited over the ten year period to Taiwan, Japan, India, Indonesia, Iran, and Thailand. All of these centers produced equine hyperimmune antiserum.

With the exception of Japan, Taiwan, and to some extent, Korea, Ceylon and Thailand, most of the vaccine produced for animal use in the Asian countries had been for post-exposure immunization of exposed animals. Single dose pre-exposure prophylaxis of dogs has played a minor role in the rabies control activities of a majority of the Asian countries. Successful demonstrations of mass canine vaccination programs have been made by countries including Japan, Malayasia, Taiwan, and the eastern province of the island of Negros in the Philippines, and to varying degrees, cities like Bangkok and Colombo. A variety of types of animal vaccines have been produced in Asia. Like the human product, most of it has been the Semple vaccine produced in sheep and goat brains. Besides the latter, Japan, for instance, has produced goat brain vaccine inactivated by ultraviolet irradiation and by thimerosal for use in animals. Afghanistan has made Fermi type sheep brain vaccine for animals. Burma, India (Coonoor), Korea and West Pakistan have produced varying quantities of LEP Flury vaccine for use in dogs.

In 1958 a preponderence of areas in Asia reported using the Sellers stain and tissue-impression technique, along with animal innoculation, usually the mouse, as the standard techniques for laboratory diagnosis of rabies. In the early 60s a few institutes experimented with complement fixation and gel-diffusion techniques. Some began to add the serum-virus neutralization test for ultimate confirmatory diagnosis. By the time the tenth report was made available, a good many of the major institutes and laboratories in Asian countries had begun to use the fluorescent antibody test for identification of the rabies virus in tissue specimens submitted for diagnosis.

It seems appropriate to note in closing that one of the greatest contributing factors of the past in the standardization and adoption of effective techniques of diagnosis, vaccine production, immunization practices and control methods was the highly successful WHO working conference on rabies for countries of Asia held at Coonoor, India, in July 1952.

## RABIES QUESTIONNAIRE NO. 11

(covering the year 1969)

Last date for completion and return (one copy only) to the following address, 31 October: 1970:

Chief, Veterinary Public Health
World Health Organization
Avenue Appia
1211 Geneva 27
Switzerland

1. Name and address of laboratory, institute, medical or veterinary service:

2. (a) Is rabies now present in your country? . . . . . . . . . . .
   (b) If present, does this represent an introduction during 1969?
   If so, how was it introduced? . . . . . . . . . . . . .
   . . . . . . . . . . . . . . . . . . . . . . . . . . . . . . . . . . . . . .

3. If rabies is present in your country
   (a) Which animal species have been found rabid in 1969? Please indicate the number of reported cases in each species, if known.

| Name of animal | No. | Name of animal | No. |
|---|---|---|---|
| . . . . . . | . . . | . . . . . . | . . . |
| . . . . . . | . . . | . . . . . . | . . . |
| . . . . . . | . . . | . . . . . . | . . . |

   (b) Which animals were the most important sources of bite wounds for man that required rabies prophylactic treatment?

| Name of animal | No. of humans who received rabies treatment | Name of animal | No. of humans who received rabies treatment |
|---|---|---|---|
| . . . . . . | . . . . . . | . . . . . . | . . . . . . |
| . . . . . . | . . . . . . | . . . . . . | . . . . . . |
| . . . . . . | . . . . . . | . . . . . . | . . . . . . |
| . . . . . . | . . . . . . | . . . . . . | . . . . . . |
| . . . . . . | . . . . . . | . . . . . . | . . . . . . |

4. What has been the trend in the spread of rabies in your country? (Please add recent maps indicating the prevalence of the disease, with reference to dogs, cats and wildlife vectors if you have not submitted these within the last five years.)

5. Human exposures:
   (a) Number of human beings who received the following specific antirabies treatment:
      Vaccine alone . . . . . . . . .
      Vaccine and serum . . . . . . . .
      Serum alone . . . . . . . . .
   (b) Number of serious systemic reactions to biological prophylaxis:
      Paralytic accidents (vaccine) . . . . . . . .
      Serum sickness . . . . . . . .
   (c) Total number of human deaths from rabies . . . . . . . . . .
      (specify animal giving fatal bite, if known)

| | Incubation period | | |
|---|---|---|---|
| | 0–30 days | 31–90 days | Over 91 days |
| (i) Number of deaths in untreated individuals (no vaccine or serum) | . . . | . . . | . . . |
| (ii) Number of deaths in individuals receiving: | | | |
| vaccine alone | . . . | . . . | . . . |
| vaccine and serum | . . . | . . . | . . . |
| serum alone | . . . | . . . | . . . |

(For treatment failures, we would welcome any further information such as interval of delay in beginning treatment, number of vaccine doses received, etc., on separate sheets.)

6. Type(s) and amount of vaccine for animals and/or man produced in your laboratory (e.g. Fermi Sheep brain, etc.); specify as requested below. State also for each type of vaccine produced which potency test, if any, is used:

Animal vaccine

| Type | Quantity produced in doses | Tissue concentration | Potency test |
|---|---|---|---|
| . . . . . . | . . . . . . . . . . | . . . . . . . | . . . . . . . |
| . . . . . . | . . . . . . . . . . | . . . . . . . | . . . . . . . |
| . . . . . . | . . . . . . . . . . | . . . . . . . | . . . . . . . |

Human vaccine

| Type | Quantity produced in doses | Tissue concentration | Potency test |
|---|---|---|---|
| . . . . . . | . . . . . . . . . . | . . . . . . . | . . . . . . . |
| . . . . . . | . . . . . . . . . . | . . . . . . . | . . . . . . . |
| . . . . . . | . . . . . . . . . . | . . . . . . . | . . . . . . . |

7. Species of animal in which antirabies serum or gamma-globulin for specific treatment is produced in your laboratory; specifythe amount in millilitres.

| Species of animal | Amount in ml | Number of international units per ml |
|---|---|---|
| . . . . . . . | . . . . . . . | . . . . . . . . . . |
| . . . . . . . | . . . . . . . | . . . . . . . . . . |
| . . . . . . . | . . . . . . . | . . . . . . . . . . |

8. To be answered only if the situation has changed in 1969 as compared with 1968; if not, state "as in 1968".

What is the schedule of vaccine inoculations used in your institute for exposed human beings? Please specify mild, moderate and severe exposure; schedules; amounts of dose used for each type of exposure.

| Type of exposure | Schedule of inoculation | Amount of dose in ml |
|---|---|---|
| Mild | . . . . . . . . . . | . . . . . . . |
| Moderate | . . . . . . . . . . | . . . . . . . |
| Severe | . . . . . . . . . . | . . . . . . . |

9. Give any changes in the routine diagnostic methods used in your institute in 1968; otherwise state "same as in 1968".

. . . . . . . . . . . . . . . . . . . . . . . . .
. . . . . . . . . . . . . . . . . . . . . . . . .
. . . . . . . . . . . . . . . . . . . . . . . . .

10. Give any changes in the requirements in your country, with respect to rabies, for the importation of the following animals: (otherwise state "same as in 1968").

Dogs: . . . . . . . . . . . . . . . . . . . . . . . .
Cats: . . . . . . . . . . . . . . . . . . . . . . . .
Other animals (please give species): . . . . . . . . . . .
. . . . . . . . . . . . . . . . . . . . . . . .
. . . . . . . . . . . . . . . . . . . . . . . .

For Discussion, see page 29.

# The Last Rabies Outbreak in Japan

KOUJI SHIMADA

*Yakult Institute for Microbiological Research, Tokyo*

It is not known when the first invasion of rabies into Japan took place. According to the records of the Ministry of Welfare, there were canine rabies cases every year from 1906 to 1956. During this period there were recurrent epizootics with interlude years having only a few reported cases (Fig. 1). In 1948, in the midst of postwar confusion and social unrest, there was a mass outbreak of canine rabies all over the Kanto district, including the Tokyo metropolis (Fig. 2). After reaching a peak in 1950, the number of rabies cases gradually decreased until rabies was eradicated in Japan, with the last six cases recorded in 1956.

Tokyo also has a long history of animal rabies and its pattern of epizootics resembles that of the rest of the country. The last known rabies cases in Tokyo were three reported in 1955 (Fig. 1).

In Japan, the diagnosis of rabies in dogs had traditionally been made principally on the basis of clinical symptoms, but, with the 1948 outbreak, the Tokyo metropolitan government decided to

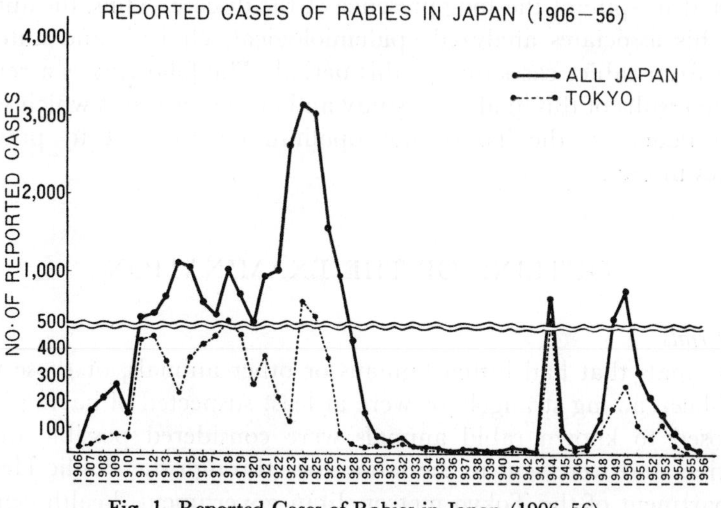


Fig. 1. Reported Cases of Rabies in Japan (1906–56).

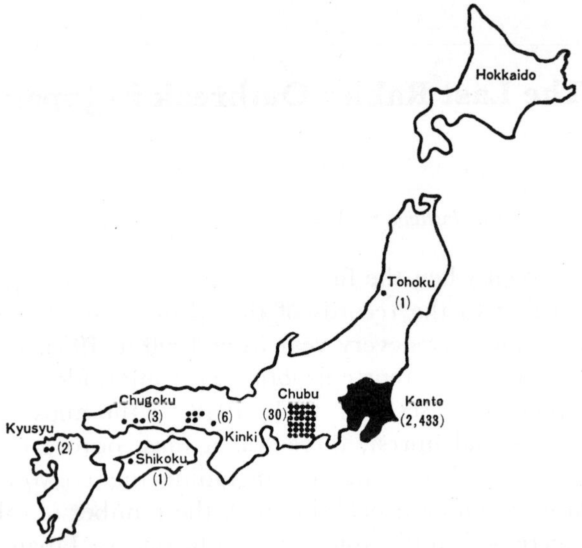


Fig. 2. Geographical Distribution of Rabies Cases (1948–56).

carry out laboratory diagnoses. Thus, from 1948 to 1955, the Tokyo Laboratories for Medical Sciences tested 2,032 suspected animals of which 904 were found to be genuine carriers of rabies (Shimada, 1949; Shimada *et al.*, 1951; Shimada *et al.*, 1953; Shimada *et al.*, 1954a). The data from these examinations contributed greatly to the study of rabies epizootics in this country, which had been neglected in spite of the long presence of the disease. Thus, the author and his associates analyzed epidemiological, clinical, and autopsy data from rabies cases during this period. The following is a report of the results of this analytical study and of the measures which were undertaken by the Tokyo metropolitan government to prevent rabies in dogs.

## OUTLINE OF THE EXAMINATION

### *Materials*

Animals that had bitten humans or other animals, or those that had been acting strangely or were at least suspected of having been exposed to known rabid animals were considered possible rabies carriers and were sent to the laboratory through the Public Health Department of the Tokyo metropolitan government, health centers or dog pounds. Usually the complete cadavers of dead or sacrificed animals were used, but in some instances only the heads cut off from the atlas were used after autopsy by rabies control officers or by veterinary practitioners. The 2,032 animals were received during the period 1948 to 1955, including 1,925 dogs, 95 cats, 2 horses, 1 goat, 2 llamas (Shimada *et al.*, 1954b) and 7 monkeys (Table 1).

*Methods*

Table 1. Animal Species Suspected of Rabies Infection and Those Diagnosed as Having Rabies (1948–55)

| Year | No. of specimens received | | | | | Positive rate |
|---|---|---|---|---|---|---|
| | Dogs | Cats | Horse | Others | Sum | |
| 1948 | 105 ( 92) | 4 (2) | | | 109 ( 94) | 86.2% |
| 1949 | 213 (183) | 5 (1) | 1 (1) | | 219 (185) | 84.5% |
| 1950 | 352 (260) | 19 (4) | | 1 | 372 (264) | 71.0% |
| 1951 | 258 (112) | 9 | 1 (1) | | 268 (113) | 42.2% |
| 1952 | 206 ( 70) | 16 (1) | | | 222 ( 71) | 32.0% |
| 1953 | 359 (124) | 18 (4) | | | 377 (128) | 33.9% |
| 1954 | 251 ( 43) | 20 (1) | | 9 (2) | 280 ( 46) | 16.4% |
| 1955 | 181 ( 3 ) | 4 | | | 185 ( 3 ) | 1.6% |
| Total | 1,925 (887) | 95 (13) | 2 (2) | 10 (2) | 2,032 (904) | 44.5% |

Note: The figures in parentheses represent the number of animals diagnosed as having rabies. The diagnosis was made when virus isolation was positive. In a few cases in 1948 to 1950, these tests could not be carried out because of advanced putrefaction, and the diagnosis was made solely on a clinical basis.

Upon receiving a specimen, the accompanying specimen forms filled out by a rabies control officer or veterinary practitioner were checked and an autopsy was carried out to check for abnormalities in various organs. Then the brain was removed and the following examinations were made.

1. Negri body detection: For rapid detection of Negri bodies in the Ammon's horn of the brain, impression specimens were prepared and stained by a modified Seller's method.

Modified Seller's stain:

Methylene blue methanol solution (methanol 100: methylene blue 1.5 g)................................... 0.5 m*l*

Basic fuchsin methanol solution (methanol 100: fuchsin appr. 6 g)..................................................... 0.55 m*l*

50% glycerine in distilled water..................... 100 m*l*

Staining Method:

Air-drying

Fixation for 1–2 minutes with any of the following:
methanol, alcohol, ether
Stain for 5–6 minutes with the modified Seller's solution
Cover with a cover glass without discarding the fluid
Place between filter papers, apply light pressure to
spread the nerve cell granules

Paraffin sections were also prepared and stained using Mann's method and the haematoxylin eosin method for histological examination. Simultaneously, nonpurulent inflammations of the medulla oblongata were examined for reference.

2. Virus isolation (Webster & Dawson, 1935): In 1948, as it was difficult to obtain mice, rabbits and guinea pigs were used, and the tests were carried out only with animal brains in which Negri bodies were not detected. After 1949, commercial mice were used. A 10% saline emulsion of the brain was made and centrifuged at 2,000 rpm for 15 minutes. Five mice weighing 8–10 g were inoculated intracerebrally with 0.03 m*l* of the supernatant fluid. The inoculated animals were observed for 30 days. The brains of all the mice that died on the fifth day after inoculation or later were examined histologically, regardless of the presence or absence of clinical symptoms.

3. Complement fixation test (CF) (Ando *et al.*, 1953a, b): Studies on the use of this test to detect rabies antigen in brain tissues of the suspected animal were carried out previously by K. Ando of the National Institute of Health and others. Brains that had been histologically examined were used. As the results were satisfactory, the test was officially adopted for rabies diagnosis in January, 1953. Details of the test can be found in K. Ishii's paper in this volume.

4. Final confirmation: Specimens positive for Negri bodies and/or CF antigen were diagnosed as rabies, but final confirmation was always made by virus isolation.

## RESULTS OF LABORATORY EXAMINATIONS

The results are summarized in Tables 1 and 2. When virus isolation was positive, the case was diagnosed as rabies. However, several specimens received during the summer were extremely putrid and could not be examined. Those cases were treated as positive merely on a clinical basis for the safety of the human victims because they occurred in the first three years of the epizootic when there was the greatest incidence of rabies. Of 2,032 animals received for examination, 904 animals, or 44.5%, were diagnosed as rabid (Table 1). These animals include 887 dogs, 13 cats, 2 horses, and 2 llamas. The positive rate was very high in the first two years, and declined in the subsequent years with a sudden drop to a very low level in 1955. This decline is most probably due to the increasing awareness of the danger of rabies.

1. Virus isolation: This test was more sensitive than the tests for Negri bodies and CF antigen. Virus isolation showed numerous cases positive which had not been detected by the Negri body or CF tests. On the other hand, there were no cases positive for Negri body or CF antigen showing negative virus isolation (Table 2). Thus, virus isolation is an indispensable method in rabies diagnosis.

2. Negri body: In 1948 animal experiments were done only on Negri body negative cases (Table 2). Therefore, the results of that year are excluded. For the following years, the Negri body incidence among virus positive cases varied between 67% and 90% according to year (Table 2). This variation may be due to the strain difference or the time of sacrifice of the suspected animals, although no direct evidence is available.

Figure 3 illustrates the results of our experiments regarding the viral replication and the time of appearance of Negri bodies and CF

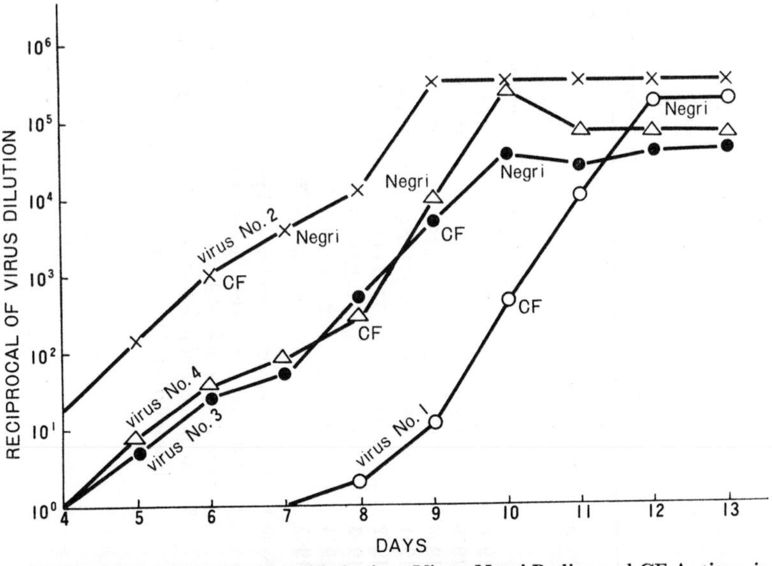


Fig. 3. Time of Appearance of Infectious Virus, Negri Bodies and CF Antigen in Mouse Brains Experimentally Infected with Rabies Street Virus

Table 2. Summarized Results of Diagnostic Tests (1948–55)

| Year | No. of specimens received | Number and per cent of positives | | | | | Rabies diagnosis | |
|---|---|---|---|---|---|---|---|---|
| | | Negri body | Virus isolation | CF antigen | Nonpurulent encephalitis | Not done | Positive | Negative |
| 1948 | 109 | 78 (86.7%) | 12* | | | 4 | 94 | 15 |
| 1949 | 219 | 149 (83.7%) | 178 (100%) | | 156 (87.6%) | 7 | 185 | 34 |
| 1950 | 372 | 177 (68.3%) | 259 (100%) | | 202 (77.9%) | 5 | 264 | 108 |
| 1951 | 268 | 81 (71.6%) | 113 (100%) | | 101 (89.3%) | | 113 | 155 |
| 1952 | 222 | 53 (74.6%) | 71 (100%) | | 66 (92.9%) | | 71 | 151 |
| 1953 | 377 | 115 (89.8%) | 128 (100%) | 119 (92.9%) | 119 (92.9%) | | 128 | 249 |
| 1954 | 280 | 32 (69.5%) | 46 (100%) | 40 (86.9%) | 39 (84.7%) | | 46 | 234 |
| 1955 | 185 | 2 (66.7%) | 3 (100%) | 3 (100%) | 3 (100%) | | 3 | 182 |

Note 1) *Only the Negri-negative specimens were tested for virus isolation.

2) "Not done" represents the cases which were not tested due to extreme putrefaction of the specimen, but were taken administratively as rabies-positive solely on a clinical basis for the safety of human victims.

3) The percent of positives for each test shown in parentheses represents the rate of positives by the respective test over positives for virus isolation. There were no cases positive for Negri body or CF antigen and negative for virus isolation.

antigen in the brains of mice infected with street virus. (Ueki *et al.*, 1957) Four groups of mice weighing 10–11g received 0.03 m*l* of 10% emulsions of four rabid dog brains intracerebrally. Negri bodies were first detected one or two days later than CF antigen, which became positive two to four days after the initial appearance of active virus (Fig. 3). These findings would suggest the importance of the stage of infection in detection of Negri bodies in infected dogs or other species of animals.

3. Complement fixation test: This method was used only in the last three years of the epizootic. Rabies CF antigen was present and was detected in 87% to 100% of the animals positive for virus isolation (Table 2). The method is evidently more sensitive than the Negri body test. It should be emphasized that the complement fixation test enables very quick (five-six hours) diagnosis.

4. Non-purulent cerebral inflammation: This is not pathognomonic for rabies, but seems to be of value in the diagnosis, as it was found in 78% to 100% of our virus-positive cases (Table 2).

Needless to say, there were almost always human victims involved in these cases, and it was necessary to arrive at a decision on whether to administer prophylactic vaccination or not. The diagnosis was made as quickly and accurately as possible, and extreme care was taken in deciding whether or not an animal was rabid.

## EPIDEMIOLOGICAL, CLINICAL AND OTHER OBSERVATIONS ON 904 RABID ANIMALS

### *Monthly Incidence*

From 1948 to 1955, with the exception of 1955, confirmed cases occurred in every month, but some seasonal variation is discernible (Table 3). Higher incidences were observed from May to October. The total number of cases during these months was 568 (63%). This is probably due to greater mobility of dogs during these months which provides a greater opportunity for contact with rabid dogs. In the first two to three years of the epizootic, however, the incidence did not decline in the winter months and seemed to foretell the greater outbreak occurring every year at that time.

### *Age Distribution*

The estimated age was available for 786 confirmed cases (Table 4). The majority of the confirmed rabid dogs were one to three years old. This age group had 773 animals, or 98% of the total. One-

Table 3. Monthly Incidence of Reported and Confirmed Rabid Animals in Tokyo (1948–55)

| Year \ Month | Jan. | Feb. | March | April | May | June | July | Aug. | Sept. | Oct. | Nov. | Dec. | Total |
|---|---|---|---|---|---|---|---|---|---|---|---|---|---|
| 1948 | 7 (5) | 4 (4) | 3 (3) | 7 (5) | 8 (8) | 7 (6) | 5 (5) | 10 (7) | 10 (9) | 21 (20) | 14 (12) | 13 (10) | 109 (94) |
| 1949 | 11 (10) | 9 (9) | 16 (13) | 9 (7) | 23 (22) | 20 (18) | 27 (22) | 21 (19) | 17 (16) | 23 (22) | 19 (12) | 24 (15) | 219 (185) |
| 1950 | 17 (12) | 19 (17) | 26 (20) | 23 (18) | 51 (39) | 40 (28) | 38 (28) | 35 (21) | 37 (28) | 31 (21) | 33 (19) | 22 (13) | 372 (264) |
| 1951 | 13 (2) | 25 (12) | 24 (13) | 20 (11) | 29 (14) | 27 (16) | 32 (13) | 26 (12) | 24 (8) | 14 (3) | 17 (5) | 17 (4) | 268 (113) |
| 1952 | 12 (4) | 10 (2) | 15 (4) | 14 (4) | 31 (11) | 21 (8) | 20 (9) | 24 (5) | 23 (8) | 15 (6) | 18 (6) | 19 (4) | 222 (71) |
| 1953 | 12 (2) | 14 (5) | 30 (8) | 24 (9) | 31 (10) | 39 (17) | 55 (22) | 44 (16) | 38 (11) | 34 (12) | 32 (10) | 24 (6) | 377 (128) |
| 1954 | 22 (5) | 19 (5) | 30 (5) | 25 (1) | 36 (9) | 24 (4) | 20 (5) | 22 (3) | 19 (5) | 12 (1) | 24 (2) | 27 (1) | 280 (46) |
| 1955 | 20 | 19 (2) | 13 | 13 | 20 | 22 (1) | 15 | 13 | 13 | 11 | 12 | 14 | 185 (3) |
| Total | 114 (40) | 119 (56) | 157 (66) | 135 (55) | 229 (113) | 200 (98) | 212 (104) | 195 (83) | 181 (85) | 161 (85) | 169 (66) | 160 (53) | 2,032 (904) |

Note: The figures in parentheses represent the number of confirmed cases.

Table 4. Age of Confirmed Rabid Dogs in Tokyo (1949–54)

| Year | Presumed age of infected dog | | | | | | | Sum |
|---|---|---|---|---|---|---|---|---|
| | Less than 90 days | 1 Year | 2 Years | 3 Years | 4 Years | 5 Years | 6 Years | 7 Years or more | |
| 1949 | 27 | 98 | 39 | 17 | 1 | 0 | 0 | 1 | 183 |
| 1950 | 45 | 145 | 48 | 13 | 1 | 1 | 0 | 1 | 254 |
| 1951 | 23 | 61 | 20 | 7 | 1 | 0 | 0 | 0 | 112 |
| 1952 | 13 | 39 | 14 | 3 | 0 | 1 | 0 | 0 | 70 |
| 1953 | 21 | 65 | 28 | 7 | 2 | 1 | 0 | 0 | 124 |
| 1954 | 5 | 22 | 9 | 4 | 3 | 0 | 0 | 0 | 43 |
| Total | 134 | 430 | 158 | 51 | 8 | 3 | 0 | 2 | 786 |

year-old dogs were especially numerous, numbering 564 (72%). The major cause of this fact may be that there was a great number of one-year-old dogs in Tokyo at the time. It is also worth noting that 134 dogs, or 24%, were less than 90 days of age and not required to be registered and vaccinated according to the Japanese rabies prevention law.

*Legal Classification*

Legal status was available for 786 rabid dogs (Table 5). About 50% of those were unregistered dogs, and about 30% stray dogs. There were only 140 registered dogs, or 18%, during this period. Over the period the percentage of cases of unregistered dogs increased, and that of strays also increased rapidly after 1950, whereas cases of registered dogs decreased. These patterns seem to reflect a large, increasing number of unregistered and stray dogs in Tokyo which were usually not vaccinated.

Table 5. Legal Classification of Confirmed Rabid Dogs in Tokyo (1949–54)

| Year | Registered | Unregistered | Stray | Total |
|---|---|---|---|---|
| 1949 | 43 (23.5%) | 83 (45.4%) | 57 (31.1%) | 183 |
| 1950 | 56 (22.0%) | 128 (50.4%) | 70 (27.6%) | 254 |
| 1951 | 21 (18.7%) | 53 (47.3%) | 38 (34.0%) | 112 |
| 1952 | 6 ( 8.6%) | 37 (52.9%) | 27 (38.5%) | 70 |
| 1953 | 10 ( 8.1%) | 65 (52.4%) | 49 (39.5%) | 124 |
| 1954 | 4 ( 9.3%) | 23 (53.5%) | 16 (37.2%) | 43 |
| Total | 140 (17.8%) | 389 (49.5%) | 257 (32.7%) | 786 |

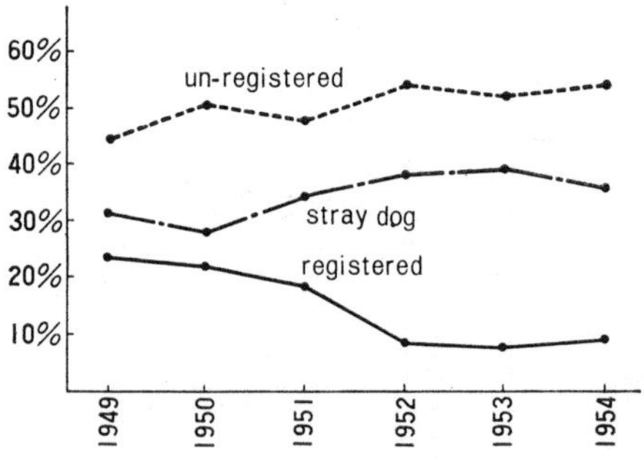


*Sex*

Of 786 rabid dogs detected during the period 1949 to 1954, 460 (58.5%) were male and 326 (41.5%) were female (Table 6). Furthermore, the preponderance of male cases became greater every year after 1950. Whether this is because there was a greater number of male dogs or because male dogs move around over a broader area than female dogs is not known.

Table 6. Sex of Confirmed Rabid Dogs in Tokyo (1949–54)

| Year | Male | Female | Total |
|---|---|---|---|
| 1949 | 107 (58.5%) | 76 (41.5%) | 183 |
| 1950 | 142 (55.9%) | 112 (44.1%) | 254 |
| 1951 | 64 (57.1%) | 48 (42.9%) | 112 |
| 1952 | 41 (58.6%) | 29 (41.4%) | 70 |
| 1953 | 78 (62.9%) | 46 (37.1%) | 124 |
| 1954 | 28 (65.1%) | 15 (34.9%) | 43 |
| Total | 460 (58.5%) | 326 (41.5%) | 786 |

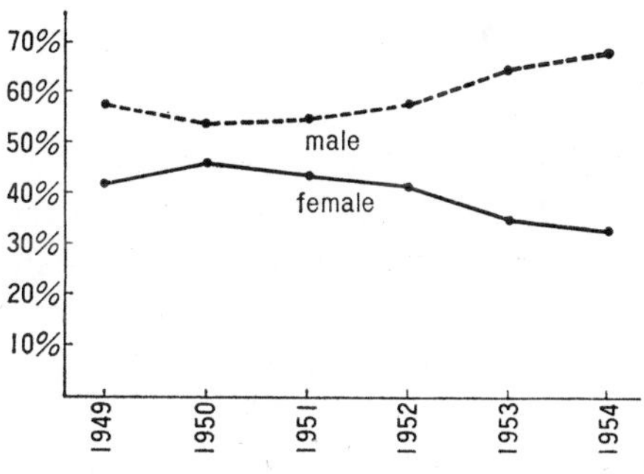


*Incubation Period*

Of the 884 dogs and 13 cats which were found to be rabid during the period 1948–1954, it was stated by owners or neighbors on the forms accompanying the cadavers, that in 98 cases, 92 dogs and 6 cats they had been bitten by rabid dogs before developing rabies. These data are summarized in Table 7. The minimum period was 6 days and the maximum, 150 days. The incubation period was 6 to 30 days in 78 cases (79.6%), 31 to 60 days in 15 cases (15.2%), and over 61 days in only 5 cases (5.1%).

The incubation period of rabies is subject to various conditions, and in this investigation, the relationship between the incubation period and the bite site could not be studied because of lack of information.

*Clinical Symptoms*

The forms filled out by rabies control officers or veterinarians were analyzed for clinical symptoms in 898 confirmed cases from 1948 to

Table 7. Incubation Period of Confirmed Rabid Animals in Tokyo (1948–54)

| Day | Dogs | Cats | Sum | |
|---|---|---|---|---|
| 6～10 | 11 | 1 | 12 (12.2%) | 78 (79.6%) |
| 11～20 | 35 | 2 | 37 (37.8%) | |
| 21～30 | 29 | | 29 (29.6%) | |
| 31～40 | 5 | 1 | 6 ( 6.1%) | 15 (15.2%) |
| 41～50 | 6 | 1 | 7 ( 7.1%) | |
| 51～60 | 2 | | 2 (2.0%) | |
| 61～150 | 4 | 1 | 5 ( 5.1%) | |
| Total | 92 | 6 | 98 | |

1954. Typical symptoms were observed in 394 cases (43.9%); slight symptoms in 246 (27.4%); and no apparent symptoms but only evidence of having been bitten by, or having come in contact with, a rabid animal, in 126 cases (14%); distemper-like symptoms in 16 cases (1.7%), and unknown or not specified in 116 cases (12.9%). In less than 50% of these cases the clinical symptoms coincided with the results of laboratory examinations. Because there are paralytic and furious types of rabies, clinical symptoms differ according to the form and the stage in which the diagnosis is made. However, it was found that there were many dogs which were strongly suspected of rabies from clinical symptoms but which were later found to be non-rabid. Thus, clinical symptoms are of value in suggesting rabies, but the final diagnosis should be based on specific diagnostic procedures.

*Autopsy Findings and Contents of Stomach*

It is a well-known fact that rabies does not have any anatomically specific lesions. However, cerebral cloudy swelling, congestion, vascular congestion of the liver and kidneys, and oral and dental injury were frequently observed. There were also many cases of cerebral anemia among puppies less than 90 days old.

It has been said that the presence of foreign materials in the stomach is extremely significant in the diagnosis of animal rabies. An investigation of the contents of the stomachs of 660 rabid animals during the period 1948 to 1954 showed that 85 animals (12.9%) had only food in their stomachs, 94 (14.2%) had a mixture of food and foreign materials, and 256 (38.8%) had only foreign elements (Table 8). It is noteworthy that 225 (34%) had completely empty stomachs. The foreign elements in order of frequency were straw, stones, wood, grass, sand, clods and fur.

Table 8. Contents of the Stomach of Infected Animals in Tokyo (1948–54)

| | |
|---|---|
| Food | 85 (12.9%) |
| Foreign materials | 350 (53.0%) |
| Straw | 178 |
| Grass | 51 |
| Stones and Clods | 43 |
| Fur | 89 |
| Wood | 46 |
| Other | 56 |
| Empty | 225 (34.0%) |
| Total | 660 |

Note: When more than 2 kinds of foreign materials were found in a stomach, they were classified separately

*Intracerebral Virus Titers of Infected Dogs*

One hundred and one brain specimens of dogs confirmed to be rabid during the period 1951–1952 were studied for virus titers. A 10% saline emulsion of the brain was made and centrifuged at 2,000 rpm for 15 minutes. Tenfold serial dilutions were made from $10^{-2}$ to $10^{-6}$. Five mice weighing 10–11g were inoculated intracerebrally with 0.03 m*l* of the dilutions in and observed for 30 days. The $LD_{50}$ was calculated by means of the Reed and Muench method (Reed & Muench, 1938). The virus titers ranged from $10^{-2.3}$ to $10^{-5.7}$, being most frequent in the range $10^{-3}-10^{-3.99}$, followed by the range $10^{-4}-10^{-4.99}$. Seventy-seven cases or 76% were found in these two ranges (Table 9).

*Human Victims*

During the period 1948–1955 the 904 confirmed rabid animals were reported to have bitten a total of 1,848 persons. It was not known whether these people had received prophylactic vaccine or not, but there were 53 (2.8%) deaths. In the first three years, the number of victims was 1,240 (67%) and the number of deaths, 50 (94%). Incidentally, 50,171 persons were bitten by non-rabid dogs during the entire epizootic period (Table 10).

Table 9. Virus Content of Rabid Dog Brains in Tokyo (1951~52)

| $Log_{10}$ $LD_{50}$ | No. of dog | sum |
|---|---|---|
| −2.0~2.49 | 4 | 14 |
| −2.5~2.99 | 10 | (13.8%) |
| −3.0~3.49 | 13 | 44 |
| −3.5~3.99 | 31 | (43.5%) |
| −4.0~4.49 | 23 | 33 |
| −4.5~4.99 | 10 | (32.6%) |
| −5.0~5.49 | 8 | 10 |
| −5.5~5.99 | 2 | ( 9.9%) |
| Total | 101 | |

Note: Assay was made by inoculating 5 mice with 0.03 *ml* of each of ten-fold serial dilutions of 10% dog brain suspension.

Table 10. Human Victims of Rabid Animals in Tokyo (1948–55)

| Year | No. of rabid animals | Bitten by rabid animals | No. of fatal rabies cases | Bitten by non-rabid animals |
|---|---|---|---|---|
| 1948 | 94 | 290 | 22 | 415 |
| 1949 | 185 | 419 | 19 | 1,747 |
| 1950 | 264 | 531 | 9 | 22,284 |
| 1951 | 113 | 181 | 1 | 3,571 |
| 1952 | 71 | 134 | 1 | 4,386 |
| 1953 | 128 | 195 | 1 | 6,916 |
| 1954 | 46 | 94 | 0 | 5,571 |
| 1955 | 3 | 4 | 0 | 5,281 |
| Total | 904 | 1,848 | 53 | 50,171 |

*Rabies Incidence and Prophylactic Vaccination*

In Tokyo, registered dogs were vaccinated according to the dog control ordinance up to 1949 and according to the rabies prevention law after 1950. The total doses of vaccine given to those dogs during the period 1949–1954 was 973,294 (Table 11). This number includes not only the doses given regularly twice a year but also emergency vaccinations. This would mean that some of the dogs received the vaccine several times. However, most dogs are supposed to have received the vaccine twice a year, and hence the number of dogs vaccinated is estimated at about one half of the number of the total doses. Of the rabid dogs during this period, 140 were registered dogs. The number of registered rabid dogs gradually diminished after 1951, since the number of vaccinated dogs increased. Thirty-eight of the 140 rabid dogs had received vaccinations. Of these vaccinated dogs, only 18 had received vaccination 21 to 180 days before the onset of their clinical symptoms. During this period after vaccination, immunity is considered to be high. These results indicate that the vaccination was extremely effective, especially after 1952, when the phenol inactivated vaccine came into use.

Table 11. Survey of Vaccinated Dogs Which Died of Rabies in Tokyo (1949–54)

| Year | Doses given registered dogs | Registered dogs which died of rabies | Vaccinated dogs which died of rabies | No. of dogs rabid within 21∼180 days of vaccination |
|---|---|---|---|---|
| 1949 | 27,887 | 43 | 7 | 3 |
| 1950 | 105,470 | 56 | 18 | 8 |
| 1951 | 164,015 | 21 | 10 | 5 |
| 1952 | 199,272 | 6 | 2 | 2 |
| 1953 | 240,151 | 10 | 0 | 0 |
| 1954 | 236,499 | 4 | 1 | 0 |
| Total | 973,294 | 140 | 38 | 18 |

## RABIES CONTROL MEASURES IN TOKYO

The Tokyo Metropolitan government had its own ordinance for catching of stray dogs and registration and vaccination of registered dogs. In 1950, the rabies prevention law was established and helped to reinforce the measures which had existed up to that time (Table 12).

Each health center in Tokyo had to have a full-time rabies control officer (veterinarian) for the general work of preventing animal rabies in the area.

Catching stray dogs, previously the work of the private companies, was placed under the direct supervision of the Tokyo city government and, at the same time, more dog catchers were employed, new dog pounds were established and dog catchers were given more freedom of movement. Dog owners had to keep their dogs chained and all registered dogs found running loose were caught in the same way as the unregistered and stray dogs. Dogs that were abandoned or had lost their status as registered dogs were also caught. The number of dogs caught increased yearly but decreased from 1954, around the end of the epizootic period.

It became the duty of all dog owners to register their dogs once every year if the dogs were over 91 days old. At the same time various propaganda measures such as the establishment of a rabies prevention week every year and dissemination of information through communications media were also carried out. All registered dogs had to wear a special tag on their collars so that they could be easily identified,

Table 12. Rabies Control Measures Taken and Their Results in Tokyo (1949–55)

| Year | Estimated no. of dogs in Tokyo | No. of stray dogs captured | No. of dogs registered | No. of vaccine doses given | No. of dog pools (capacity of detaining dogs | No. of rabies control officers | No. of dog catchers |
|---|---|---|---|---|---|---|---|
| 1949 | 50,000 | 21,664 | 37,481 | 27,887 | | | |
| 1950 | 100,000 | 42,382 | 65,315 | 105,470 | 6 (1,250) | 61 | 30 |
| 1951 | 140,000 | 48,997 | 110,255 | 164,015 | 6 (1,250) | 61 | 30 |
| 1952 | 200,000 | 64,737 | 127,653 | 199,272 | 6 (1,250) | 61 | 30 |
| 1953 | 250,000 | 87,168 | 146,669 | 240,151 | 7 (2,250) | 61 | 40 |
| 1954 | 250,000 | 59,055 | 141,939 | 236,499 | 7 (2,250) | 61 | 40 |
| 1955 | 200,000 | 48,759 | 144,407 | 242,153 | 7 (2,250) | 62 | 50 |

and the detection and catching of dogs not bearing the tag were reinforced.

Because of the financial burden of owning a dog including registration fee, taxes, and vaccination fee it was difficult to enforce these regulations thoroughly in the beginning, but after these measures began to take effect, the number of registrations grew to two to four times what it was in the beginning.

Prophylactic vaccination was carried out by each health center, with the cooperation of practicing veterinarians in the area under its jurisdiction, in the spring (April-June) and fall (October-December) and also for any emergency situations. Regularly vaccinated dogs were issued certificates to wear on their collars for each vaccination. The number of vaccinations grew in parallel to the number of registered dogs and eventually covered 70%–80% of the number of registered dogs for every vaccination period.

Other measures were enforced, such as the killing of stray dogs with drugs, muzzling of biting dogs, and castration and spaying operations to prevent the increase of mongrel dogs.

These are the results of examinations and preventive measures undertaken by the Tokyo metropolitan government at the time of the last animal rabies outbreak in Japan. The author considers that these systematic examinations and measures contributed, both directly and indirectly, to the eradication of rabies in Tokyo.

As for areas other than Tokyo, each prefecture also established a system of examinations and enforced preventive measures based on the rabies prevention law. Furthermore, the fact that there were no rabies reported in wild animals and bats, as is the case in some other countries, has enabled Japan, which had a long history of animal rabies, to eradicate rabies.

## REFERENCES

Ando, K., Ishii, K., Oka, Y., Irisawa, J., Shimada, K. and Kato, T. (1953a). Studies on the immunological diagnosis of the animals suspected of rabies. *Jap. J. Med. Sci. Biol.*, **6**, 221.

Ando, K., Ishii, K., Oka, Y., Irisawa, J., Shimada, K., Kato, T. and Murakami, H. (1953b). Studies on the immunological diagnosis of the animals suspected of rabies. II. *Jap. J. Med. Sci. Biol.*, **6**, 659.

Reed, L. J. and Muench, H. (1938). A simple method of estimating fifty percent endpoints. *Am. J. Hyg.*, **27**, 493.

Shimada, K. (1949). Examination results of rabies in 1949. *Ann. Rep. Tokyo-to Laboratories for Medical Sciences*, **1**, 68. (in Japanese)

Shimada, K., Kato, T. and Ueki, H. (1951). Examination results of rabies in 1951. *Ann. Rep. Tokyo-to Laboratories for Medical Sciences*, **3**, 105. (in Japanese).

Shimada, K., Kato, T. Ueki, H., Oishi, J. and Murakami, H. (1953). Examination results of rabies in 1953. *Ann. Rep. Tokyo-to Laboratories for Medical Sciences*, **5**, 154. (in Japanese)

Shimada, K., Kato, T., Ueki, H., Oishi, J. and Murakami, H. (1954a). Examination results of rabies in 1954. *Ann. Rep. Tokyo-to Laboratories for Medical Sciences*, **6**, 131.(in Japanese)

Shimada, K., Kato, T., Ueki, H., Oishi, J., Murakami, H. and Noda, M., (1954b). Examination results of rabies in llama. *Ann. Rep. Tokyo-to Laboratories for Medical Sciences*, **6**, 137. (in Japanese)

Ueki, K., Kato, T., Oishi, J., Murakami, H. and Shimada, K. (1957). Observation of the time of appearance of Negri bodies, complement-fixing antigen and virulence in mouse brains inoculated with rabies street virus. *Am. J. Vet. Res.*, **18**, 66. Jan. 216–218.

Webster, L. T. and Dawson, J. R. (1935). Early diagnosis of rabies by mouse inoculation. *Proc. Soc. Exp. Biol. and Med.*, **32**, 570.

For Discussion, see page 29.

# Discussion*

HAMMON: Dr. Shimada, this was a very interesting presentation of the story of rabies control in Tokyo during that period of time. I found it difficult, however, to interpret the fact that from 1950 on there were much more dogs vaccinated than were registered. How did that occur? The stray dogs, I understand, were killed, but were some of those vaccinated and released or were some dogs vaccinated that were not registered?

SHIMADA: As I mentioned, dogs are inoculated twice a year, in the spring and fall. Therefore, if all the registered dogs are vaccinated, the vaccinations would come to exactly double the number of registered dogs. But actually the number of vaccinated dogs is less than this, as the actual percentage of registered dogs that receive vaccination is 70% to 80% each time.

HAMMON: Did you see any incidence of rabies in cats?

SHIMADA: Yes. We examined them in the same way as we examined the dogs. The number of cats examined during this eight-year period was 95, and 13 were found to be rabid.

LENNETTE: Did you actually have llamas, and where did they come from? Were they from a zoo?

SHIMADA: I think I had better explain this incident of the llamas. They were in Ueno Zoo and became rabid, presumably having been bitten by a rabid dog. One died and the other was killed. They were found to be rabid on examination. These llamas were imported to the zoo from Germany and Holland.

BERAN: Dr. Tierkel, are there any countries in South Asia and Southeast Asia that report incidence of rabies in animals as compared to the figures you gave for incidence in man?

---

* This Discussion refers to the reports by Tierkel and Shimada.

TIERKEL: First of all, the reports which I outlined are those based on the questionnaires sent out from Geneva. And these sometimes go to the centrally located reporting organization on communicable diseases in the country; sometimes, in areas where this sort of thing is not done, they are to the individual institutes where this activity goes on. There may be three or four Pasteur Institutes in one country. But the problem is that there is no uniform reporting of animal rabies in Asian countries at the local level and, as I pointed out in the review, the only areas that are fairly well reported are those in the vicinity of the diagnostic laboratories.

BERAN: In any of the countries in South and Southeast Asia where they do not have extensive rabies control programs what is happening to the incidence of human rabies, is it going up or down?

TIERKEL: It fluctuates; it goes up and down. There are outbreaks in one part of the country and then in another. There seems to be no real depression in the number of human rabies cases as far as I can see. For instance, the ones that have created an impact on most of us are India and the Philippines, and this seems to be the story year after year. There are always a great many cases which are reported. Of course, these are numbers of cases, not rates. When you consider a country like India with a population of 525 million, the "guesstimate" of 15,000 human deaths does not seem as large. But it is a huge problem, of course, and it is only in certain well-organized areas such as the state of Tamilnadu, around Coonoor where Dr. Veeraraghavan has taken as active interest in the control of rabies, that there is a great deal being done. In other areas, little or nothing is being done.

BERAN: Dr. Shimada, one of your tables listed the clinical symptoms of rabies in animals, including 126 cases there where the virus was apparently asymptomatic or inapparent. Were those dogs killed and rabies found, or did they die and were subsequently examined, or what is the status?

SHIMADA: Some of them died naturally and some were killed. These were sent in from the various health centers without any record of symptoms on the forms that accompanied the dogs' bodies. They were probably sent without any consideration as to symptoms, and the forms were left blank.

DAVENPORT: Dr. Shimada, I did not understand why the incidence of rabies was so high in dogs under three years of age. Are there more free running or wild dogs in Japan between the ages of one and three after which time they are either caught or they die? I would have expected that the Japanese dog born and surviving for one year would have a longer life span than three years and that, therefore, there would be many older four and five-year-old dogs. I should like to ask Dr. Tierkel what he estimates the number of rabid deaths in the Philippines is, if the number for India is thought to be 15,000.

SHIMADA: The majority of the dogs in Tokyo was of that age group, 1 to 3 years old, and the number decreased with increasing age. This is, in my opinion, the reason why we found more rabid dogs from this age group.

TIERKEL: I want to defer to Dr. Beran who has just come from the Philippines. Maybe he can give us something better than a "guesstimate."

BERAN: The reports to the Department of Health on human rabies deaths in the Philippines range from about 150 to 350 cases each year. I really have no explanation for the fact that the number in the last couple of years has been about half what it was the decade before. In other words, we are down in the 150 range now where we used to have 300 and more recorded deaths. The reporting of all deaths in man in the Philippines is fairly developed for a Southeast Asian country and rabies is probably about the best reported of all communicable diseases. I would say that the actual number of human deaths is certainly not more than twice the number that is reported. That is rather a close figure for a country in Southeast Asia.

SIKES: One comment and one question to Dr. Shimada. First I wish to acknowledge our appreciation for your summarizing so beautifully the rabies experience in Japan. I think this again proves that where you do not have the wildlife reservoir, you can eradicate rabies in the dog and the urban situation. This is a wonderful experience. Perhaps I misunderstood, but my question is: at what age do you vaccinate your dogs? You alluded once to one year. Do you not vaccinate sooner?

SHIMADA: In Japan, we start vaccination of dogs when they are 91 days or three months old. I would also like to add that we did see several cases of rabies in dogs which were only 1.5 months old in our study.

MATUMOTO: Dr. Shimada, the dogs start to receive vaccination when they are over 91 days of age. They henceforth receive the vaccination every spring and fall. How long do they continue to be vaccinated?

SHIMADA: Until they die. That is the regulation.

TIERKEL: I would like to know whether this is still being carried out. Is it still required every six months in spite of the fact that you have eradicated the disease?

SHIMADA: That is correct. This is still being carried out. There are some who say it is no longer necessary because we have eradicated rabies, but this precaution is still taken because we have no guarantee that rabies will not appear again.

HAMMON: I would like to ask a question of Dr. Lennette. I am surprised that Dr. Lennette questioned the interpreter regarding the llama, for, if I recall, about twenty-five years ago I heard him report that he isolated a rabies virus from a giraffe in California. I believe this was at the San Diego Zoo, but at the same time I recall that he described the height of the fence around the giraffe. I have seen that fence; it has very small mesh near the ground and reaches almost to the neck of the giraffe. He seemed at that time quite sure that no dog had jumped that fence. Dr. Shimada indicated, however, that it might have been a dog that bit the llama. Has Dr. Lennette ever decided what rabid animal bit the giraffe?

LENNETTE: No, we have never unequivocally determined what vector was involved. When we reported the recovery of rabies virus from the brain of this giraffe, there was considerable skepticism that this actually was rabies virus—both the curator of the zoo and his associates were quite firm in their opinion that access of any rodent into the enclosure was precluded by the wire fence and other precautionary measures that existed. The possibility of vampire bat transmission was broached, because about this time Dr. Harald N. Johnson had shown in Mexico that derriengue represents vampire bat transmitted rabies. This did not seem very probable, however, since vampire bats are not present in Southern California. In retrospect, however, and with the knowledge that rabies can be transmitted by fruit-eating and insect-eating bats, this could conceivably have represented a case of bat-transmitted rabies.

WIKTOR: I would like to ask Dr. Shimada for more information concerning the type of vaccine used in Japan for immunization of animals and how the vaccine is applied.

SHIMADA: Up to 1951 in Japan, we had been using mainly phenol-attenuated vaccine with glycerine added. In 1952 a new law was promulgated and only the phenol inactivated vaccine was permitted to be used. The vaccine is usually injected subcutaneously. Large dogs of, say, 10 to 15 kg receive 5 to 7 m*l*, dogs of 5 to 9 kg receive 3 to 4 m*l* and very small dogs weighing 4 kg or less receive 2 to 3 m*l*.

SHIRAKI: I would like to ask Dr. Shimada a question concerning the histological diagnosis. I understood from your presentation that you rely principally on Negri body formation in diagnosis, and that you consider inflammation secondary. I have seen several autopsies of rabid dogs and found that the inflammatory reactions were extremely severe whereas Negri bodies were rarely noticeable. I therefore doubt whether it is correct to place so much weight on Negri body formation alone. We may also encounter the opposite: marked Negri body formation with very little inflammation. I would like to have your, or anyone else's opinion on this question.

SHIMADA: I am speaking from the standpoint of administrative examinations and I have never investigated the kind of problem you are talking about. We always carried out animal inoculation and examined inoculated animals for Negri bodies and inflammation. We have never delved any further into this question.

HARWOOD: I would like to ask Dr. Shimada why they use phenolized instead of a modified live virus vaccine.

SHIMADA: This is stipulated by Japanese law. At the time the law was promulgated, this was a measure to advance the vaccination one step further.

CABASSO: Dr. Shimada, in your answers on your vaccine, you did not mention the source of tissue. I thought, however, that you said in your main presentation it was rabbit brain. If so, I wonder whether the high frequency of injection does not induce neuro-paralytic accidents in dogs in Tokyo, and whether such have been observed.

TAKAMATSU: As Dr. Tierkel mentioned in his paper, the live vaccine was made from rabbit brain by Umeno, Doi and Kondo, and this was used up to 1951. However, it was difficult to maintain the stability of the virus. Because there were some problems to the safety of the vaccine, the advances made elsewhere were introduced here, influencing our use of the Semple vaccine and the Semple modified vaccine in Japan from 1952. This was first made from dog brain, and later from goat brain. With greater advances being made—progress in Japan was also made in this field the ultra-violet irradiated vaccine and the methiolate inactivated vaccine, vaccines other than the Semple type, began to be used although I do not recall the exact year. These were all made from goat brain. The tissue concentration ranged from 10% to 20%. In Japan also there were many surveys, and may still being carried out, on post-vaccinal encephalitis, yet there is no literature proving that there was a case of post-vaccinal encephalitis in a dog. There is one case only which seems to be post-vaccinal encephalitis, but there is no proof there either.

KOPROWSKI: I think we need to clarify why the chick-embryo-adapted live virus vaccine is not used in Japan. Dr. Shimada mentioned that in Japan, legislation that restricted the type of vaccine used to phenolized vaccine was based on the premise that experience in other countries showed phenolized vaccine to be more effective than live virus vaccine. If anything, experience in other countries showed chick-embryo-adapted live virus vaccine to be more effective.

SHIMADA: Dr. Koprowski, you may think it more effective perhaps because you are a specialist in the chick embryo vaccine, but

Japanese law stipulates that we use the phenolized inactivated vaccine and, as far as I know, chick embryo vaccine is still not authorized.

TAKAMATSU: This is a question of administration and it is difficult for me, as an investigator, to try to answer this question. Dr. Nomura, from my laboratory, will present a paper later on experiments with Flury virus, live vaccine and inactivated vaccine. As you know, we have been rabies-free since 1952. Administrators probably think that there is no need to go to the trouble of changing vaccines. I think there are some representatives of the authorities present here, so I would like to ask them why this vaccine is not being used.

KOPROWSKI: I should like to ask if one of the representative authorities present would explain why the killed virus vaccine rather than the live virus vaccine receives official sponsorship. I agree that, using this vaccine, you have done a wonderful job of eradicating rabies in Japan. But the entire dog population must be vaccinated twice a year. This procedure could be reduced to once a year or even to once in a dog's lifetime by using the live virus vaccine, which would be much more economical.

HUMPHREY: I want to point out that during the period Dr. Shimada covered in his report, even in the United States there were some reservations about the utilization and efficiency of the live virus vaccine. I really think the only question that occurs in many of our minds is why at the present time they are continuing to use nerve tissue vaccine and vaccinating at twice a year interval in Japan, whereas in the United States, the trend has been towards using the live virus vaccine. For example, in California we recognize it for a maximum period of 30 months.

# Nature and Properties of Rabies Virus*

T. J. Wiktor

*The Wistar Institute of Anatomy & Biology, Philadelphia, Pennsylvania 19104*

The basic characteristics of rabies virus and its relationship to the host cell were poorly defined until, during the past few years, modern virological techniques were applied to the study of rabies. Important advances have been made possible through adaptation of the virus to tissue culture systems and subsequent application of immunofluorescence staining, complement-fixation and hemagglutination techniques, electron microscopy and physicochemical studies of concentrated and purified virus.

## VIRAL CLASSIFICATION

Rabies virus is included in the newly classified family of viruses tentatively designated either Stomatoviridae (Provisional Committee for Nomenclature of Viruses, 1965) or Rhabdoviruses (Melnick & McCombs, 1966).

This group, comprising several virions with distinctive morphological features not shared by other animal virions, includes vesicular stomatitis virus (VSV) and rabies virus. The rabies virion is a cylinder, flat on one end and round at the other, consisting of an inner helical component which resembles the nucleoprotein helix of the paramyxovirus group, and an envelop with surface projections. In addition to the members of this virus family infecting animals, several plant and insect viruses with similar structures have recently been described (Kitaoka & Murphy, 1969).

The principal Rhabdoviruses infecting animals are listed in Table 1. Although the Marburg virus may not fulfill all the criteria for final inclusion in the group, it was included in this table, nevertheless, for the sake of completeness and because of the interest created by the tragic circumstances surrounding the discovery of this agent.

* Supported, in part, by Public Health Service Research Grant AI-02954 from the National Institute of Allergy and Infectious Disease and by funds from the World Health Organization

Table 1. Rhabdoviruses of Animals

| Virus | Morphological description |
|---|---|
| Vesicular Stomatitis-Indiana type | Howatson & Whitmore, 1962 |
| Cocal | Ditchfield & Almeida, 1964 |
| Argentina-Brazil type | Federer *et al.*, 1967 |
| Vesicular Stomatitis-New Jersey type | Hackett, 1964 |
| Piry-Chandipura | Shope & Murphy, unpublished |
| Bovine Ephemeral Fever | Ito *et al.*, 1969 |
| Flanders-Hart Park | Murphy *et al.*, 1966 |
| Mount Elgon | Murphy *et al.*, 1970 |
| Rabies | Matsumoto, 1962 |
| Lagos bat | Shope *et al.*, 1970 |
| IbAn 27377 | Shope *et al.*, 1970 |
| M 1056 | Johnson, unpublished |
| Marburg | Siegert, 1967 |

## MORPHOLOGY

External dimensions of a typical rabies virus particle are 75 × 180 m$\mu$. The surface has a honeycomb-configuration with surface protrusions 60–70 m$\mu$ long, having knoblike structures at their distal end; these protrusions are generally not found at the end of the particle.

In cross section the virus appears to consist of a core surrounded by a dense membrane. This core, with an average diameter of 40 m$\mu$, usually appears empty, but occasionally some material can be found inside. The dense membrane is always surrounded by a fringe of surface projections.

When preparations were stained with ammonium molybdate instead of phosphotungstic acid, the fringe of surface protrusions could also be seen on the base of the virus particle.

At the base of whole viruses there is usually a "tail" which resembles a flattened balloon. This "tail" is sometimes visibly hollow; it is seen both on particles with apparently intact bases and attached directly to capsids with broken bases. Most particles with "tails" also have visible axial canals, but this is not always the case. It is difficult to determine whether the "tail" represents "leakage" from the virions or an extension of the capsid base.

Free nucleocapsids can be isolated from purified rabies virus preparations, (Hummeler *et al.*, 1968) and from rabies virus-infected cells (Sokol, unpublished data). They appear as single-stranded helixes, 1 $\mu$ long, with an average outside diameter of 150 Å and a periodicity of 75 Å. The length of the uncoiled strand is about 4.2 $\mu$ and its width varies from 20 to 65 Å.

## CHEMICAL COMPOSITION

Extracellular rabies virus of tissue culture origin can easily be concentrated and purified by a simple procedure worked out in our laboratory, involving precipitation of the virions by zinc acetate,

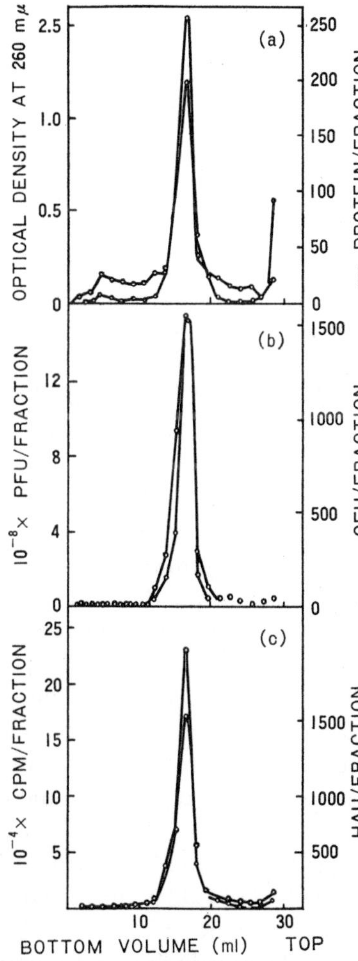


Fig. 1. Centrifugation in Sucrose Density Gradient of Concentrated and Partially Purified Rabies Virus (strain HEP).

A linear gradient of sucrose (10 to 55%, w/w) was used.
(a) Symbols: ○, protein content; ●, optical density at 260 nm.
(b): ○, CFU; ●, PFU.
(c) Symbols: ○, HAU; ●, radioactivity of $^3$H-uridine.

The three parts of the figure represent the same centrifugation experiment. The virus was grown in BHK cells in the presence of BSA.

(Reprinted with permission from Sokol *et al.*, 1968.)

desalting on a Sephadex column, additional concentration by high-speed centrifugation and banding in a sucrose density gradient (Sokol *et al.*, 1968). The virus has a high degree of purity, as shown in Figure 1. The precipitation of the virus by zinc acetate can be replaced by concentrating the infectious tissue culture fluid through ultrafiltration (Wiktor *et al.*, 1969).

The properties of a purified rabies virus preparation (Flury HEP) are listed in the following table (Sokol *et al.*, 1968).

| | |
|---|---|
| Specific infectivity | $10^{10}$PFU/mg protein |
| Specific HA activity | $10^4$ HAU/mg protein |
| Specific CF activity | $5 \times 10^3$ CFU/mg protein |
| Buoyant density in sucrose solution at 20°C | 1.17 g/cm$^3$ |
| Sedimentation coefficient | 550–650 S |
| Antibody types induced after immunization | Virus-neutralizing, HAI, CF and lytic |

## ISOLATION AND CHARACTERIZATION OF VIRION COMPONENTS

The different components of rabies virions can be separated from concentrated and purified rabies virus by treatment with sodium deoxycholate (DOC) and by combined velocity and equilibrium gradient centrifugation (Sokol *et al.*, 1969). The viral coat falls apart into relatively slowly sedimenting components, whereas the nucleocapsid is released in essentially intact form and sediments at 200S. Thus the components of the viral coat can be separated from the nucleocapsid which contains all the viral ribonucleic acid (RNA) by rate zonal centrifugation in a sucrose density gradient. The nucleocapsid can then be further purified by isopycnic centrifugation in a CsCl solution.

The pure nucleocapsid contains 96% protein and 4% RNA; it has a buoyant density in CsCl of 1.32 g/cm$^3$, a sedimentation constant of 200S and a molecular weight of $1.2 \times 10^8$ daltons. It is noninfectious, exhibits complement-fixing (CF) activity and induces the formation of CF antibodies. The rabies virus RNA is a single-stranded molecule with a molecular weight of about $4.6 \times 10^6$ daltons per nucleocapsid and is noninfectious. Only the viral RNA and the nucleocapsid have thus far been isolated in a pure form from preparations of disrupted virus.

The coat of the rabies virus consists of proteins, lipids, and possibly carbohydrates. Procedures are now being developed for the fractionation of rabies virus coat proteins.

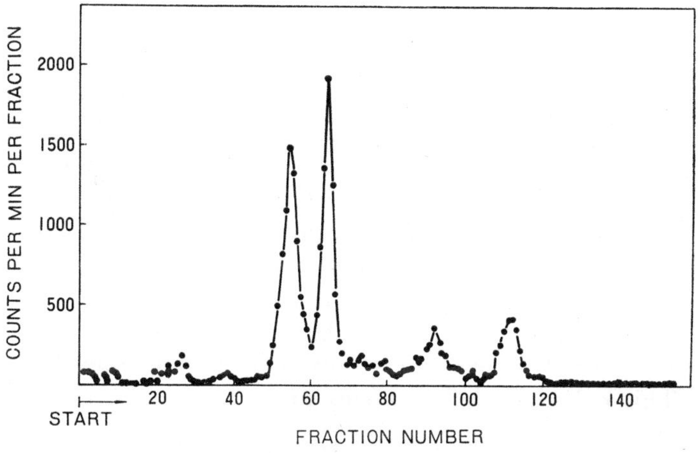


Fig. 2. Electrophoresis in Polyacrylamide Gel of Purified Rabies Virus Decomposed by Treatment with Sodium Dodecylsulfate and 2-Mercaptoethanol.

When purified rabies virions decomposed by treatment with sodium dodecylsulfate and 2-mercaptoethanol were analyzed by electrophoresis in polyacrylamide gel (Fig. 2) (Sokol *et al.*, 1971) four major components could be detected. The polypeptide with the second largest molecular weight ($\pm$ 82,000 daltons) corresponds to the protein component of the nucleocapsid whereas that with the largest molecular weight ($\pm$ 100,000 daltons) is a glycoprotein, and the remaining two components (Molecular weight $\pm$ 48,500 and 13,500 daltons) are constituents of the viral coat.

## VIRUS-HOST CELL INTERACTION

The difficulties encountered in propagating rabies virus in various tissue culture systems were related to the inability of the virus to either adsorb onto or penetrate the cell membrane. These difficulties have now been overcome by the addition of polycations to the virus inoculum (Kaplan *et al.*, 1967). Small amounts of DEAE-dextran or protamine sulfate facilitate the penetration of the virus into cells in which it subsequently replicates. The exact mechanism of this action is not known; the polycations may serve as receptor sites for the virus after binding to the cell surface, or they may form complexes with the virion which are then easily adsorbed onto the cell.

With the use of this technique various strains of rabies virus can be grown in many different tissue culture systems, not only in cells from warm-blooded animals, but also in cells from at least four reptile cell lines originated from a viper snake, gecko lizard, and turtle (Clark, unpublished data).

Although all mammalian tissue cultures are susceptible to infection with either street or fixed virus, the degree of susceptibility varies from that of the highly susceptible hamster fibroblast BHK-21 or Nil-2 cultures to that of the highly resistant L or MK-2 cell cultures. The susceptibility of human embryonic fibroblasts (human diploid cell strains) falls somewhere in the middle.

Infection of cells in culture by rabies virus is enhanced when they are exposed simultaneously to lymphocytic choriomeningitis (LCM) virus. This enhancing effect seems to be specific for rabies virus, since no other virus has been found to be enhanced by LCM virus (Wiktor *et al.*, 1966).

In ideal conditions, using tissue-culture-adapted strains of virus and a highly susceptible cell system, adsorption and penetration of the virus are extremely rapid events (Wiktor, 1966). A few seconds of contact are sufficient for the virus to become attached so that it can not be removed even by multiple washings, and "penetration" of the attached virus beyond the influence of antibody occurs within minutes after exposure.

The highest yields of rabies virus are obtained from cells maintained at 31–33°C and the lowest from those kept at 40°C. The virus can replicate at temperatures as low as 20°C. Experiments to determine the stability of rabies virus in tissue culture have shown that the growth medium should contain a low concentration of serum or serum components, such as albumin, and have a slightly alkaline pH (7.4–7.6).

## DYNAMICS OF VIRUS REPLICATION

The time needed for the production of viral antigens in rabies virus-infected cells has been investigated by immunofluorescence, CF and hemagglutination (HA) techniques (Wiktor & Kuwert, unpublished data). The results obtained were correlated with the production of intracellular and extracellular infectious virus in BHK-21 cells infected with the HEP strain of rabies virus at various input multiplicities (IM).

At an IM of 20 plaque-forming units (PFU)/cell, immunofluorescence was first observed 8 hours after infection in 24% of the cells (Fig. 3). Two hours later 68% of the cells showed fluorescent antibody (FA) antigen and this level of infection persisted for the next 6 hours. The second cycle of virus replication began at this time, and by 24 hours after infection 100% of the cells showed FA antigen.

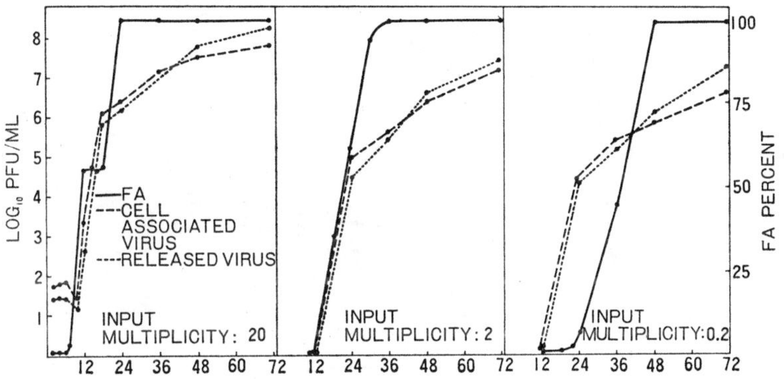


Fig. 3. Dynamics of Rabies Virus (HEP) Replication in BHK-21 Cell Culture. Production of FA antigen, cell associated and released virus. Three input multiplicities.

A small amount of residual virus persisted in the cultures during the first 7 hours after infection. The eclipse phase lasted for the next 5 hours. The newly produced virus was detected in cell homogenates, as well as in the tissue culture fluid, at 12 hours after infection. The level of infectious virus increased rapidly during the next 6 hours and continued to rise with prolonged incubation. At first most of the virus was present in the cell homogenates, but after the 30th hour post infection, the medium contained the higher level of infectivity, indicating continuous production in the cells and accumulation of infectious virions in the medium.

The input of infectivity had no effect on the final yield of virus (Fig. 4). The peak of infectivity was obtained in four days with an IM of 20 PFU/cell whereas 6 days were required to achieve the same level with a lower IM, i.e., 2 or 0.2 PFU/cell.

No specific cytopathic effect could be observed in rabies-infected cultures, regardless of the IM used.

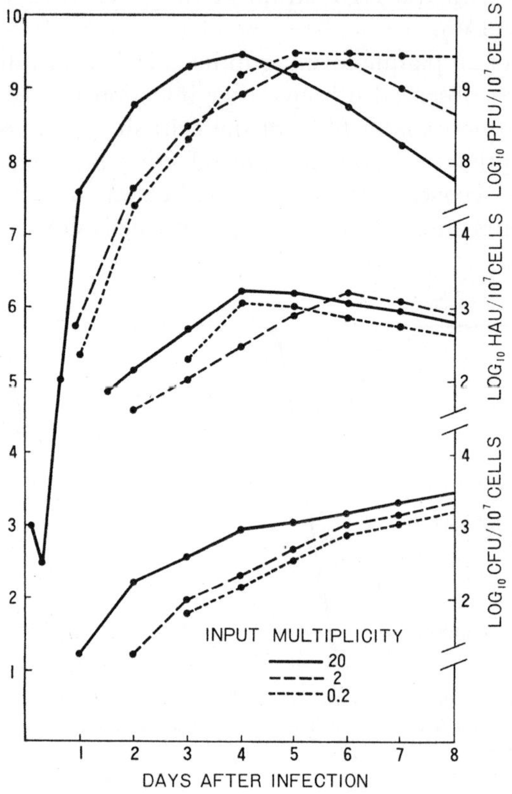


Fig. 4. Dynamics of Rabies Virus (HEP) Replication in BHK-21 Cell Culture. Production of infectious virus, HA and CF antigen. Three input multiplicities.

Practically all HA activity occurred in the tissue culture fluid. Cell-associated virus contained very little of this activity, even though in the early stage of infection, concentration of infectious virus was higher in the cell homogenates than in the tissue culture fluid.

Hemagglutinin could first be detected 30 hours after infection with an IM of 20 PFU/cell and later with lower IM's. The level of hemagglutinin increased with that of infectivity, and both reached a peak at approximately the same time.

CF antigens were detected 24 hours after infection and before the appearance of hemagglutinin. The dynamics of their formation followed the pattern of the production of infectious virus. At the start of the infection higher activity was observed in the cell homogenates whereas later more activity was present in the infected culture fluid. CF activity appears to be more resistant to heat inactivation than infectivity and hemagglutinin.

The cytoplasm of rabies-infected cells in tissue culture contain inclusions which can be demonstrated by several staining procedures for protein-bound groups. These inclusions correspond to the Negri bodies found in nerve cells of animals infected with street rabies virus. Comparative cytochemical studies (Lowe *et al.*, 1967) indicate that the protein in the matrix of the inclusions produced by infection with rabies virus *in vivo* is cytochemically indistinguishable from that of the *in vitro* inclusions.

The sequential events of rabies virus replication on the cellular level were studied by electron microscopy (Hummeler *et al.*, 1967). In this study it was seen that virus particles adsorbed to the surface were attached to it by fine fibers. The particles passed into the cytoplasm by phagocytosis. Phagocytotic vesicles were formed, enclosing one or more particles, 15 to 30 minutes after infection.

Eight to nine hours after infection the normal structure of the cytoplasm was replaced by a granular mass containing occasional fine fibers. The ribosomes in the unaltered cytoplasm surrounding these areas showed distinct polyribosomal aggregates. Virus particles became visible at the edges of some matrices at 24 hours after infection, and, later, within them.

Virus also appeared to be formed or released by the process of budding into intracytoplasmic vacuoles and, to a lesser degree, from the cell surface. Thus it seems that rabies virus, in a unique fashion, may be assembled either like myxovirus at the cell surface or like vaccinia virus at the intracellular matrix.

Judging by the disproportionately large ratio of virions present inside the infected cell to the amount of virus released, it seems possible that a large portion of the synthesized virus either was not released from the infected cells, or did not reach complete maturation.

## ACTION OF ARABINOSYL CYTOSINE ON RABIES VIRUS REPLICATION

Like other RNA viruses, the rabies virus is only slightly inhibited by actinomycin D and not at all by mitomycin C, fluorodeoxyuridine or bromodeoxyuridine (Wiktor, 1966). An unexpected finding, therefore, was the inhibition of rabies virus by 1, beta-*p*-arabinofuranosylcytosine (ara-C), a potent inhibitor of DNA synthesis (Maes *et al.*, 1967; Campbell *et al.*, 1968).

When actinomycin D, nogalomycin, cyclohexamide or puromycin is added during the first 3 hours of rabies virus replication in the presence of ara-C, the inhibitory action of ara-C is partially or completely reversed, supporting the hypothesis that ara-C requires the induction of a cellular protein for its specific inhibitory action on rabies virus growth. This action is completely different from the mode of ara-C inhibition of another RNA virus, Rous sarcoma virus, which has a transitory need for DNA synthesis, and it is likely that ara-C inhibits the replication of Rous sarcoma virus by interfering with this stage.

## TYPES OF VIRUS–CELL INTERACTION

Rabies virus-infected cells can generally be maintained in tissue cultures for extensive periods of time without showing any noticeable cytopathic effect. Different types of chronic infection take place, depending on the cell system used.

Two exceptions, however, should be mentioned. Agarose-suspended BHK-13S cell cultures are sufficiently affected by several strains of rabies virus to allow production of plaques (Sedwick & Wiktor, 1967) and a strain of street rabies virus (R–205) adapted to growth in primary dog kidney cells (Hronovsky & Benda, 1970) developed stabilized cytopathic properties which can be used in direct titration as an indicator system suitable for quantitative assay for antirabies serum antibody, based on a specific neutralization of the viral cytopathic effect.

Several types of chronic cell-virus infection have been described:

*Endosymbiotic infection*, as found with rabbit endothelial cells infected with the CVS strain of virus (Fernandes *et al.*, 1964), is characterized by the accumulation in cells of only small intracytoplasmic inclusions. During prolonged cultivation for more than two years, such infected cultures appear to have suffered no interference with the mechanism of cellular replication. The growth rate, plating efficiency, and morphology of infected and uninfected, control cultures are identical, although viral antigen is present in the cytoplasm of each cell of the infected cultures.

The synthesis of DNA and RNA in CVS-infected and uninfected rabbit endothelial cell populations could not be differentiated by labeling experiments with tritiated thymidine or uridine. The presence of antirabies serum in the endosymbiotic system did not prevent the persistence of infection, unless complement was added to mediate cell lysis (Wiktor *et al.*, 1968).

*In carrier-type infection*, after infection with rabies virus of cultures of hamster fibroblasts (stable line, Nil-2) (Fig.5) (Wiktor & Koprowski, 1967) the production of new virus reaches its peak in 3 to 4 days and falls off sharply in the course of the following six to seven cell transfers. In contrast, intracytoplasmic inclusion bodies containing rabies antigen detectable by immunofluorescence remain present in all the cultured cells even when the synthesis of new virus is minimal. At that time cultures became resistant to superinfection with VSV and an inhibitor with interferon-like properties can be recovered from the culture medium. After this phase of infection, there is a marked decrease in the number of antigen-containing cells during subsequent cell transfers, followed by a gradual rise in the proportion of these cells and an increase of infectious virus production. These cycles of high and low levels of rabies infection and corresponding resistance to challenge recur periodically.

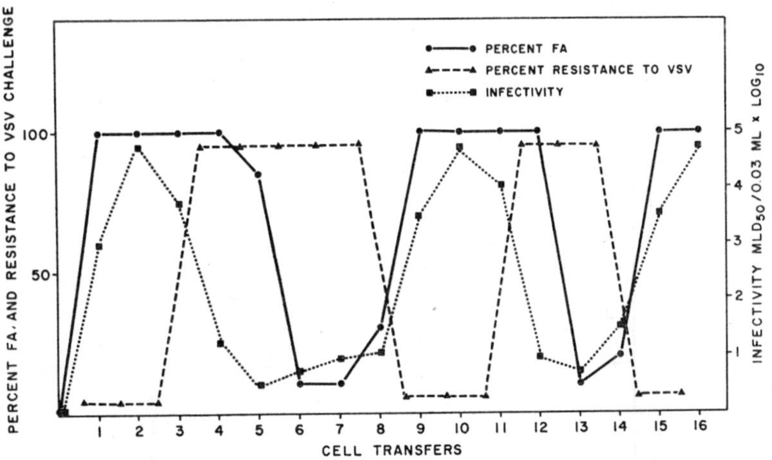


Fig. 5. Carrier-type of Rabies Virus Infection (PM strain) in Hamster Cell Culture (Nil-2).

## BY-PRODUCTS OF RABIES VIRUS INFECTION IN TISSUE CULTURE

The existence of virion-free proteins occurring as "soluble antigens" in infected cells has been demonstrated by differential centri-

Table 2. Biologic Activities of Fractions Obtained after Differential Centrifugation of Infectious Tissue Culture Fluid (Strain PM)

| Fraction | Infectivity (PFU $\times 10^{-7}$) | | | CF Activity | | | Protective Activity | | | |
|---|---|---|---|---|---|---|---|---|---|---|
| | | | | | | | $ED_{50}$ | | | AV |
| | Per m*l* | Total | % recovery | Per m*l* | Total | % recovery | Per m*l* | Total | % recovery | Per m*l* |
| Tissue culture fluid concentrated by ultrafiltration ($\times 14.5^a$) | 20 | 3,400 | 100 | 64 | 10,900 | 100 | 370 | 62,900 | 100 | 9.2 |
| 13,600 $\times$ G sediment ($\times 117$) | 190 | 4,000 | 117 | 128 | 2,700 | 24.8 | 2,100 | 44,000 | 70.0 | 52.5 |
| 23,300 $\times$ G sediment ($\times 223$) | 11 | 120 | 3.5 | 64 | 680 | 6.2 | 720 | 7,600 | 12.1 | 18.0 |
| 34,900 $\times$ G sediment ($\times 223$) | 0.4 | 4.2 | 0.12 | 32 | 340 | 3.1 | 109 | 1,150 | 1.8 | 2.7 |
| 64,400 $\times$ G sediment ($\times 223$) | 0.00002 | 0.0001 | 0.001 | 32 | 340 | 3.1 | 74 | 790 | 1.3 | 1.85 |
| 64,400 $\times$ G supernatant ($\times 14.5$) | 0.0003 | 0.05 | 0.0014 | 64 | 10,900 | 100 | 9 | 1,530 | 2.4 | 0.23 |

[a] Concentration factor: Ratio of the original tissue culture fluid to the fraction volume. (Reprinted with permission from Schlumberger *et al.*, 1970.)

fugation of concentrated tissue culture fluid infected with different strains of rabies virus (Schlumberger *et al.*, 1970).

The results (Table 2) indicate that the terminal supernatant fluid ($64,400 \times g$) obtained after sequential differential high-speed centrifugation of the concentrate derived by ultrafiltration of rabies virus-infected tissue culture fluids, was essentially virion-free and contained most of the CF activity of the original preparation. The $13,600 \times g$ fraction which contained essentially all the virions showed less CF activity.

In spite of the high CF activity, the virion-depleted, $64,400 \times g$ supernatant fluid showed poor protective activity in the mouse potency test. In rabbits, however, the same fractions elicited formation of significant levels of virus-neutralizing antibody. Moreover, a booster injection of these preparations caused a much greater rise in antibody level than did a booster injection of a virion-rich fraction.

## CONCLUSIONS

Significant progress has been made during the last few years in our fundamental understanding of the virus itself and its relation to the cell host, but much remains to be learned. Such knowledge, accompanied by modern quantitative techniques, is needed before any worthwhile advance can be made in the prophylaxis of rabies, as well as in the other biological and epidemiological aspects of the disease that still remain obscure.

## REFERENCES

Campbell, J. B., Maes, R. F., Wiktor, T. J. and Koprowski, H. (1968). Inhibition of rabies virus by arabinosyl cytosine. Studies on the mechanism and specificity of action. *Virology*, **34**, 701–708.

Defendi, V. and Wiktor, T. J. (1966). Metabolic and autoradiographic studies of rabies virus-infected cells. *In* International Rabies Symposium, Talloire, 1965, Vol I, pp. 119–124 (Basel: Karger).

Ditchfield, J. and Almeida, J. D. (1964). The fine structure of cocal virus. *Virology*, **24**, 232–235.

Federer, K. E., Burrows, R. and Brooksby, J. B. (1967). Vesicular stomatitis virus—The relationship between some strains of the Indiana serotype. *Res. Vet. Sci.*, **8**, 103–117.

Fernandes, M., Wiktor, T. J. and Koprowski, H. (1964). Endosymbiotic relationship between animal viruses and host cells. *J. Exp. Med.*, **120**, 1099–1116.

Hackett, A. J. (1964). A possible morphologic basis for the auto-interference phenomenon in vesicular stomatitis virus. *Virology*, **24**, 51–59.

Howatson, A. F. and Whitmore, G. F. (1962). The development and structure of vesicular stomatitis virus. *Virology*, **16**, 466–478.

Hronovsky, V. and Benda, R. (1970). Kinetics of reaction of rabies virus with specific antibodies in conditions of *in vitro* virus neutralization test. *Acta Virol.*, **14**, 209.

Hummeler, K., Koprowski, H. and Wiktor, T. J. (1967). Structure and development of rabies virus in tissue culture. *J. Virol.*, **1**, 152–170.

Hummeler, K., Tomassini, N., Sokol, F., Kuwert, E. and Koprowski, H. (1968). Morphology of the nucleoprotein component of rabies virus. *J. Virol.*, **2**, 1191–1199.

Ito, Y., Tanaka, Y., Inaba, Y. and Omori, T. (1969). Electron microscopic observations of bovine epizootic fever virus. *Nat. Inst. Animal Health, Tokyo, Quarterly*, **9**, 35–44.

Kaplan, M. M., Wiktor, T. J., Maes, R. F., Campbell, J. B. and Koprowski, H. (1967). Effect of polyions on the infectivity of rabies virus in tissue culture: Construction of a single-cycle growth curve. *J. Virol.*, **1**, 145–151.

Kitaoka, M. and Murphy, F. (1968). Bullet-shaped viruses. *In* Proc. 1st Intl. Cong. Virol., Helsinki, 1968 (J. L. Melnick, ed.), *Intl. Virol.* Vol. I (Basel: Karger).

Love, R., Fernandes, M. V. and Wiktor, T. J. (1966). The response of the cell to infection with rabies virus. *Rev. Path. Comp.*, **66**, 533–541.

Maes, R. F., Kaplan, M. M., Wiktor, T. J., Campbell, J. B. and Koprowski, H. (1967). Inhibitory effect of a cytidine analogue on growth of rabies virus. Comparative studies with other metabolic inhibitors. *In* Symposium on Molecular Biology of Viruses, pp. 449–462 (New York: Academic Press).

Matsumoto, S. (1962). Electron microscopy of nerve cells infected with street rabies virus. *Virology*, **17**, 198–202.

Melnick, J. L. and McCombs, R. M. (1966). Classification and nomenclature of animal viruses. *Progr. Med. Virol.*, **8**, 400–408.

Murphy, F., Coleman, P. H. and Whitfield, S. G. (1966). Electron microscopic observations of Flanders virus. *Virology*, **30**, 314–317.

Murphy, F. A. and Fields, B. N. (1967). Kern Canyon virus: Electron microscopic and immunological studies. *Virology*, **33**, 625–637.

Murphy, F., Shope, R. E., Metselaar, D. and Simpson, D. I. H. (1970). Characterization of Mount Elgon bat virus, a new member of the Rhabdovirus group. *Virology*, **40**, 288–297.

Provisional Committee for Nomenclature of Viruses. (1965). Proposals and recommendations. *Ann. Inst. Pasteur*, **109**, 625–635.

Schlumberger, H. D., Wiktor, T. J. and Koprowski, H. (1970). Antigenic and immunogenic properties of components contained in rabies virus-infected tissue culture fluids. *J. Immunol.*, **105**, 291–298.

Sedwick, W. D. and Wiktor, T. J. (1967). Reproducible plaquing system for rabies, lymphocytic choriomeningitis and other ribonucleic acid viruses in BHK-21/13S agarose suspensions. *J. Virol.*, **1**, 1224–1226.

Shope, R. E., Murphy, F., Harrison, E. A. K., Causey, O. R., Kemp, G. E., Simpson, D. I. H. and Moore, D. L. (1970). Two African viruses serologically and morphologically related to rabies virus. *J. Virol.*, **6**, 690–692.

Siegert, R. H., H. L. Shu, W. Slenczka, D. Peters, and G. Muller, (1967). Zur Atiologie einer unbekannten von Affen ausgegangen menschlichen Infectionskrankheit. *Deutsch. Med. Wschr.*, **92**, 2341–2343.

Sokol, F., E. Kuwert, T. J. Wiktor, K. Hummeler, and H. Koprowski. (1968). Purification of rabies virus grown in tissue culture. *J. Virol.*, **2**, 836–849.

Sokol, F., Schlumberger, D., Wiktor, T. J., Koprowski, H. and Hummeler, K. (1969). Biochemical and biological studies on the nucleocapsid and the RNA of rabies virus. *Virology*, **38**, 651–665.

Sokol, F., D. Stančekk, and H. Koprowski. (1971). Structural proteins of rabies virus. *J. Virol.,* 7, 241–249.

Wiktor, T. J. (1966). Kinetics of rabies virus in tissue culture. National Rabies Symposium, Atlanta, Ga.

Wiktor, T. J., Kaplan, M. M. and Koprowski, H. (1966). Rabies and lymphocytic choriomeningitis virus (LCMV) infection of tissue culture: Enhancing effect of LCMV. *Ann. Med. Exp. Fenn.*, **44**, 290–296.

Wiktor, T. J. and Koprowski, H. (1967). Cyclic appearance of viral inhibitor in tissue cultures chronically infected with rabies virus. *Bact. Proc. Abstracts,* 1967, p. 166.

Wiktor, T. J., Kuwert, E. and Koprowski, H. (1968). Immune lysis of rabies virus-infected cells. *J. Immunol.*, **101**, 1271–1282.

Wiktor, T. J., Sokol, F., Kuwert, E. and Koprowski, H. (1969). Immuno-genicity of concentrated and purified rabies vaccine of tissue culture origin. *Proc. Soc. Exp. Biol. Med.*, **131**, 799–805.

For Discussion, see page 57.

# Rabies and Serologically-Related Viruses from Africa*

ROBERT E. SHOPE
AND
GREGORY H. TIGNOR

*The Yale Arbovirus Research Unit, Department of Epidemiology and Public Health, Yale University School of Medicine, New Haven, Connecticut 06510*

The evolutionary process mitigates against the existence of organisms without relatives. Rabies virus has kept its family secrets longer than most. There has been tacit agreement that rabies virus was a unique antigenic type (Bell, 1967) until recently, when as a result of our collaborative studies with investigators at the National Center for Disease Control (NCDC), the University of Ibadan and Porton, England, two viruses were shown to be serologically and morphologically related to rabies virus (Shope *et al.*, 1970).

One of these, Lagos bat virus, was isolated from the brains of fruit bats, *Eidolon helvum* on Lagos Island, Nigeria, in 1956 by Boulger and Porterfield (Boulger & Porterfield, 1958). The virus was re-isolated from the original brain suspension, and was pathogenic for baby and weanling mice intracerebrally, but not for weanling mice intraperitoneally, guinea pigs or rabbits intramuscularly, or *Cercocebus torquatus* monkeys subcutaneously. *Aedes aegypti* which fed upon mouse brain suspension did not become infected. Negri bodies were not seen in infected mouse brain preparations. Weanling mice infected intracerebrally with non-mouse-adapted virus died with an average survival time of 14.8 days which shortened, using seventh mouse passage virus, to 7.2 days. There is only one existing strain of Lagos bat virus.

The other rabies-related virus is Ib An 27377, isolated during 1968

* This study was supported by The Rockfeller Foundation and by the United States-Japan Cooperative Medical Science Program administered by the National Institute of Allergy and Infectious Diseases of the National Institutes of Health, Department of Health, Education, and Welfare, under Grant No. 1-R22-AI-08215-01A1.

from pooled viscera of shrews (*Crocidura* sp.) captured near Ibadan, Nigeria (Shope *et al.*, 1970). The Ibadan shrew virus had mouse pathogenicity similar to the Lagos bat virus. At the fifth mouse passage level, weanling mice infected intracerebrally died with an average survival time of 6 days. Virus has been demonstrated in fluid phase of VERO cell cultures infected from mouse brain material, and plaques appeared under agar overlay in 8 to 11 days. Three strains from shrews have been characterized.

Both the Lagos bat and the Ibadan shrew virus appeared as bullet-shaped particles in thin section electron microscopy done at the NCDC (Shope *et al.*, 1970).

By complement-fixation (CF) test (Table 1) there were marked cross-reactions among the 3 viruses. The Lagos bat ascitic fluid appeared specific although it was less potent than the other immune reagents. The ascitic fluids were produced by immunizing mice with 4 intraperitoneal injections of mouse brain mixed with Freund's complete adjuvant and thus represent hyperimmune reagents.

Table 1. Complement-fixation Reactions of Rabies-related Viruses[a]

| Antigen | Hyperimmune Rabies | ascitic fluid Lagos bat | IbAn 27377 | Control |
|---|---|---|---|---|
| Rabies (Pasteur) | 512/512[b] | 0/0 | 128/512 | 0/0 |
| Lagos bat | 32/128 | 64/128 | 128/512 | 0/0 |
| IbAn 27377 | 32/32 | 0/0 | 512/512 | 0/0 |
| Control | 0/0 | 0/0 | 0/0 | 0/0 |

*a* From Shope, R.E. *et al.*

*b* Titer expressed as reciprocal of dilution: ascitic fluid/antigen
0=<4

Table 2. Serum-dilution Neutralization Test of Rabies-related Viruses[a]

| Virus | Inoculum: mouse $LD_{50}$ | Serum (S) or mouse ascitic fluid (MAF) | | | |
|---|---|---|---|---|---|
| | | Rabies burro S | Lagos bat MAF | IbAn 27377 MAF | Control MAF (M-1056) |
| Rabies, strain CVS | 160 | 15,625[b] | 11 | 0[c] | 0 |
| Rabies, vampire bat | 200 | 15,625 | 11 | 1 | 0 |
| Lagos bat ....... | 50 | 5 | 280 | 18 | 0 |
| IbAn 27377 ..... | 100 | 3 | 3.5 | 320 | 0 |
| Control (M-1056) | 125 | 0 | 0 | 0 | 25 |

*a* From Shope *et al.*

*b* Reciprocal of 50% neutralization endpoint of serum or ascitic fluid; five-fold serum dilutions vs. constant virus dilution

*c* No survivors

Results of serum dilution neutralization tests done in mice at NCDC (Shope *et al.*, 1970) are illustrated in Table 2. The vampire bat and CVS strains of rabies appeared similar. Lagos bat and the Ibadan shrew viruses were distinct from rabies and from each other. Sera and ascitic fluids cross-reacted with heterologous viruses only when used in concentrated form.

Results of virus-dilution neutralization tests using undiluted hyperimmune mouse ascitic fluids and rabies virus (Pasteur strain) approximated the CF results. Log neutralizing indices were $\geq 5.3$ for rabies ascitic fluid, 3.1 for Ibadan shrew, and 4.1 for Lagos bat ascitic fluid. Another less potent Lagos bat ascitic fluid did not neutralize rabies virus.

Three hamsters were immunized intramuscularly (i.m.) with 100 suckling mouse i.c. $LD_{50}$ of the Ibadan shrew agent and challenged i.m. after one month with 100 $LD_{50}$ of Pasteur strain rabies virus. One of 3 survived. This rabies virus dose was uniformly lethal for 8 unimmunized control hamsters.

A serological survey of human residents of the Western Region and the Benue River area of northern Nigeria has been carried out with the Ibadan shrew agent using undiluted serum and from 4 to 30 suckling mouse i.c. $LD_{50}$ of Ibadan shrew virus. Of 468 sera tested, only two protected all of the mice in spite of the very low virus dose. There is thus no evidence for significant numbers of humans immune to the Ibadan shrew virus, although it may be that the population sampled is not representative of the population at risk.

What are the implications, to future research and to our conceptual thinking about rabies, of the discovery of rabies-related viruses? One of these viruses might serve as a basis for development of a heterologous rabies vaccine. Alternatively, it may be possible to take advantage of group cross-reactivity to develop a successful combined vaccination schedule.

We are thinking in terms of possible biological exclusion of rabies virus from a geographical area or from a potential host population. Bat rabies is not known in Africa (Kaplan, 1967). Could Lagos bat virus, apparently a natural parasite of fruit bats, be responsible, through the mechanism of a heterologous antibody, for maintaining these bats free of rabies virus infection? Could rabies biological control be accomplished by introduction of a rabies-related virus into a given wild-life population?

We are also concerned that infection with a rabies-related virus may be erroneously diagnosed as rabies, thus leading to unnecessary treatment or unrealistic control measures.

There appears to be little chance of documenting the development and spread of rabies infection prior to historical times. Nevertheless finding 2 rabies-related viruses in West Africa favors the hypothesis that an ancestral virus evolved in Africa; that rabies as we know it today spread widely because it evolved into a neuropathic organism capable of inducing its host to bite and ensuring its spread via dogs and wild animals; and that Lagos bat and Ibadan shrew viruses remain focalized in West Africa as nontransported evolutions of the ancestral virus.

The search for additional rabies-related viruses continues. It has not been fashionable to support the nontargeted internationally oriented research of a survey nature which has led to the finding of the rabies-related viruses. The foresight of The Rockfeller Foundation, the World Health Organization, and the United States-Japan Cooperative Medical Science Program of the National Institutes of Health should be recognized in this regard.

## ACKNOWLEDGMENTS

Human survey sera of the Benue River area, Northern Nigeria, from the WHO Trepanematoses Survey (1965–1966) were obtained through the courtesy of Dr. Thorsten Guthe, and those from the Western Region through the courtesy of Dr. Robert Williams, NAMRU III, Cairo, Egypt.

## REFERENCES

Bell, J. F. (1967). Present concepts of the epidemiology of rabies. First International Conference on Vaccines. PAHO Scientific Publication 147, pp. 481–487.

Boulger, L. R. and Porterfield, J. S. (1958). Isolation of a virus from Nigerian fruit bats. *Trans. Roy. Soc. Trop. Med. Hyg.*, **52**, 421–424.

Kaplan, M. M. (1967). First International Conference on Vaccines. PAHO Scientific Publication 147, p. 496.

Shope, R. E., Murphy, F. A., Harrison, A. K., Causey, O. R., Kemp, G. E., Simpson, D. I. H. and Moore, D. L. (1970). Two African viruses serologically and morphologically related to rabies virus. *J. Virol.* Vol. **6**, 690–692.

For Discussion, see page 57.

# Discussion*

OKUNO: Let me ask a simple question of Dr. Robert Shope. What is the reason for your careful handling of the title, "Rabies-related viruses"? Could it not be the "strains of rabies virus"? I would like to know the criteria of differentiating the strain of rabies virus from the rabies-related viruses. According to your complement fixation test, I think one can hardly tell that this is not a rabies virus. Even with the neutralization test, which you probably performed by the intracerebral route in mice, I wonder, if we see about the same degree of the strain variation among the many strains of rabies virus.

SHOPE: I think that this may be a moot point. It is a matter of degree, obviously, and I would say that, certainly in my experience, which is not as great as many of the other people sitting around this table, the amount of variation that one sees from one strain of rabies to another is not as great as we see among rabies in the Lagos bat and Ibadan shrew agent. I would also be very interested in hearing comments from other people on this point.

KOPROWSKI: This question is the subject of the panel discussion "Strain variation of rabies virus and cross reaction with other viruses." I suggest that we defer discussion of this point until that time.

DAVENPORT: What is known about the pathogenicity for animals of the strains of Rhabdovirus, which are grown in plants, and do they share any antigens with the strains isolated from man? I should like to know if your inclusion in that family is based only on their morphology and if so, I wish to express my prejudice and also question the value of including them.

WIKTOR: Some plant and insect viruses were included in the rhabdo virus group solely according to their morphology. The Egtvet virus of hemorrhagic fever of trout, included in this group, was

* This Discussion refers to the reports by Wiktor and Shope *et al.*

studied in our laboratory. It exhibited no pathogenicity for small laboratory animals; and no cross reaction with rabies virus could be detected by any of the serological methods used. To my knowledge, no comparative studies were performed with plant and rabies viruses.

OKUNO: Are there any cell lines or primary cells derived from a warm-blooded animal which are entirely unable to absorb all the 13 rabies virus strains you have tested?

WIKTOR: All mammalian cells seem to be susceptible to rabies virus infection. Some are more easily infected than others, but by using DEAE-dextran during virus adsorption, we were able to propagate rabies virus in cells from any warm-blooded animal and in some cells from cold-blooded animals.

HAMMON: You had a chart which indicated that the complement fixing antigen was effective in protecting, I believe the rabbit but not the mouse. Did I understand correctly?

WIKTOR: The role of the so-called soluble antigen in protecting animals against rabies is under investigation in our laboratory. Preparations depleted of virions but showing high activity in the complement fixation test, demonstrated a low protective activity when tested in mice by the standard NIH potency test for rabies vaccines. The same preparations, however, induced high levels of neutralizing antibody in rabbits and protected them from virulent challenge. It may be that mice are not the best animals in which to study the protective activity of soluble antigens.

# The Pathogenesis of Experimental Rabies

RICHARD T. JOHNSON

*The Johns Hopkins University School of Medicine,*
*Baltimore, Maryland 21205*

## INTRODUCTION

In 1769 Morgagni recorded that the onset of clinical rabies was often heralded by paresthesias in the area of the original wound and postulated that the "virus did not seem to be carried through the veins but by the nerves up to their origins" (Morgagni, 1769). Early experimental studies in the late 19th century lent support to this hypothesis. In 1888 Roux (Roux, 1888) isolated rabies from nerves in experimental rabies; in 1889 DiVestea and Zagari (DiVestea & Zagari, 1889) demonstrated initial central nervous system (CNS) infection at the spinal cord level corresponding to the inoculation site; and in 1889 Helman (Helman, 1889) showed removal of the tail 24 hours after distal inoculation gave protection. More sophisticated studies after the turn of the century provided further support of the hypothesis of neural spread; Nicolau and his colleagues (Nicolau & Meteiesco, 1928; Nicolau & Serbanescu, 1928) showed that interruption of the appropriate nerve protected against disease; Goodpasture (Goodpasture, 1925) found histologically that initial cytopathic changes in ganglia and CNS segments corresponded to sites of peripheral inoculation; and Schweinburg and Windholz (Schweinburg & Windholz, 1930) noted the failure of spread of infection between parabiotic rats. Certainly, these and other early studies of rabies biased subsequent work on the pathogenesis of other neuropathic viruses and were a major factor in formulating the doctrines of the 1930s that 1) all viruses invading the CNS spread along peripheral or olfactory nerves, and 2) that the blood-brain barrier was impervious to virus particles (Friedemann, 1943; Hurst, 1936).

With the demonstration of the importance of viremia and the hematogenous spread of poliomyelitis and arthropod-borne viruses to CNS, a reversal of dogma developed. Searching for universal mechanisms in nature, though biological systems are notorious for their lack of uniformity, many abandoned the notion that any virus could move centripetally in structures of peripheral nerves, despite prior studies to the contrary.

Leaving bias and personal taste aside, newer evidence for mechanisms of pathogenesis must be evaluated utilizing criteria not appreciated in older studies.

*A sequential study of the incubation period is essential*

Few conclusions can be drawn from the distribution of virus after the onset of symptoms or even late in the incubation period. For example, following subcutaneous inoculation of mice, California virus has been shown to replicate in several extraneural tissues; a high titered plasma viremia develops; and infection of the vascular endothelial cells of the CNS precedes infection of the parenchymal cells of the brain. Following cerebral infection, virus spreads centrifugally in nerves with infection of endoneural cells (Johnson & Johnson, 1968). However, demonstration of this "neural infection" is little more than a curiosity, since the sequential studies showed it played no evident role in CNS invasion.

*Virus growth in a tissue must be documented by showing significant increases in titer*

The presence of high titers of virus in tissues may only represent blood-borne virus in transit. Indeed, a higher titer of virus in liver than blood can be achieved by virus concentration in Kupfer cells clearing the viremia and may not represent active virus replication by any cells of that organ (Mims, 1964).

*Cell types supporting virus growth need to be determined by immunofluorescent staining or electron microscopy*

Virus growth in an organ may not indicate growth in the dominant cell type. For example, virus growth in the brain does not necessarily represent neuronal infection or even infection of parenchymal cells of the brain. Such growth may represent infection of only meningeal or ependymal cells, and even histological changes may not disclose this selectivity of infection (Johnson, 1968; Johnson & Mims, 1968).

*Generalizations must be made with caution*

Different viruses or different strains of virus have different cellular affinity; the route of spread of the same virus may differ in different species of hosts or even within the same species at different ages; and some viruses are capable of pursuing multiple pathways simultaneously within the same host animal (Johnson, 1964; Johnson & Mims, 1968).

## PATHOGENESIS AFTER INTRAMUSCULAR OR SUBCUTANEOUS INOCULATION

Most new evidence supports the centripetal spread of rabies virus along peripheral or cranial nerves as the major mechanism of CNS penetration following intramuscular or subcutaneous inoculation. However, this ingress of virus appears to occur without replication at the site of inoculation or in the nerve. CNS invasion occurs promptly, and the infection of salivary glands or other selective tissues may represent subsequent centrifugal neural dissemination. The evidence for this seemingly curious sequence of events follows.

*Fate of virus at inoculation site*

Habel (1941) noted in mice and guinea pigs that street virus may persist at the site of inoculation for 4 days, and questioned whether multiplication in muscle might occur. Isolations of fixed or street rabies viruses from tissues at the site of inoculation have been reported ranging from several hours to 6 days (Baer *et al.*, 1965; Kligler & Bernkopf, 1943; Petrovic & Timm, 1969; Schindler, 1961). However, increasing virus titers in muscle have not been reported. Indeed, Schindler (1961) showed a fall in titer over 2 days, and recently Petrovic and Timm (1969) reported fixed virus in the inoculated footpads of hamsters during the entire 6 day incubation period, but daily quantitation showed a clearcut decline of virus content (>99%) over this interval. Furthermore, fluorescent antibody staining has failed to show any development of virus antigen in the cells of subcutaneous or muscle tissues prior to CNS invasion (Baer *et al.*, 1968; Fischman, 1969; Johnson, 1965).

*Evidence for neural spread*

Prior to virus replication in the CNS, virus is usually not recoverable from peripheral nerves (Baer *et al.*, 1965, 1968; Kligler & Bernkopf, 1943; Schindler, 1961; Webster, 1937), and high titers of virus or detectable virus antigen in nerve have not been found (Baer *et al.*, 1965, 1968; Dean *et al.*, 1963; Johnson, 1965; Yamamoto *et al.*, 1965). Despite these findings, the initial CNS invasion, as demonstrated by virus isolation, occurs in the lumbar spinal cord following hindleg inoculation, the upper cord after foreleg inoculation, and the brainstem after masseter inoculation (Baer *et al.*, 1965, 1968; Huygelen & Mortelmans, 1959; Johnson, 1965; Kligler & Bernkopf, 1943; Otani, 1965; Petrovic & Timm, 1969; Webster, 1937). Immunofluorescence studies of fixed rabies have indicated earliest replication in appropriate ipsilateral dorsal root ganglia cells following hind footpad inoculations (Johnson, 1965) (Fig. 1). Using a street rabies virus, Yamamoto *et al.* (1965) have shown initial fluorescence in ipsilateral 2nd cervical dorsal root ganglia following masseter inoculation, and Otani (1965) has reported initial virus antigen in ipsilateral gasserian ganglion and basis pontis after masseter inoculation.

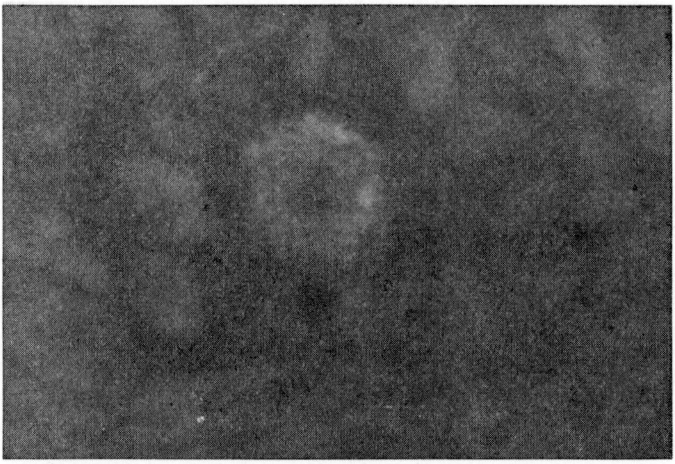

Fig. 1. Section of Mouse Lumbar Dorsal Root Ganglion Stained with Fluorescent Antibody 4 Days after Ipsilateral Hindfoot Subcutaneous Inoculation with CVS Strain of Fixed Rabies Virus.
The initial granules of cytoplasmic fluorescence are shown in one ganglion cell; no fluorescence was detectable in subcutaneous tissue, muscle, or peripheral nerve. X

Whether CNS invasion is dependent on an initial cycle of growth in the ganglia is unknown. When studies were done, this seemed an inconsequential point, but subsequent controversy regarding the efficacy of interferon in the postexposure treatment of rabies may make it germaine (Vieuchange, 1967). Unlike the CNS, the dorsal root ganglia of rabbits and guinea pigs have been shown to be readily permeable to large molecular weight dyes and proteins (Waksman, 1961); therefore, circulating interferon, which is largely excluded from CNS (Subrahmanyan & Mims, 1966), should have ready access to these ganglia. The recent report of a protective effect of Poly-I-poly C within 24 hours after intramuscular injection of street virus (Fenje & Postic, 1970) could be explained by an inhibition of replication in the afferent ganglia.

Initial virus replication in ganglia and cord segments corresponding to the central connections of nerves innervating the inoculation site is solid evidence for a neural pathway, but it is not conclusive. In view of studies showing reflex vasodilitation in cord segments corresponding to sites of peripheral trauma (Field *et al.*, 1951), the argument could be advanced that if virus were in blood, it might preferentially localize to these areas.

However, the evidence that integrity of the nerve is necessary for CNS invasion provides confirmatory evidence for a neural pathway. In agreement with older studies, recent investigations with street and fixed rabies viruses have shown that amputation of limbs or sectioning of nerves proximal to inoculation prevent CNS infection (Baer *et al.*, 1965, 1968; Dean *et al.*, 1963b; Johnson, 1965). The argument that denervation might hinder growth in muscle at the inoculation site (Schindler, 1961) is unconvincing, since neurectomy up to 24 hours after inoculation can have a sparing effect and, as discussed above, there is no evidence for replication in normally innervated muscle prior to CNS invasion. Lack of movement alone may, in some way, retard virus dissemination, since anesthetics with no virocidal effects provide some protection when injected proximal to the inoculation wound (Dean *et al.*, 1963a; Kaplan *et al.*, 1962). However, effects of neurectomy cannot be explained solely on the basis of lack of motor function, since Dean *et al.* (1963b) cut motor or sensory roots selectively and found that sectioning of either roots failed to protect while cutting the composite nerve gave complete protection.

The data on the sites of initial virus localization in CNS and on the necessity of neural integrity for CNS invasion provide almost incontrovertible evidence that fixed and street rabies virus spread to the nervous system along peripheral nerves following subcutaneous or intramuscular inoculation.

*Mechanisms of neural spread*

In 1960 Burnet (1960) reviewed the data on the neural spread of virus and concluded "it is quite impossible to review the literature without accepting the existence of such movement and almost equally impossible to believe in its physical reality." One mechanism was demonstrated with immunofluorescence studies when herpes simplex virus inoculated subcutaneously in suckling mouse was shown to spread to the CNS by ascending infection of endoneural cells (Johnson, 1964). This was confirmed by electron microscopic studies (Rabin *et al.*, 1968).

One might assume a similar mechanism for rabies; however, rabies virus antigen has not been shown to develop in endoneural cells during the neural spread to CNS (Baer *et al.*, 1965; Johnson, 1965; Yamamoto *et al.*, 1965), and the rapidity of ascent, in contrast to herpes simplex virus, suggests some mechanism not necessitating replication. Electron microscopic studies again confirmed fluorescent antibody studies failing to demonstrate particles in endoneural cells, axons, or interspaces prior to their development in the appropriate ganglia (Jenson, 1967). Dean *et al.* (1963b) calculated a rate centripetal virus transmission of about 3 mm/hour, and results of other studies employing amputation and nerve section at intervals after inoculation would be consistent with this rate (Baer *et al.*, 1965; Johnson, 1965). Considering a lag for the first CNS replication cycle, the initial recovery of virus from cord, 24 to 72 hours later, is consistent with this rapid centripetal movement (Baer *et al.*, 1965, 1968; Dean *et al.*, 1963b; Huygelen & Mortelmans, 1959; Johnson, 1965). The spread of fixed virus may be slightly more rapid than that of street (Baer *et al.*, 1965; 1968; Dean *et al.*, 1963b).

The movement of virus in nerves without replication suggests passage through some "conduit"—perineural lymphatics, axoplasm, or interspaces—might be involved (Wright, 1953). Baer *et al.* (1965, 1968), removed the perineural structures from nerve and caused demyelination but found no decrease in mortality; they concluded that neither perineural cells nor myelin were involved in the neural progression of fixed or street rabies viruses. In view of the viscosity of axoplasm and its alleged centrifugal flow, virus spread via tissue interspaces within the nerve has seemed the reasonable conclusion (Baer *et al.*, 1965, 1968; Johnson, 1965; Wright, 1953). This conclusion may have been premature, however, since recent studies of axoplasm have shown it to be metabolically active and a remarkably fascile transport system. Active contractions of myelin have recently been described (Singer & Bryant, 1969), and high speed, differential interference cinemicrographic studies of nerve cells *in vitro* have shown rapid bidirection particle movement within axons (Burwood, 1965). Goodpasture's theory of centripetal movement of virus particles within axis cylinders (Goodpasture, 1925), discarded by many of us, must again be given serious consideration.

*Centrifugal spread of virus*

Infection of the salivary glands appears to develop after CNS infection with street and occasionally fixed strains of rabies virus (Dean *et al.*, 1963b; Fischman, 1969; Otani, 1965; Yamamoto *et al.*, 1965). The assumption has been made that virus moves centrifugally in nerves to infect the glands. Why this peripheral spread is more evident with street than fixed strains is unknown. An interesting possibility is suggested by comparing the fluorescent antibody studies of Yamamoto *et al.* (1965), with street virus where, after neuronal infection, antigen was shown in the axons, and my studies with fixed virus where fluorescence in axons was carefully looked for but not found (Johnson, 1965; Johnson & Mercer, 1964). Centrifugal spread in axons or replication in axoplasm might be a characteristic of street virus causing greater centrifugal dissemination.

Few studies have been done on the pathogenesis of salivary gland infection. Dean *et al.*, (1963b) removed one lingual nerve and cranial cervical ganglion in dogs and foxes and showed an impedence of transmission of virus to the salivary gland on that side. However, the effects of atrophy of the gland following denervation must be considered.

Since the amounts of virus in the salivary gland may exceed those in the brain (Parker & Wilsnack, 1966; Vaughn *et al.*, 1965), street rabies virus must have the capacity to grow in salivary glands. Yamamoto, Otani, and Shiraki (Otani, 1965; Yamamoto *et al.*, 1965) first demonstrated antigen in acinar cells. More recently, Dierks *et al.* (1969) reported immunofluorescence and electron microscopic studies of infected fox salivary glands and showed virus development only in acinar epithelium with release of particles into the lumens.

Virus may also be recovered or demonstrated by immunofluorescence in a variety of areas late in disease. Virus isolations from lacrimal glands (Leach & Johnson, 1940), peripheral nerves and ganglia, lens, vitreous, cornea (Kitselman & Mital, 1968), and blood (see below) may represent centrifugal spread of virus. Following intramuscular inoculation of fixed rabies in mice, Fischman (1969) showed virus antigen in muscle spindles terminally suggesting a centrifugal spread similar to that demonstrated with California virus in mice (Johnson & Johnson, 1968). However, the isolation of rabies virus from bat brown fat which had been previously denervated

(Sulkin, 1962) raises the question of other pathways as do several studies sited below.

## PATHOGENESIS AFTER ORAL AND RESPIRATORY TRANSMISSION

The early literature contained assorted references to the respiratory and oral transmission of rabies, but these were largely anecdotal and appeared of little importance with dog and wolf bites being the major obvious route of inoculation. With a shift of rabies to a sylvatic ecology, the possible importance of respiratory transmission in bat caves and oral transmission via breast milk or cannibalization of dead rabid animals has become evident. A variety of recent experimental studies have demonstrated the potential of respiratory and oral transmission (Atanasiu, 1965, 1966; Constantine, 1962, 1967; Correa-Giron *et al.*, 1970; Fischman, 1969; Fischman & Schaeffer, 1970; Fischman & Ward, 1968; Hronovsky & Benda, 1969a, b; Jenson *et al.*, 1967; Reagan *et al.*, 1955; Sims *et al.*, 1963; Soave, 1966; Svet-Moldavskaya, 1958). The argument that oral transmission might be dependent on breaks in the integrity of the oral mucosa are largely met by Fischman and Ward's (1968) use of stomach tube inoculation.

The pathways of CNS penetration following these routes of inoculation are less clear. In view of studies of herpes simplex virus in suckling mice where different mechanisms of virus dissemination followed different routes of inoculation (i.e., neural after subcutaneous, hematogenous after intraperitoneal, and both after intranasal inoculation) (Johnson, 1964), the data on pathogenesis after intramuscular and subcutaneous inoculation of rabies virus cannot be assumed to apply to other portals of virus entry.

After intranasal inoculation, Jenson *et al.* (1967), in an electron micrographic study found virus matrices in the trigeminal ganglion but particles were not seen until 6 to 8 days and could represent centrifugal neural infection or blood-borne virus. Atanasiu (1965, 1966) isolated virus in high titers from the lung following aerosol infection suggesting virus growth in the lungs as well as CNS, but unfortunately sequential growth curves or virus localization were not reported. A recent fluorescent antibody study in suckling guinea pigs by Hronovsky & Benda (1969) demonstrated antigen in nasal mucosal cells 6 days after intranasal inoculation, a day before antigen was found in the brain. Initial CNS infection was prominent in olfactory bulbs, suggesting an olfactory pathway, but simultaneous antigen was found in unidentified cells in the kidney. Terminally, antigen was also found in unidentified cells in the lungs and trachea, but no antigen or virus was found in other organs or blood. A dog kidney adapted strain was used introducing the possibility of unusual adaptation to extraneural cells. However, Fischman and Schaeffer (1970) recently reported intranasal inoculation of 5 strains of rabies in mice with similar results. The sequence of infection was not determined, but terminally, in addition to CNS, virus antigen was found in nerves and nerve plexes of the nasal and tracheal submucosa, lung, adrenal and bladder and in a few nonneural cells including hair follicles, lingual papillae nasal mucosa and acinar cells of salivary glands.

Following oral inoculation, there is a similar paucity of data. Employing the less physiological intraperitoneal route of inoculation in mice, Kligler and Bernkopf (1943) isolated virus from liver, spleen and lymph nodes for up to 6 hours, initial evidence that infection occurred in the cervical cord at 72–96 hours consistent with a neural pathway. Otani (1965) after intraperitoneal inoculation of mice and hamsters found virus antigen first in sympathetic and celiac ganglia and Auerbach's plexus after 2–3 days with subsequent infection of the spinal cord.

Recently, Correa-Giron *et al.* (1970) reported a more detailed study of mice after eating brain infected with a vampire bat strain of rabies. Virus appeared surprisingly resistent to digestive pH and enzymes: it was isolated from stomach and gut for 6 hours. No tissues yielded virus at 12 hours, but virus was isolated from pooled lungs at 2 days. Fluorescent antibody staining showed virus only in the brain at 2 days, but at 6 days, antigen was found in heavily innervated epithelial cells of buccal mucosa, tongue, and stomach, Bellini ducts of kidney, salivary glands and probable nerves and ganglia in lung, heart, esophagus and trachea. Fischman and Schaeffer (1970) in a similar study of oral transmission failed to show virus antigen in buccal or gastric epidermis but found antigen in the stratum granulosum and stratum Malpighii of cheek mucosa and mucosa and papillae of tongue. Specific fluorescence in esophagus, trachea and gut was limited to nerve bundles and nerve cells of Auerbach and Meissner plexuses. Antigen was not found in other nonneural tissues. This fluorescence was found 3 days after virus was eaten but was synchronous with antigen development in CNS. Both of these studies demonstrate new sites of extraneural infection and potential new pathways of virus invasion, but infection of mucosa prior to

CNS infection and the route of CNS invasion were not demonstrated.

One can only conclude that after experimental intranasal or oral transmission the distribution of virus growth appears to differ from that after intramuscular inoculation. There is little evidence for or against a different pathway of CNS penetration.

## ROLE OF VIREMIA IN THE PATHOGENESIS

Wong and Freund (1951) showed the presence of virus in the blood of mice up to 3 hours after intracerebral inoculation of several strains of virus, but such transient overflow into blood and subsequent clearance by the reticuloendothelial system would be anticipated with the intracerebral inoculation of any particulate material (Mims, 1960). Early spillage of virus into blood after other routes of inoculation might also be anticipated. In a number of studies, virus has been irregularly isolated from blood (Dean *et al.*, 1963b; Johnson, unpublished data; Krause, 1957, 1966), but a consistent and high titered viremia has never been documented except in chick embryos (Koprowski & Cox, 1948a, b). The recent claim of rabies virus antigen in circulating leucocytes of rabbits after intramuscular inoculation needs confirmation, since it is in marked contradiction to other studies; possibly this finding is explicable by the fact that a porcine kidney adapted strain of virus was employed (Baratawidjaja, 1965). The simple presence of virus in the blood does not, of course, imply that it is relevant to the pathogenesis.

Rabies can be transmitted by intravenous inoculation but incubation period is prolonged as compared with intramuscular inoculation of comparable doses (Fischman & Schaeffer, 1970). Rabies is rapidly cleared from the blood of mice after intravenous inoculation ($<99.9\%$ clearance in one hour) (Johnson, unpublished data), so administration by this route is essentially an inoculation of the reticuloendothelial system.

In contrast to earlier studies (Schweinburg & Windholz, 1930; Zunker, 1963; Yamamoto *et al.*, 1965 recently demonstrated transmission of street and fixed rabies in parabiotic rats to the non-inoculated partners. This finding does not, however, prove that virus spreads to the nervous system from the blood; that transient viremia can occur and that rabies is transmissible by intravenous inoculation have previously been established. Furthermore, the time of transmission was not determined, and, as Dean (1966) noted, virus might spread to the brain in the inoculated animal and then centrifugally in nerves to blood or cutaneous tissues shared by the partner.

To prove hematogenous spread of rabies to CNS, a sequential study documenting viremia followed by initial CNS infection around cerebral vessels is needed (Johnson & Mims, 1968). Unlike neural spread, evidence for the hematogenous dissemination of rabies viruses lacks critical data.

## DEVELOPMENT OF INFECTION AND DISEASE WITHIN THE CNS

Following the initial CNS invasion via ganglia and corresponding CNS segments or by other routes, there appears to be a rapid dissemination of virus throughout the CNS. By fluorescent antibody staining, granules of cytoplasmic fluorescence were found in susceptible neurons throughout the CNS 24 hours after initial lumbar cord infection resulting from footpad inoculation of fixed rabies virus (Johson, 1965). This finding suggests dispersion within spinal fluid, and rabies virus has been isolated from CSF during life (Blattner, 1961).

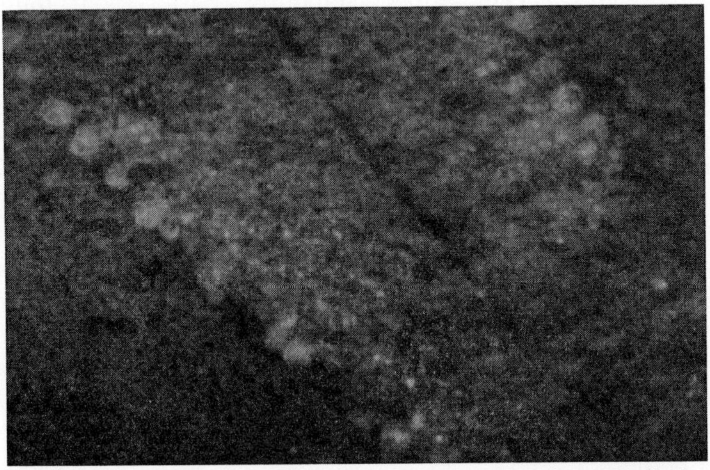

Fig. 2. Section of Mouse Cerebellum Stained with Fluorescent Antibody 7 Days after Intracerebral Inoculation with CVS Strain of Fixed Rabies Virus. Fluorescence is limited to perikaryon and dendrites of Purkinje cells in two adjacent folia. No specific fluorescence is present in granular layers (upper right and lower left) or in white matter (extreme lower left) through which Purkinje cell axons pass. Fluorescence in molecular layers (center) is limited to dendrites of Purkinje cells extending to the meningeal surface (diagonally across center).

The selectivity of susceptibility of CNS cells to rabies infection is unique. Meningeal, ependymal, vascular endothelial and glial cells show no antigen, and neurons of spinal cord, brainstem, hypocampus, septal nuclei and limbic cortex appear selectively vulnerable. In the cerebellum, only the Purkinje cells are infected, as demonstrated by immunofluorescence (Fig. 2) and electron microscopic studies (Fischman, 1969; Johnson, 1965; Johnson & Mercer, 1964; Yamamoto *et al.*, 1965). However, Matsumoto (Matsumoto, 1963) has published convincing electron micrographs of virus matrices in astrocytic cytoplasms, so neuronal selectivity must not be absolute.

The greater localization to limbic system with relative sparing of neocortex provides a fascinating clinicopathologic correlate with the alertness, loss of natural timidity, aberrant sexual behavior and aggressiveness that may occur in clinical rabies. No other virus is so diabolically adapted to selective neuronal populations that it can drive the host in a fury to transmit the virus to another host animal.

The relatively long incubation periods of rabies in experimental rodents appear related to a slow development of virus in the neurons rather than rapid growth causing cell lysis. Indeed, the pathology of rabies usually lacks the cytolysis and inflammation which characterize most viral encephalitides (Dupont & Earle, 1965; Johnson, 1965).

The beautiful electron microscopic studies of Miyamoto and Matsumoto (1967) on rabies infected neurons may provide some clues to the prolonged incubation period, paucity of pathology, and differences between fixed and street strains. Neurons infected with street virus showed little ultrastructural changes except the development of matrices, which became so large as to form Negri bodies. Neurons infected with fixed virus showed vesicles in the cytoplasm, increased lysosomes and necrotic alterations. Identical matrices were present, but they were smaller than those discernable with the light microscope as Negri bodies. Fixed virus development appeared to cause greater intracellular injury, possibly explaining the shorter incubation period as well as the incomplete development of the Negri bodies.

The noncytopathic infection of tissue culture cells with rabies is well recognized. The question has been raised whether the paucity of neuropathologic changes *in vivo* is analogous, with disease in the animal resulting from chronic cellular dysfunction not discernable in cultured cells (Johnson, 1967). However, chronically infected tissue culture cells can be lysed by antirabies serum (Fernandes *et al.*, 1964); an *in vivo* analogy to immune lysis is not evident. In studies of the 6–10 day incubation period of the CVS strain in mice, no fixation of mouse gamma globulin could be detected by immunofluorescence on mouse neurons. Furthermore, intracerebral or intravenous injections of immune serum in infected mice did not alter the pathologic changes—there was no increase in cell lysis or inflammation (Johnson, unpublished data).

The slow and relentless noncytolytic enlargement of virus matrices interfering with cell function may not be the sole explanation for very long incubation periods and disease pathogenesis. Several groups of studies suggest a more complex host-parasite relationship can be operative. The natural history of chronic rabies infections of bats certainly suggests alternative mechanisms of pathogenesis (Sulkin, 1962). In mice, Bell and his colleagues (Bell, 1964; Bell *et al.*, 1966; Lodmell *et al.*, 1969) have produced abortive rabies and have found virus antigen in brains 30 days after intraperitoneal inoculation; virus could not be isolated at this time and high virus-neutralization titers were present in the brain as well as serum. Svet-Moldavskaya (1958) reported rabies virus recovery from brains of healthy rats 2 months after oral and intranasal street virus inoculation even though animals had virus in salivary glands during the first 3 weeks following inoculation. Similar persistent infection was suggested by Soave *et al.* (1961), when they induced rabies by giving ACTH to a guinea pig that had survived for 20 weeks after intramuscular street rabies and had antibody when given the drug. Persistent and chronic infections of the brain with rabies may occur, and the late development of rabies in some host animals may well be dependent upon alterations in the immune defenses.

## SUMMARY

There is not *one* pathway by which viruses spread through the host animal, and there is not *one* mechanism by which viruses cause disease. If one seeks "laws of nature" governing the pathogenesis of viral infections, one will only discover the folly of making generalizations. Animal hosts are complex biological systems, and the adaptations achieved by different viruses or even by the same virus in different hosts are diverse.

Rabies was the first virus with which the pathogenesis of CNS infection was investigated in the laboratory, yet after almost 100 years of experimental work, questions remain unanswered. Rabies virus can spread via the nerves, yet the mechanism is unknown. Rabies virus may enter the host by multiple portals, yet the relative importance of oral and respiratory transmission in the natural ecology is still uncertain. Rabies virus may, at times, be in the blood, yet the relation of this to disease is unclear. Rabies virus spreads rapidly within the nervous system showing a remarkable specificity of cellular infections, but the route of this spread and the mechanisms of selective vulnerability remain uninvestigated. Rabies virus can cause disease after a long latent period, yet the intricate host-parasite interrelationships during this period are still an enigma.

## REFERENCES


Atanasiu, P. (1965). Transmission de la rage par la voie respiratoire aux animaux de laboratoire. *Compt. Rend. Acad. Sci.*, **261**, 277.

Atanasiu, P. (1966). Transmission de la rage par la voie aerienne aux animaux de laboratoire. Internat. Symp. Rabies, Talloires, 1965. *Symp. Series Immunobiol. Standard*, **1**, 159.

Baer, G. M., Shanthaveerappa, T. R. and Bourne, G. H. (1965). Studies on the pathogenesis of fixed rabies virus in rats. *Bull. Wld. Hlth. Org.*, **33**, 783.

Baer, G. M., Shantha, T. R. and Bourne, G. H. (1968). The pathogenesis of street rabies virus in rats. *Bull. Wld. Hlth. Org.*, **38**, 119.

Baratawidjaja, R. K., Morrissey, L. P. and Labzoffsky, N. A. (1965). Demonstration of vaccinia, lymphocytic choriomeningitis and rabies viruses in the leucocytes of experimentally infected animals. *Arch. Ges. Virusforsch.*, **17**, 273.

Bell, J. F. (1964). Abortive rabies infection. I. Experimental production in white mice and general discussion. *J. Infect. Dis.*, **114**, 249.

Bell, J. F., Lodmell, D. L., Morre, G. J. and Raymond, G. H. (1966). Brain neutralization of rabies virus to distinguish recovered animals from previously vaccinated animals. *J. Immunol.*, **97**, 747.

Blattner, R. J. (1961). Rabies infection transmitted by insectivorous bats: human case with virus isolation from spinal fluid during life. *J. Pediat.*, **58**, 433.

Burnet, F. M. (1960). Principles of Animal Virology. Second Edition, Academic Press, New York.

Burwood, W. O. (1965). Rapid bidirectional particle movements in neurons. *J. Cell Biol.*, **27**, 115A.

Constantine, D. G. (1962). Rabies transmission by non-bite route. *Public Health Rep.*, **77**, 287.

Constantine, D. G. (1967). Rabies transmission by air in bat caves. U.S. Government Printing Office, Washington, D.C.

Correa-Giron, E. R., Allen, R. and Sulkin, S. E. (1970). The infectivity and pathogenesis of rabies virus administered orally. *Am J. Epid.*, **91**, 203.

Dean, D. J. (1966). Discussion. Internat. Symp. Rabies, Tallories, 1965. *Symp. Series Immunobiol. Standard*, **1**, 209.

Dean, D. J., Baer, G. M. and Thompson, W. R. (1963a). Studies on the local treatment of rabies-infected wounds. *Bull. Wld. Hlth. Org.*, **28**, 477.

Dean, D. J., Evans, W. M. and McClure, R. C. (1963b). Pathogenesis of rabies. *Bull. Wld. Hlth. Org.*, **29**, 803.

Dierks, R. E., Murphy, F. A. and Harrison, A. K. (1969). Extraneural rabies virus infection. Virus development in fox salivary gland. *Am. J. Path.*, **54**, 251.

DiVestea, A. and Zagari, G. (1889). Sur la transmission de la rage par voie nerveuse. *Ann. Inst. Pasteur*, **3**, 237.

Dupont, J. R. and Earle, K. M. (1965). Human rabies encephalitis: Study of forty-nine fatal cases and review of the literature. *Neurology*, **15**, 1023.

Fenje, P. and Postic, B. (1970). Protection of rabbits against experimental rabies by Poly 1-poly C. *Nature*, **226**, 171.

Fernandes, M. V., Wiktor, T. J. and Koprowski, H. (1964). Endosymbiotic relationship between animal viruses and host cells: Study of rabies virus in tissue culture. *J. Exp. Med.*, **120**, 1099.

Field, E. J., Grayson, J. and Rogers, A. F. (1951). Observations on the blood flow in the spinal cord of the rabbit. *J. Physiol.*, **114**, 56.

Fischman, H. R. (1969). Fluorescent antibody staining of rabies infected tissue embedded in paraffin. *Am. J. Vet. Res.*, **30**, 1213.

Fischman, H. R. and Schaeffer, M. (1970). Pathogenesis of experimental rabies as revealed by immunofluorescence. *Ann. New York Acad. Sci.* In press.

Fischman, H. R. and Ward, F. E. (1968). Oral transmission of rabies virus in experimental animals. *Am. J. Epid.*, **88**, 132.

Friedemann, U. (1943). Permeability of blood-brain barrier to neurotropic viruses. *Arch. Path.*, **35**, 912.

Goodpasture, E. W. (1925). A study of rabies with reference to a neural transmission of the virus in rabbits and the structure and significance of Negri bodies. *Am. J. Path.*, **1**, 547.

Habel, K. (1941). Tissue factors in antirabies immunity of experimental animals. *Weekly Pblc. Hlth. Rpts.*, **53**, 692.

Helman, M. C. (1889). Action du virus rabique. Introduit, soit dans le tissu cellulaire. Sous-cutané, soit dans le autre tissus. *Ann. Inst. Pasteur*, **3**, 15.

Hronovsky, V. and Benda, R. (1969a). Experimental inhalation infection of laboratory rodents with rabies virus. *Acta Virol.*, **13**, 193.

Hronovsky, V. and Benda, R. (1969b). Development of inhalation rabies infection in suckling guinea pigs. *Acta Virol.*, **13**, 198.

Hurst, E. W. (1936). Newer knowledge of virus diseases of nervous system: Review and interpretation. *Brain*, **59**, 1.

Huygelen, C. and Mortelmans, J. (1959). Quantitative determination of Flury rabies virus in the central nervous system of the guinea pig after intramuscular innoculation in the hind leg. *Antonie Leeuwenhoek*, **25**, 265.

Jenson, A. B., Rabin, E. R., Bentinck, D. C. and Melnick, J. L. (1967). Rabies virus neuronitis. *J. Virol.*, **3**, 265.

Johnson, K. P. and Johnson, R. T. (1968). California encephalitis. II. Studies of experimental infection in the mouse. *J. Neuropath. Exp. Neurol.*, **27**, 390.

Johnson, R. T. (1964). The pathogenesis of herpes virus encephalitis. I. virus pathway to the nervous system of suckling mice demonstrated by florescent antibody. *J. Exp. Med.* **119**, 343.

Johnson, R. T. (1965). Experimental rabies. Studies of cellular vulnerability and pathogenesis using fluorescent antibody staining. J. Neuropath. *Exp. Neurol.*, **24**, 662.

Johnson, R. T. (1967). Chronic infectious neuropathic agents: possible mechanisms of pathogenesis. *Current Topics Microbiol. Immunol.*, **40**, 3.

Johnson, R. T. (1968). Mumps virus encephalitis in the hamster. Studies of the inflammatory response and noncytopathic infection of neurons. *J. Neuropath. Exp. Neurol.*, **27**, 80.

Johnson, R. T. and Mercer, E. H. (1964). The development of fixed rabies virus in mouse brain. *Australian J. Exp. Biol. Med. Sci.*, **42**, 449.

Johnson, R. T. and Mims, C. A. (1968). Pathogenesis of viral infections of the nervous system. *New England J. Med.*, **278**, 23 and 84.

Johnson, R. T., Unpublished data.

Kaplan, M. M., Cohen, D., Koprowski, H., Dean, D. and Ferrigan, L. (1962). Studies on the local treatment of wounds for the prevention of rabies. *Bull. Wld. Hlth. Org.*, **26**, 765.

Kitselman, C. H. and Mital, A. K. (1968). Terminal dissemination of rabies virus in selected rat tissues. *Canad. J. Comp. Med.*, **32**, 461.

Kligler, I. J. and Bernkopf, H. (1943). The path of dissemination of rabies virus in the body of normal and immunized mice. *Brit. J. Exp. Path.*, **24**, 15.

Koprowski, H. and Cox, H. R. (1948a). Occurrence of rabies virus in the blood of developing chick embryo. *Proc. Soc. Exp. Biol. Med.*, **68**, 612.

Koprowski, H. and Cox, H. R. (1948b). Studies on chick embryo adapted rabies virus. *J. Immunol.*, **60**, 533.

Krause, W. W. (1957). Kritische experimentelle uber die Prufung von Tollwutimpfstoffen, die Pathogenese der Lyssa und das Geschehen in der Inkubationsperiode. *Zbl. Bakt. I. Orig.*, **167**, 481.

Krause, W. W. (1966). The pathogenesis of rabies. Internat. Symp. Rabies, Tallories, 1965. *Symp. Series Immunobiol. Standard.*, **1**, 153.

Leach, N. and Johnson, H. N. (1940). Human rabies, with special reference to virus distribution and titer. *Am. J. Trop. Med.*, **20**, 335.

Lodmell, D. L., Bell, J. F., Moore, G. J. and Raymond, G. H. (1969). Comparative study of abortive and nonabortive rabies in mice. *J. Infect. Dis.*, **119**, 569.

Matsumoto, S. (1969). Electron microscope studies of rabies virus in mouse brain. *J. Cell. Biol.*, **19**, 565.

Mims, C. A. (1960). Intracerebral injections and the growth of viruses in mouse brain. *Brit. J. Exp. Path.*, **41**, 52.

Mims, C. A. (1964). Aspects of pathogenesis of virus diseases. *Bact. Rev.*, **28**, 30.

Miyamoto, K. and Matsumoto, S. (1967). Comparative studies between pathogenesis of street and fixed rabies infection. *J. Exp. Med.*, **125**, 447.

Morgagni, J. B. (1769). The seats and causes of disease investigated by anatomy, (quoted by Wright, G. P. Movement of neurotoxins and neuroviruses in the nervous system. *In*: Modern Trends in Pathology [edited by D. H. Collins], New York, Hoeber, 1959).

Nicolau, S. and Meteiesco, E. (1928). Septinévrites à virus rabique des rue. Preuves de la marche centrifuge du virus dans les nerfs peripheriques des lapins. *Compt. Rend. Acad. Sci.*, **186**, 1072.

Nicolau, S. and Serbanescu, V. (1928). Septinévrite expérimentale a virus rabique fixe dans l'organisme du lapin. *Compt. Rend. Soc. Biol.*, **99**, 294.

Otani, S. (1965). Studies on rabies encephalitis by means of fluorescent antibody staining. *Jap. J. Exp. Med.*, **35**, 42.

Parker, R. L. and Wilsnack, R. E. (1966). Pathogenesis of skunk rabies virus: Quantitation in skunks and foxes. *Am. J. Vet. Res.*, **27**, 33.

Petrovic, M. and Timm, H. (1969). Experimenteller Beitrag zur Pathogenese der Tollwut. *Zentralblatt Bakt., Parasit., Infekt., Hyg., Erste Abt. Orig.*, Bd. **211**, 149.

Rabin, E. R., Jenson, A. B. and Melnick, J. L. (1968). Herpes simplex virus in mice: electronmicroscopy of neural spread. *Science*, **162**, 126.

Reagan, R. L., Yancy, F. S., Chang, S. C. and Brueckner, A. L. (1955). Transmission of street rabies virus strain (V308) to suckling hamsters during lactation. *Proc. Soc. Exp. Biol. Med.*, **90**, 301.

Roux, E. (1888). Notes de laboratoire. Sur la presence du virus rabique dans les nerfs. *Ann. Inst. Pasteur*, **2**, 18.

Schindler, R. (1961). Studies on the pathogenesis of rabies. *Bull. Wld. Hlth. Org.*, **25**, 119.

Schindler, R. (1966). Pathogenesis of rabies infection. International Symposium on Rabies, Talloires, 1965. *Sym. Series Immunobiol. Standard.*, **1**, 147.

Schweinburg, F. and Windholz, F. (1930). Ueber den Ausbreitungsweg des Wuterregers von der Eintrittspforte aus. *Virchows Arch. f. Path. Anat.*, **278**, 23.

Sims, R. A., Allen, R. and Sulkin, S. E. (1963). Studies on the pathogenesis of rabies in insectivorous bats. III. Influence of the gravid state. *J. Inf. Dis.*, **112**, 17.

Singer, M. and Bryant, S. V. (1969). Movements in the myelin Schwann sheath of the vertebrate axon. *Nature*, **221**, 1148.

Soave, O. A., Transmission of rabies to mice by ingestion of infected tissue. (1966). *Am. J. Vet. Res.*, **27**, 44.

Soave, O. A., Johnson, H. N. and Nakamura, K. (1961). Reactivation of rabies virus infection with adrenocorticotropic hormones. *Science*, **133**, 1360.

Subrahmanyan, T. P. and Mims, C. A. (1966). Fate of intravenously administrated interferon and distribution of interferon during virus infections in mice. *Brit. J. Exp. Path.*, **47**, 168.

Sulkin, S. E. (1962). The bat as a reservoir of viruses in nature. *Progr. Med. Virol.*, **4**, 157.

Svet-Moldavskaya, I. A. (1958). Experimental study of the infectivity of salivary glands of laboratory animals in the latent form of street rabies. *Acta Virol.*, **2**, 228.

Vaughn, J. B., Gerhardt, P. and Newell, K. W. (1965). Excretion of street rabies virus in the saliva of dogs. *J. Am. Med. Ass.*, **193**, 363.

Vieuchange, J. (1967). Interference entre le virus vaccinal et le virus rabique; role éventuel d'un interféron. *Arch. ges. Virusforsch.*, **22**, 87.

Waksman, B. H. (1961). Experimental study of diphtheritic polyneuritis in the rabbit and guinea pig. III. The blood-nerve barrier in the rabbit. *J. Neuropath. Exp. Neurol.*, **20**, 35.

Webster, L. T. (1937). Epidemiologic and immunologic experiments on rabies. *New England J. Med.*, **217**, 687.

Wong, D. H. and Freund, J. (1951) Fixed rabies virus in blood following intracerebral inoculations into mice and rabbits. *Proc. Soc. Exp. Biol. Med.*, **76**, 717.

Wright, G. P. (1953). Nerve trunks as pathways in infection. *Proc. Roy. Soc. Med.*, **46**, 319.

Yamamoto, T., Otani, S. and Shiraki, H. (1965). A study of the evolution of viral infection in experimental herpes simplex encephalitis and rabies by means of fluorescent antibody. *Acta Neuropath.*, **5**, 288.

Zunker, M. (1963). Ergebnisse und Probleme der Tollwutforschung. *Zbl. Veterinärmed.*, **3**, 271.

For Discussion, see page 91.

# The Laboratory Diagnosis of Rabies: Review and Prospective

EDWIN H. LENNETTE
AND
RICHARD W. EMMONS

*Viral and Rickettsial Disease Laboratory, California State Department of Public Health, Berkeley, California 94704*

## INTRODUCTION

Perhaps more than any other disease, rabies has stimulated investigators to attempt development of accurate and rapid laboratory diagnostic methods. In man, factors which make laboratory diagnosis the key to rabies prevention and control are: the virtual inevitability of death, once clinical illness appears; the lack of specific treatment for the disease, but the availability of effective *preventive* measures for persons exposed to the virus; and the need to accurately assess the significance of exposure of the individual to an animal, or the risk of exposure of the population to various animal species in the community.

Diagnostic methods for rabies have been presented in detail elsewhere, and are readily accessible and well known to public health workers (World Health Organization, 1966; H. N. Johnson, 1969; H. N. Johnson, 1970). In addition, detailed reviews of the epizootiology of rabies in California, including extensive statistical data on animals tested in our laboratory and in local public health laboratories in the state, will be presented to this conference by Dr. Johnson and Dr. Humphrey of our department. It is not our purpose, therefore, to describe in detail laboratory methods or compilations of laboratory test results, nor to discuss all aspects of the subject. And, we have included only a few references for general information or to document specific points. Rather, we wish to (1) briefly view past and present diagnostic techniques; (2) emphasize certain practical aspects and implications of laboratory procedures which will best support a rabies control program, based on our experience in California; (3) review newer developments and innovations in diagnostic methods and present a few of our current studies; and (4) suggest important areas for future research.

Many of the points we wish to emphasize may seem simple or obvious. However, it has been our experience that even in an area where rabies is common and well known to the medical community, some of the simplest precautions and methods are still overlooked or wrongly applied. Therefore, we wish to place greatest emphasis on these practical aspects of diagnosis.

Our topic is perhaps of particular importance for countries free of rabies at present, but in which early recognition of the introduction of the disease will enable prompt and complete control and eradication.

## DIAGNOSTIC PROGRAM

A good rabies diagnostic program should include the following essential elements.

(1) Accurate epidemiologic data must be collected and permanently recorded regarding all animal species tested by the laboratory. These data should include accurate genus and species identification, sex, age, exact location, date collected, all persons or animals exposed to or bitten by the animal, rabies vaccination status of the animal, a description of the animal's behavior and circumstances surrounding the exposure, and the medical personnel to be informed of the test results. This information should be recorded on the same form used for recording results of laboratory tests, so that all pertinent information is readily accessible in one place. Such data are of great importance to control programs, and to understanding the epizootiology of rabies, as well as for making decisions about the treatment of individuals exposed to the animal. The information may not be obtained or recorded unless the laboratory insists that it be done.

(2) There must be proper collection, labelling, storage, and transport to the laboratory of the appropriate tissue specimens for testing. Separate, sterile autopsy instruments must be used for removing each tissue and for each animal, to avoid cross-contamination. Adequate safety precautions must be used to avoid laboratory accidents. Accurate labelling of the tissue to be tested, including an identifying code number (not duplicated elsewhere), and separate and careful packaging to prevent cross-contamination, mix-up, or leakage of specimens during transport are essential. If the specimen

can be tested within a day or two, it should be kept at 4°C. If longer delay or transport over a long distance are unavoidable, the specimen may be kept frozen on dry ice or liquid nitrogen, or the brain tissue preserved in sterile 50% glycerine in saline. We have found the latter method quite simple and satisfactory if care is taken to wash the tissue free of the glycerine solution prior to the fluorescent antibody test. The full cooperation of postal services or other messenger and delivery services is essential, to expedite receipt of the specimen in the laboratory. If possible, a portion of the tissue to be tested should be retained by the submitter in case the first package is lost in shipment to the laboratory.

(3) Accurate, permanent records must be maintained by the laboratory of test procedures and results on each specimen. Portions of the original whole tissue and of all passage materials must be stored (frozen at −20°C or colder) in case reisolation of virus must be attempted, or for referral to another laboratory to confirm test results. It is desirable to maintain indefinitely selected viral isolates for use as reference strains, particularly any strains showing unusual characteristics (such as in the incubation period, pathogenicity, or host susceptibility spectrum).

(4) Laboratory tests must be properly conducted by well-trained personnel, using standard methods, adequate controls on the specificity and accuracy of the tests, and adequate precautions to avoid cross-contamination, laboratory accidents, or mix-up of specimens tested. Results of one test method (for example, Negri body staining or fluorescent antibody staining) should be confirmed by virus isolation in mice. When sufficient experience has been gained with the fluorescent rabies antibody (FRA) method, that method may be used as the routine test procedure. In our laboratory, this method is relied on as the best single test, but mouse inoculation is also routinely performed if results of the FRA test are inconclusive, or if special circumstances (such as an animal species of particular interest, an unusually severe bite exposure or referral of the specimen from another laboratory for confirmation) warrant it (Lennette *et al.*, 1965).

(5) There must be accurate, permanent recording of test results and prompt reporting to the medical authorities responsible for treatment of exposed persons or animals and for rabies control programs. In addition, the laboratory should prepare periodic summary reports of test results, to assist in epidemiologic surveillance.

(6) There must be adequate financial support and efficient

direction of the laboratory effort towards the most important areas of public health concern regarding rabies. Thus, as mentioned above, rabies diagnosis is equally important for epidemiologic surveillance, assessment of public health risks and guidance of control programs as it is for individual decisions regarding treatment of exposed persons.

## METHODS

### *Histopathologic Methods*

Histopathologic methods such as staining fresh brain tissue smears or fixed sections for the presence of specific cytoplasmic inclusion bodies of rabies (Negri bodies) still have merit and are commonly used in laboratories throughout the world. Experience with such methods should be maintained by the laboratory staff. However, they must be supplemented by the more reliable FRA method as a routine diagnostic tool. Nonspecific inclusion bodies or those formed during viral infections other than rabies may be confused with Negri bodies. On the other hand, Negri bodies may not be detectable in a high percentage of rabid animals, particularly in feral species such as skunks or bats, the commonest hosts of rabies in California. In a series of 363 rabies-positive specimens, out of 4,200 specimens tested during a special comparative study in our laboratory, only 239 (65.8%) were detected by the presence of Negri bodies (Lennette *et al.*, 1965).

### *Fluorescent Antibody Staining Methods*

Fluorescent rabies antibody staining (FRA), as mentioned previously, is the best method for providing rapid, reliable results. Specific conjugates may be obtained from commerical sources, or may be prepared by an experienced laboratory. Problems of non-specificity of staining, poor titer or other technical difficulties have been encountered with some of the commercial products available on the market. We have had the best results with our own conjugate, prepared with rabies immune serum from hamsters hyperimmunized with the CVS strain of fixed rabies virus grown in suckling hamster brain (Lennette *et al.*, 1965). It is important to pay careful attention to preparation methods, immunization of the animals with virus grown only in homologous tissue and proper conjugation procedures. Animals used for immunization should be free of antibodies to other viruses or bacteria, as far as possible. Proper controls must be used with each staining procedure, demonstrating that freshly prepared rabies-positive brain smears are properly stained and that normal brain smears do not stain. Specificity of staining may further be shown by: (1) isolation of the virus in mice; (2) the absorption test, in which the FRA conjugate prepared as a working dilution in 20% suspension of rabies-infected mouse brain fails to stain the brain tissue smear under study, while a dilution of the conjugate in normal mouse brain suspension does stain properly; (3) the heterologous staining test in which the rabies-positive brain smears are not stained by fluorescent conjugates for other viruses (for example, distemper or herpes simplex viruses); (4) the blocking test in which flooding of tissue smears with unconjugated rabies immune serum prevents subsequent staining by conjugated antiserum, because attachment sites for the conjugate are already preempted (this test does not actually work very well and is little used); (5) and finally, submission of a portion of the animal brain tissue to another reference laboratory for independent confirmation of results.

In addition to good reagents and careful procedures, a good microscope and accessory equipment are required. We cannot present detailed specifications here, but the need for quality equipment and careful standardization of it cannot be overemphasized.

Finally, as mentioned above, there is no substitute for good training and extensive experience in performing and interpreting the FRA test. The technician or microbiologist should receive bench training from qualified persons before undertaking independent diagnostic work, since diagnostic acumen is difficult to obtain through written descriptions or photographs alone. The FRA test should be performed frequently (preferably daily) to maintain technical and interpretive skills. The same safety precautions used in virus isolation procedures should be used in the FRA staining procedures, since even acetone-fixed tissue smears still contain live virus.

Two other points about the FRA test should be emphasized. An animal actually suspected of having rabies should be promptly killed and the brain immediately examined for rabies antigen. Any wild animal biting a person should be so treated. The only possible exceptions are domestic or pet animals of definite value in which there are no signs of illness nor real reason to suspect rabies. There is no longer any need or justification for holding the animal until the disease has progressed sufficiently to produce Negri bodies. Fluorescent antigen will be present and detectable in the brain at any stage of the disease in which the animal could possibly have transmitted rabies.

The other point which corresponds with this is that if a properly performed FRA test of the brain tissue is negative, we are confident that no danger of rabies *transmission* existed. We have no data or evidence from our own experience, nor have we seen convincing evidence from elsewhere, that a true "carrier" state exists in any animal species, although we realize that the controversy over this issue has not been completely settled. Aberrant rabies in vampire bats is the one possible exception that must be reassessed in light of modern laboratory techniques and it will be discussed further by Dr. Harald Johnson. There is evidence, however, that *recovery* from rabies may occur, at least in experimental animals and perhaps under natural conditions in a few special instances. This will be discussed later by others at this Conference. Prolonged incubation periods are also well known in rabies, the onset of disease apparently having been precipitated by various forms of "stress" to the organism (Soave *et al.*, 1961). Although study in this very interesting area must continue, it is important to reiterate the two points mentioned above, since unnecessary delay in serum and vaccine treatment, on the one hand, and unnecessary treatment, on the other, are still all too common.

*Virus Isolation Methods*

The white laboratory mouse is the best host for the isolation of rabies virus. Certain rabies virus strains (wild or vaccine strains) are more pathogenic for infant mice than adult mice, so it may be desirable to use infant mice in addition to weanling mice for isolation attempts, or to use infant mice alone. Mice should be obtained from a colony kept as free as possible from infection with microbial and viral agents. Details of methods used are available elsewhere (World Health Organization, 1966; H. N. Johnson, 1969; H. N. Johnson, 1970). The most important points to emphasize here are: (1) inoculated animals must be carefully observed for signs of illness for a sufficient period of time (28 days in our laboratory) some of the test animals, however, may be sacrificed at any stage, even before signs of illness appear, and examined by the FRA technique to facilitate more rapid confirmation of virus isolation; (2) identification of viruses isolated in mice must be conclusive, based on an FRA test known to be reliable; a neutralization test in mice, using specific rabies immune serum; or a cross-protection test. In the latter test, vaccination of mice intracerebrally with HEP Flury strain of rabies virus will protect against intracerebral challenge one month later with rabies virus, but not against challenge with other viruses. Identification of Negri bodies in inoculated mice is also commonly used as a specificity test, but the more reliable steps outlined above are preferable. No reliable cell culture methods have as yet been developed for primary isolation and identification of rabies virus.

*Electron Microscope Methods*

Electron microscopy has been used as a research tool for the most part, but may find increasing usage in diagnosis, as experience with it is gained. Its greatest value at present is in determining the structure and morphologic relationships of rabies virus with other viruses, and the pathogenesis of rabies (Jenson *et al.*, 1967; Matsumoto and Kawai, 1969; Morecki and Zimmerman, 1969; Rabin and Jenson, 1967).

*Serologic Methods*

Serologic methods are used to determine the antibody status of animals or persons immunized against rabies, or in some instances for the diagnosis of the clinical disease in man prior to death. Antibody levels in persons immunized against rabies are usually measured by neutralization tests in mice and by the indirect FRA staining method. Other newly developed methods include: (1) *in vitro* neutralization tests in cell cultures (inhibition of cytopathic effect, inhibition of plaque formation, or inhibition of immunofluorescent focus formation); (2) lytic rabies antibody test; (3) hemagglutination-inhibition test; (4) gel-diffusion precipitation test; and (5) complement-fixation test.

The hemagglutination-inhibition (HI) and complement-fixation (CF) tests (Halonen *et al.*, 1968; Kuwert *et al.*, 1968) will be discussed in detail by Dr. Ishii at this conference. Problems of nonspecific inhibitors, cross-reactions with other viral antibodies, and other technical difficulties in the preparation and use of antigens have prevented practical application of these tests to diagnostic virology or serologic surveys in animal populations.

Similarly, gel-diffusion methods and the immune-lysis test (Wiktor *et al.*, 1968) have contributed to further understanding of the antigenic and immunologic characteristics of rabies virus, and the pathogenesis of rabies in man and other animal hosts, but the tests have not yet been generally applied in the diagnostic laboratory.

We have made some progress recently in adapting cell culture methods to routine serologic procedures for rabies. Although cell cultures have not yet been found useful for the primary isolation and identification of rabies virus, many cell culture types support virus growth, detectable by FRA staining, or in a few instances by cytopathic effect (H. N. Johnson, 1970; Habel, 1964). Cultures of a baby hamster kidney cell line (0853), derived in our laboratory, have given better results than infected mouse brain smears in performing the indirect FRA test. Bottle cultures infected with the LEP Flury strain of rabies virus are trypsinized and harvested when approximately 50% of the cells contain viral antigen. A concentrated cell suspension is then prepared, and drops are pipetted onto microscope slides to form small, circular cell monolayers. Normal cells can be mixed with the infected cells to adjust the proportion of antigen-containing cells if needed. Sera may then be titrated for antibody content by the indirect FRA method. A large number of slides with identical proportion and pattern of antigen-containing cells may be prepared, fixed in acetone, and stored at −70° C for ready use. The antigenicity is well preserved for many months. The clear distinction between antigen-containing cells or clusters of cells and the completely normal adjacent cells on the slides, and the absence of any background or nonspecific fluorescence make this method preferable to the use of mouse brain smears.

One advantage of the indirect FRA test is its ability to distinguish between the individual's own antibody response to vaccination and antibodies present as a result of administration of hyperimmune rabies antiserum (equine). We have found no significant cross-reaction between equine and human gamma globulins in the indirect FRA test. From 1968 to the present, we have performed 571 indirect FRA tests for rabies antibody (364 positives). Good agreement is usually obtained between replicate tests on the same samples, indicating the reliability of the test.

We have also recently developed a new plaque-reduction neutralization test and compared it with the standard neutralization test in mice and the indirect FRA test. The test is relatively rapid, economical, and quite accurate, and the results compare favorably with other methods. It is similar to the method described by King *et al.* (1965) which utilized coverslip cultures, but has certain technical advantages. Detailed methods and results will be reported elsewhere, but a brief description follows. Bottle cultures of the baby hamster kidney cell line (0857) are continuously maintained, with outgrowth medium consisting of Eagle's MEM in Hanks' BSS plus 10% fetal bovine serum, and the maintenance medium consisting of Eagle's MEM in Earle's BSS plus 10% fetal bovine serum. Trypsin-dispersed cells from young confluent monolayers (4 to 5 days) are then used to prepare heavily seeded microcultures on glass slides, which are then maintained in a $CO_2$ incubator at 35° C. By 48 hours, confluent monolayers ready for use have formed. The antibody titrations are performed as follows. Two-fold dilutions of heat-inactivated (56° C, 30 minutes) serum are prepared in maintenance medium and incubated 90 minutes at 37° C with equal volumes (0.2 m*l*) of stock LEP Flury rabies virus, diluted so as to contain 100 to 300 fluorescent plaque-forming units of virus per 0.1 m*l* of the final serum-virus mixture. Each serum-virus mixture is then inoculated (0.1 m*l*) onto 2 microculture monolayers, and the cultures are further incubated for 4 days. The slides are then fixed in acetone and stained with conjugated rabies immune serum by our standard FRA method. The number of foci of rabies virus-infected cells are recorded, and the neutralizing antibody titer is determined as the highest dilution of serum which is able to inhibit the development of fluorescent foci to less than 2 foci in 20 to 40 microscope fields examined. A titer of 1:4 or greater is considered positive for rabies antibody.

Thus far we have only applied this method in studying one human rabies case, and in determining the antibody status either of persons immunized against rabies or of commercially produced equine origin antiserum. The test may also prove useful in performing large-scale serologic surveys in wildlife or similar procedures. From 1968 through 1969, 1,115 antibody titrations were performed by this method (675 positive tests).

Comparison of assays of postimmunization sera by the fluorescent focus-inhibition test and by standard neutralization tests in mice has shown good agreement between the tests. Of 126 sera tested by these two methods plus the indirect FRA method thus far, 111 were positive by the fluorescent focus-inhibition test, 109 were positive by the neutralization test in mice, and 81 were positive by the indirect FRA test. Titers were reproducible by each of the methods employed. The failure of the indirect FRA method to detect as many positives as the other methods is apparently due to differences in concentration of antibody-bearing components in individual sera, not to inaccuracy of the test methods.

Preliminary results indicate that the same cell system may be useful for plaquing rabies virus. Clear, easily detectable plaques measuring 1 to 3 mm in diameter were obtained on baby hamster kidney (0853) cells infected with the LEP Flury strain of rabies virus. The cells were grown in $60 \times 15$ mm cell culture plastic petri dishes at 36° C in the $CO_2$ incubator. Outgrowth medium was Eagle's MEM in Earle's BSS plus 5% fetal bovine serum, with a final concentration of 25 micrograms/m*l* of DEAE Dextran, and 0.03 Molar concentration/m*l* of magnesium chloride. Pan-agar was used for the overlay medium. At 18 to 19 days, the second overlay medium of Ion-agar with neutral red (6 to 7% of a stock solution of 0.25% neutral red) was added, and the plaques counted. This method appears to be simpler to perform than the method described by Sedwick and Wiktor (1967). The technique must now be tried with other rabies virus strains, and studied for its usefulness in antibody titrations, comparison of viral strains, and virus titrations. Plaquing systems are currently under study in several other laboratories and we can anticipate considerable progress in this area in the next several years.

## PRECAUTIONS

To summarize briefly some of the points raised previously, the possible pitfalls in the diagnosis of rabies involve either failure to detect the virus, or making a diagnosis of rabies when the disease is not present. Missed diagnoses may occur if (1) the wrong tissue is tested (improper selection of anatomic site of the brain, mix-up of specimens), (2) the tissue is improperly preserved (loss of labile virus, bacterial overgrowth), (3) histopathologic methods alone are relied upon, (4) inoculated animals are not carefully observed for symptoms, (5) poor quality fluorescent antibody conjugates, equipment, or staining procedures are used, or there is wrong interpretation of staining results (due to color-blindness, insufficient review of the slides, inexperience), or (6) inhibitory substances (antibody, interferon, "rabies inhibitory substance," or other inhibitors) prevent the growth of the virus. For the latter reason, fluorescent antibody staining may be positive even though virus isolation is unsuccessful.

False positive diagnoses may occur (1) if specimens are inadvertently interchanged, (2) if tissue is poorly preserved (autofluorescence, nonspecific fluorescence), (3) when nonspecific cytoplasmic inclusion bodies are mistakenly identified as Negri bodies, (4) when nonspecific deaths or sickness and death in test animals due to other viruses are mistakenly attributed to rabies virus and specificity tests are not done, (5) when poor quality fluorescent antibody conjugates, equipment and staining procedures are used (overstaining, failure to use proper controls, misinterpretation of nonspecific fluorescence).

## FUTURE RESEARCH NEEDS

Important areas of research in diagnostic rabies virology now ongoing or which should be undertaken include: (1) evaluation of the significance of latent, subclinical, or "chronic" rabies in animal hosts and methods of detecting such infections; (2) methods for the rapid antemortem diagnosis of rabies in suspected human cases, coincidental with possible chemotherapeutic or seroprophylactic approaches; (3) methods to distinguish between the onset of clinical rabies and vaccine reactions in persons under treatment for rabies exposure; (4) cheaper, more reliable, and more readily available fluorescent antibody conjugates and fluorescence microscopes and equipment; (5) application of electron microscopic methods; (6) improved serologic methods; (7) new host systems (cell cultures, animal hosts) for virus isolation and study; (8) new methods for differentiating and for comparing the biologic characteristics of vaccine virus strains and "wild" strains; (9) fluorescent antibody methods or other specific diagnostic procedures which can be reliably applied to formalin-fixed tissues; (10) the classification of rabies virus and its relationship to other viruses. Many of these points have been presented in more detail in recent reviews such as that by Campbell *et al.* (1968).

We will conclude this review by describing briefly laboratory studies we performed on an unusual case of human rabies. The case history, clinical course, and laboratory findings will be reported in detail elsewhere but the problems which arose, the methods applied, and the laboratory findings are summarized here to illustrate many of the points raised above regarding future research needs.

The patient was a 2 1/2 year old boy who was severely bitten on April 1, 1969, by a rabid bobcat. He was treated with duck embryo rabies vaccine, but developed symptoms and early signs of rabies and was eventually hospitalized on the 24th day after exposure. A rapidly progressing ascending paralysis and coma developed. He was treated with large doses of rabies antiserum (equine origin) intraventricularly (after brain biopsy) and intrathecally, and was given intensive supportive care. The patient remained comatose, requiring artificial maintenance of vital functions, until death from cardiac failure finally occurred August 29, 1969, 133 days after onset of the first signs of illness. The diagnosis was established by fluorescent antibody staining of edematous brain tissue which drained from the brain biopsy site 21 days after onset of symptoms. Specificity tests and repeated staining procedures confirmed the accuracy of the finding. The tissue taken during the actual biopsy procedure on the 9th day of illness had by error been fixed in formalin before submission to our laboratory. No Negri bodies could be identified in this tissue, and attempts to stain the fixed tissue by the FRA method were unsuccessful. Electron microscopic examination of the biopsy tissue and tissues collected at autopsy revealed no virus-like particles.

Impression smears of corneal cells taken on days 17, 18, 19, 20, and 27 of the illness were stained by the FRA method, but did not reveal viral antigen. This test has been successful in detecting rabies prior to death in experimentally infected mice in our laboratory and elsewhere, but not in monkeys and some other animal species. It may also not be of benefit in human cases, as suggested by our findings in the present case, but further studies should be done.

Antirabies antibodies in the patient rose rapidly to final titers of 1:32,768 (indirect FRA method), 1:16,384 (fluorescent focus inhibition method), 1:12,000 (neutralization test in mice), and 1:1,250 (lytic antibody). Significant antibody titers also developed in saliva and cerebrospinal fluid (indirect FRA method). The neutralization titer in mice of a suspension of the patient's cerebrum and Ammon's horn tissue obtained at autopsy was greater than 1:5,120. There was no evidence (by precipitation tests with the patient's sera, other laboratory studies and the clinical findings) that the illness could be attributed to vaccine reaction or serum sickness and the autopsy findings were consistent with encephalitis due to rabies and not to an auto-allergic demyelinating process. It was believed that the high serum and tissue antibody titers prevented isolation of virus, even though antigen detectable by the FRA test was present at 22 days of the illness. Data supporting this concept have been reported previously by others (Lodmell *et al.*, 1969); Bell *et al.*, 1966; Bell, 1964; Parker and Sikes, 1966).

Virus isolation attempts on stool, throat secretions and saliva, urine, and spinal fluid obtained at intervals early in the course of illness and on over 40 tissues obtained at autopsy were also negative. All tissues tested at autopsy were negative for rabies virus antigen by the FRA test. It was felt that the very long delay before death, and the extremely high antibody levels which developed, may have allowed viral antigen to disappear from the brain and organ tissues, or that detection of the antigen by the FRA test was "blocked." In further attempts to reveal possible "latent" rabies virus, portions of the medulla, midbrain, cerebrum, kidneys, and lung were obtained fresh at autopsy and were grown *in vitro* for prolonged periods. Subcultures to other cell cultures and to mice, and FRA staining failed to yield virus.

We noted a similar situation some years ago in mice infected with a naturally attenuated strain of rabies virus originally isolated in our laboratory from a skunk. Many mice inoculated with the virus developed obvious signs of rabies, including paralysis and severe muscle atrophy, but recovered from the acute illness and survived well over a year. A large group of mice so affected was followed to 425 days, and mice were selected periodically and the brains tested for antigen, live virus, and for brain tissue neutralization titer. We had not recognized the additional value or importance of attempting *in vitro* culture of tissues at that time. Neutralizing capacity developed as early as 18 days in the mouse brains, and gradually increased, while live virus could not be detected after the 18th day. Fluorescent antigen was present in the hippocampus, cerebral cortex, and cerebellum of mice as long as a year later, but could not be detected in the longest survivors, suggesting that it had been eliminated from the brain tissue.

We present these data to illustrate some of the techiques which should be used in documenting possible recovery from rabies and in detecting the long-term maintenance hosts or "carriers" of rabies, if such do exist. The *in vitro* cell culture techniques hold particular promise in this regard. Of even greater importance to public health, however, is to further disseminate to the areas of greatest need the technical skill, routine laboratory methods, and proper laboratory equipment already proven by long experience to be effective in supporting and achieving control of rabies and prevention of the disease in man.

## REFERENCES

Bell, J. F. (1964). Abortive rabies infection. 1. Experimental production in white mice and general discussion. *J. Inf. Dis.*, **114** (3), 193–284.

Bell, J. F., Lodmell, D. L., Moore, G. J. and Raymond, G. H. (1966). Brain neutralization of rabies virus to distinguish recovered animals from previously vaccinated animals. *J. Immunol.*, **97** (6), 747–753.

Campbell, J. B., Kaplan, M. M., Koprowski, H., Kuwert, E., Sokol, F. and Wiktor, T. J. (1968). Present trends and the future in rabies research. *Bull. W. H. O.*, **38**, 373–381.

Habel, K. (1964). Advances in rabies research. *Ergebnisse der Mikrobiologie*, **38**, 39–54.

Halonen, P. E., Murphy, F. A., Fields, B. N. and Reese, D. R. (1968). Hemagglutinin of rabies and some other bullet-shaped viruses. *Proc. Soc. Exptl. Biol. Med.*, **127**, 1037–1042.

Jenson, A. B., Rabin, E. R., Wende, R. D. and Melnick, J. L. (1967). A comparative light and electron microscopic study of rabies and Hart Park virus encephalitis. *Experimental and Molecular Pathology*, **7** (1), 1–10.

Johnson, H. N. (1969). Rabies virus. Ch. 8 p. 321–353 *in* Lennette, E. H. and Schmidt, N. J., Editors, Diagnostic Procedures for Viral and Rickettsial Infections, Fourth Edition, American Public Health Association, Inc., New York, New York.

Johnson, H. N. (1970). Rabies virus. Ch. 63, p. 553–561 *in* Blair, J. E., Lennette, E. H., and Truant, J. P., Editors, Manual of Clinical Microbiology, American Society for Microbiology, Bethesda, Maryland.

King, D. A., Croghan, D. L. and Shaw, E. L. (1965). A rapid quantitative *in vitro* serum neutralization test for rabies antibody. *Canadian Vet. J.*, **6** (8), 187–193.

Kuwert, E., Wiktor, T. J., Sokol, F. and Koprowski, H. (1968). Hemagglutination by rabies virus. *J. Virol.*, **2** (12), 1381–1392.

Lennette, E. H., Woodie, J. D., Nakamura, K. and Magoffin, R. L. (1965). The diagnosis of rabies by fluorescent antibody method (FRA) employing immune hamster serum. *Health Lab. Sci.*, **2**, 24–34.

Lodmell, D. L., Bell, J. F., Moore, G. J. and Raymond, G. H. (1969). Comparative study of abortive and nonabortive rabies in mice. *J. Inf. Dis.*, **119** (6), 569–580.

Matsumoto, S. and Kawai, A. (1969). Comparative studies on development of rabies virus in different host cells. *Virology*, **39** (3), 449–459.

Morecki, R. and Zimmerman, H. M. (1969). Human rabies encephalitis. Fine structure study of cytoplasmic inclusions. *Arch. Neurol.*, **20**, 599–604.

Parker, R. L. and Sikes, R. K. (1966). Development of rabies inhibiting substance in skunks infected with rabies virus. *Public Health Reports*, **81** (10), 941–944.

Rabin, E. R. and Jenson, A. B. (1967). Electron microscopic studies of animal viruses with emphasis on in vivo infections. *Progr. Med. Virol.*, **9**, 392–450.

Sedwick, W. D. and Wiktor, T. J. (1967). Reproducible plaquing system for rabies, lymphocytic choriomeningitis, and other ribonucleic acid viruses in BHK-21/13S agarose suspensions. *J. Virol.*, **1**, 1224–1226.

Soave, O. A., Johnson, H. N. and Nakamura, K. (1961). Reactivation of rabies virus infection of animals with adrenocorticotropic hormone. *Science*, **133**, 1360.

Wiktor, T. J., Kuwert, E. and Koprowski, H. (1968). Immune lysis of rabies virus-infected cells. *J. Immunol.*, **101** (6), 1271–1282.

World Health Organization, Laboratory Techniques in Rabies, Second Edition, Geneva, 178 pp., 1966.

For Discussion, see page 91.

# Discussion*

DAVENPORT: I would like to ask Dr. Lennette two questions: 1) What are the procedures for protecting personnel who handle these diagnostic procedures in his laboratory—just who is vaccinated, and how often? 2) The failure to isolate live virus in materials that fluoresce implies that there is some antigen other than whole virus antigen which is being fluoresced by the anti-sera. Is it known which antigen is fluorescent since Dr. Wiktor told us of at least four antigens in the rabies virus?

LENNETTE: Perhaps Dr. Wiktor could tell you better than I which antigen or antigens fluoresce, because he is involved in studying this aspect.

As concerns the first part of your question, we do not try to immunize the entire laboratory staff, but only those people who are potentially exposed to rabies virus infection. These are the people who receive the specimens in the mail room, who open such specimen containers for recording purposes, and those who prepare the material for inoculation and who actually inoculate the mice or prepare smears for fluorescent antibody staining. So long as the Flury vaccine was available, we had no problems. We gave enough of the Flury strain vaccine until the inoculated individual developed neutralizing antibody. Booster inoculations were subsequently given at yearly intervals. We never felt we had to do any more than that unless there were an exposure, at which time we would give additional vaccine as well as hyperimmune serum. Now that the Flury vaccine is not licensed for human use, we use the duck embryo vaccine and, in general, get good antibody responses.

The need for preexposure prophylaxis is obvious when one thinks of the potential exposures that might occur. While we have had no accidents concerned with jabbing a needle into a finger or into a hand, we have had such exposures as cuts from broken glass vials or from glass fragments at the bottom of a dry ice box which was being emptied and cleaned.

---

* This Discussion refers to the reports by R. T. Johnson and Lennette *et al.*

WIKTOR: To answer Dr. Davenport's question, I must note that analysis of different antigens derived from rabies virus is still in the early stages of development. Four different structural proteins were isolated from purified rabies virions, but it is not known which one is responsible for the induction of antibody, as demonstrated by the fluorescing technique. We do know, however, that the neutralizing capacity of a given serum doesnot necessarily parallel its fluorescing activity. On the other hand, sera can be prepared which will be devoid of neutralizing activity. Fluorescence obtained by these sera is completely different from fluorescence obtained with serum prepared with the complete virions. Normally, the sera used for fluorescence are prepared using rabies-infected brain tissue as antigen, and it is evident that they contain all kinds of antibodies. We hope that in the near future, it will be possible to prepare sera with purified fractions derived from virions, as well as with purified soluble antigens. Analysis of these sera will probably provide more information about the structure and properties of different rabies antigens.

KOPROWSKI: We can distinguish three types of fluorescence in rabies-infected cells. One type, cytoplasmic fluorescence, corresponds to the presence of inclusion bodies (Negri body) and is associated with electron microscopic demonstration of virion material. The second type, referred to by Dr. Wiktor, is a granular fluorescence, probably associated with the presence of nucleocapsids. The third type, membrane fluorescence, relates to the presence of an antigen on the cell membrane which probably binds with the "lytic" antibody.

SIKES: I would like to partially answer the question that Dr. Davenport raised about pre-exposure immunization. I think all of us should know what the Public Health Service Advisory Committee on Immunization Practices recommends at present. Admittedly, we do not like the duck embryo vaccine; it is not as antigenic as we would like to have it. But it is a safe vaccine and if the series of doses is given including three doses of duck embryo vaccine, two a month apart, and a booster six months later, detectable antibody in 80% of the people will appear. A booster given within a month or two months to the remaining 20% who are negative, will produce a detectable antibody in about 50% of the remaining negatives. The duck embryo vaccine requires several doses for

90% to 100% of the people to get a detectable antibody. The key point is that if you develop a titer and even though you wait as much as 25 years and you give even a single dose of the duck embryo vaccine after an exposure, you get a very quick recall. Indeed, this is what we are after. If the people in the laboratory will bother to take this vaccine which is not as antigenic as we like but is the best we have got at the present time—it will provide detectable antibody and protection to those who get it. On exposure they would be requested to take from one to five additional boosters daily and another booster twenty days later if it is a severe challenge. These are the recommendations of the P.H.S. Advisory Committee on Immunization Practices and we think they are quite adequate.

KITAMOTO: Dr. Lennette, you described a very interesting case with death occurring after 133 days. I would like to ask what the symptoms were particularly at the onset of the disease.

LENNETTE: Do you mean the early onset or the initial stages of the illness? I have only an excerpt of the history here, but there were some questions as to the diagnosis. Inasmuch as this child had had inoculations of duck embryo vaccine, the physicians who saw him at the onset of his illness did not think a rabies virus infection was involved; rather, they thought it was an encephalitis. This is why, some days after onset, because of the aberrant clinical picture and one not typical of rabies, that the brain biopsy was done. It was from this biopsy that we obtained the brain material which, by fluorescent antibody staining, established the diagnosis of rabies. It was not too long after this that the child went into coma, and electroencephalograms showed very little brain activity. While the vital functions continued, there was essentially nothing cerebrally. One wonders how the child survived as long as he did. His survival is, incidentally, one of the longest on record.

KITAMOTO: You gave us comparisons of various assays of post-immunization sera and of 126 sera: 111 were positive by the fluorescent focus-inhibition test, 109 were positive by the neutralization test in mice, and 81 were positive by the indirect fluorescent antibody test. How many CF positive sere were in this group?

LENNETTE: We do not utilize the complement fixation test for antibody determinations, but rely on indirect fluorescent antibody, fluorescent focus inhibition and mouse neutralization tests.

For virus identification, we rely almost entirely on fluorescent antibody staining. We consider this to be a highly accurate method if done by experienced people and indeed have so much confidence in our own technique that only rarely do we inoculate mice for diagnostic purposes. Should other better techniques become available, we would certainly want to use them.

# Diagnosis of Rabid Animals by Means of Complement Fixation Test

Keizo Ishii

*Central Virus Diagnostic Laboratory, National Institute of Health, Tokyo*

Studies for this work were started in 1952 and reports based on these studies have already been published (Ando *et al.*, 1953a, b). An attempt was made to detect the antigenic substance in the brain of rabies-suspected animals by means of the complement fixation (CF) test. Based on the same ideas, the fluorescent antibody technique is widely adopted for the diagnosis of rabies at present. The fluorescent antibody technique is the most accurate test presently available for rabies diagnosis.

Although much of the information in this paper has been previously published, it should still be significant, in height of work done by K. Shimada on the CF test used for the detection of rabid animals, the results of which are present in this volume, and because the CF test has been, up to now, the best method employed, and the most suitable for the diagnosis of rabies under particular circumstances such as when the brain tissue is putrid.

## MATERIALS AND METHODS

*Materials tested*: Rabies-suspected animals which were sent to the Tokyo Municipal Laboratories for Medical Sciences during September of 1952 to June of 1953 were used. The brain specimens totalled 194. In addition to brain tissues, the salivary glands of some animals were also tested; except for one human and five cats, they were mostly dogs. Twenty-three healthy dogs were used as controls.

*Preparation of hyperimmune serum*: The rabies immune serum was prepared by means of immunizing guinea pigs. In order to prevent the production of antibodies against brain tissues, the brain tissues of homologous animals were used as immunogen. The guinea pigs were intraperitoneally injected two times with 10% UV-inactivated vaccine with 7-day interval, and five to seven times with the infective virus suspension in the same interval. The CF antibody titer of the hyperimmune serum was 1:32 to 1:64; no fixation was shown with the antigen of normal guinea pig brain tissue. The "no fixation" with normal brain antigen is an important factor in the diagnosis of rabies in animals.

*Preparation of CF antigen*: The CF antigen was usually prepared as follows (Casals & Palacios, 1941): the brain emulsion was extracted overnight in a refrigerator and centrifuged at 3,000 rpm for 30 minutes, and the supernatant was frozen and thawed repeatedly five times and then centrifuged at 10,000 rpm for 30 minutes. In order to save time but without loss of CF antigenicity, a modified method for CF antigen preparation was tried. Subsequently, a rapid method was found for the preparation of CF antigen which was not inferior in antigenicity to antigen prepared by the standard method. A 40% emulsion in saline solution of the brain tissues of suspected animals was prepared. The emulsion was extracted at 40°C for 2 hours and centrifuged at 10,000 rpm for 30 minutes. The supernatant was used as CF antigen during the period of study.

*CF test*: The CF test was carried out as follows: Immune serum (0.15 m*l*) was mixed with antigen (0.15 m*l*) and 2 units of complement (0.3 m*l*). The mixture was incubated at 37°C for 2 hours. Hemolytic system (0.3 m*l*) was then added and the resulting mixture was read after incubation at 37°C for 30 minutes.

In the tests, 16 units or more of immune serum was used in antibody titers and 40% emulsions of antigen was generally used, though diluted antigens were also sometimes used. Fifty percent guinea pig inactivated serum saline solution was otherwise used as a diluent. Although satisfactory results were also obtained with the CF test performed with the standard (Kolmer's) method, the method mentioned above using concentrated antigen and a short incubation time was adopted for rapid diagnostic procedures.

CF antigen exhibited little anticomplementary effect even though concentrated antigen as high as 40% was used. The majority of CF antigens prepared for the brains of truly rabid animals showed very strong antigenicity and were capable of fixing 1 to 4 units of antibody, although a few antigens could partially fix (50%) a considerably large number of units (16 units) of antibody. These antigens were judged as "positive" and the antigens fixing less "equivocal."

## RESULTS

1) Comparative results from various diagnostic procedures

Brain tissues of rabies-suspected animals were examined by Negri body detection using both stamp and section, by histopathological observation, and by virus isolation using mice at the Tokyo Municipal Laboratories for Medical Sciences. Examination by CF test and by virus isolation was also performed at our laboratory. Virus isolation in mice was also attempted using salivary glands of some suspected animals. The results obtained by these tests are summarized in Table 1.

Table 1. Findings of Various Diagnostic Measures Applied on the Brain Materials of Rabies Supected Animals

| Virus isolation | Pathological examinations: Negri body, Stamp sample | Pathological examinations: Negri body, Section sample | Pathological examinations: Nonpurulent encephalitic picture | Complement fixation test | Number of cases | | Total |
|---|---|---|---|---|---|---|---|
| | + | + | + | | 43 | | |
| | − | + | + | | 7 | | |
| + | + | − | + | + | 2 | 65 | |
| | − | + | − | | 3 | | |
| | − | − | + | | 10 | | 194 |
| | − | − | − | + | 8 | | |
| − | − | − | + | − | 6 | 129 | |
| | − | − | − | − | 115 | | |

Rabies virus was isolated from the brains of 65 out of 194 cases tested. Negri bodies were found in 55 cases (in 47 cases with stamp and in 53 cases with section). An encephalitic picture was found in 62 cases and CF antigen in all cases. CF antigenicity was "equivocal" in three of these cases. On the other hand, of 129 cases showing no virus isolation, eight were positive for CF antigen. CF antigenicity was "equivocal" in three of these cases. An encephalitic picture was observed in 6 cases. It is noteworthy that there were two dogs in which CF antigen was detected and from whose salivary glands rabies virus was also isolated, in spite of absence of virus from the brain tissues. From these findings, there is no doubt that the CF test is an excellent diagnostic method. Furthermore, diagnosis by the CF test was completed within 5 hours after the specimens were received. The CF test was used for the practical diagnosis of rabies in combination with other methods until 1955, when rabies was eradicated from Japan.

2) CF antigenicity in brain tissues of guinea pigs experimentally infected with street virus

Fourteen guinea pigs were infected with fresh street virus (No. 182

strain) which had passed through only one generation of mouse brain by means of intracerebral inoculations. The infectivity and CF antigenicity of the brains were tested in the course of time. Guinea pigs were infected with a virus dosis of 6000 $LD_{50}$, and two guinea pigs were sacrificed every day for testing. The results are shown in Table 2.

Table 2. CF Antigenicity and Virus Infectivity of the Brains of Guinea Pigs Experimentally Infected with Rabies Virus

| Days after inoculation | Guinea pig I | | | | Guinea pig II | | | |
|---|---|---|---|---|---|---|---|---|
| | Symptoms | CF test | | Virus titer | Symptoms | CF test | | Virus titer |
| | | Antigen % | Titer | | | Antigen % | Titer | |
| 0 | – | 40% | <1:2 | – | – | 40% | <1:2 | ≦0.6 |
| 1 | – | 40% | <1:2 | – | – | 40% | <1:2 | – |
| 2 | – | 40% | <1:2 | – | – | 40% | <1:2 | ≦0.6 |
| 3 | – | 40% | <1:2 | – | – | 40% | <1:2 | – |
| 4 | – | 40% | <1:2 | – | – | 40% | <1:2 | 2.3 |
| 5 | – | 40% | 1:32 | 3.3 | – | 40% | <1:2 | 3.6 |
| 6 | – | 20% | 1:32 | 4.0 | ± | 10% | 1:32 | 4.0 |
| 7 | + | 10% | 1:16 | 3.5 | + | 10% | 1:32 | 3.6 |

Virus inoculated: Street virus derived from the brain of rabid dog (No. 182). $LD_{50}=4.83$
Inoculation: Guinea pigs were intracerebrally inoculated with 0.1 m*l* of 10% brain emulsion.

Virus was first detected in the brain of a guinea pig on the 4th day after inoculation, and CF antigen on the 5th day. Virus isolation was either more or less sensitive than CF antigen in this experiment. Clinical symptoms were first detected on the 7th day.

3) CF antigenicity of antigens prepared from different parts of brains

Six different parts of brain, the frontal lobe, parietal lobe, thalamus, corpora quadrigemina, cerebellum and medulla oblongata were removed separately from six naturally infected rabid dogs. CF antigenicity and virus infectivity of these parts were compared. As shown in Table 3, it was observed that thalamus, corpora quadrigemina and medulla oblongata were always high in CF antigenicity and virus infectivity, while the other parts were sometimes low. CF antigenicities of frontal lobe, parietal lobe and cerebellum were especially lower than those of other parts in two dogs, though virus infectivities were not so low in these parts. Therefore, it was recommended that CF antigens for diagnosis should be prepared from the mixture of brain tissues containing corpora quadrigemina and medulla oblongata.

Table 3. CF Antigenicity and Virus Infectivity in Different Parts of Rabid Dog Brains

| Locality | Antigen concentration | Rabid dogs No. 119 CFT | No. 119 $LD_{50}$ | No. 129 CFT | No. 129 $LD_{50}$ | No. 135 CFT | No. 135 $LD_{50}$ | No. 140 CFT | No. 140 $LD_{50}$ | No. 141 CFT | No. 141 $LD_{50}$ | No. 151 CFT | No. 151 $LD_{50}$ |
|---|---|---|---|---|---|---|---|---|---|---|---|---|---|
| Frontal lobe | 40% | | | ± | | 4 | | 2 | | 4 | | 1 | |
| | 30% | | | 0 | 1.83 | 4 | 2.67 | | 3.0 | 4 | 3.5 | ± | 0.63 |
| | 20% | | | 0 | | 4 | | ± | | 3 | | ± | |
| | 10% | | | 0 | | 1 | | 0 | | ± | | 0 | |
| Parietal lobe | 40% | | | 1 | | 4 | | 4 | | 4 | | | |
| | 30% | 4 | 4.38 | ± | 2.77 | 4 | 3.5 | 1 | 3.39 | 4 | 4.0 | 1 | 1.63 |
| | 20% | 4 | | 0 | | 4 | | ± | | 4 | | ± | |
| | 10% | 1 | | 0 | | 4 | | 0 | | ± | | 0 | |
| Cerebellum | 40% | | | 1 | | 4 | | 3 | | 4 | | | |
| | 30% | 4 | 3.17 | 1 | 2.83 | | 3.5 | 1 | 2.0 | 4 | 2.75 | 2 | 1.5 |
| | 20% | 4 | | ± | | 4 | | ± | | ± | | 1 | |
| | 10% | ± | | 0 | | 4 | | 0 | | ± | | 0 | |
| Thalamus | 40% | | | 4 | | | | 4 | | 4 | | 4 | |
| | 30% | 4 | | | | | | | | | | | |
| | 20% | 4 | 4.68 | 1 | ≧4.5 | 4 | 3.33 | 4 | 3.33 | 4 | ≧4.25 | | 2.78 |
| | 10% | 4 | | ± | | 1 | | 1 | | 2 | | | |
| | 5% | | | 0 | | 0 | | ± | | ± | | | |
| Corpora quadrigemina | 40% | | | 4 | | 4 | | | | | | | |
| | 20% | 4 | 4.24 | 1 | ≧4.5 | 4 | 3.56 | 4 | 3.83 | 4 | 3.53 | 4 | 3.0 |
| | 10% | 4 | | ± | | 4 | | 1 | | 4 | | 3 | |
| | 5% | | | 0 | | ± | | ± | | 1 | | 1 | |
| Medulla oblongata | 40% | | | 4 | | 4 | | 4 | | | | 4 | |
| | 20% | 4 | ≧5.17 | 3 | ≧4.17 | 4 | ≧4.17 | 4 | 4.17 | 4 | 3.17 | 4 | 3.0 |
| | 10% | 4 | | ± | | 4 | | 4 | | 1 | | 4 | |
| | 5% | 2 | | 0 | | ± | | 2 | | ± | | 3 | |

16 units of immune serum were used.

4) CF antigenicity of putrid brain

It was not always possible to get fresh specimens from rabies-suspected animals sent to the laboratory. A few were dogs suspected of rabies which had died and been buried. In such occasions, testing of the putrid brain was impossible by Negri body detection and histopathological examination, and an attempt to isolate virus was the only successful diagnostic method possible. Eight such cases were tested; the virus was isolated from the brains in four and CF antigens were also detected. Moreover, CF antigens were detected in the brains tissues of two dogs from which no virus was isolated.

The brain emulsion of naturally infected dogs was exposed at room temperature for varying periods of time to detect the inactivation state of virus infectivity and of CF antigenicity. The brain before exposure contained infectivity of $10^{3.5}$ $LD_{50}$ and so much antigenicity that 30% brain emulsion completely fixed 16 units of antibody. The

Table 4. CF Antigenicity after Exposure at Room Temperature

| Period of exposure | Complement fixation test | | | | | | | | titer ($LD_{50}$) |
|---|---|---|---|---|---|---|---|---|---|
| | Antigen concentration | Serum dilution 2 | 4 | 8 | 16 | 32 | 64 | Antigen control | |
| | 40% | | 4 | 2 | 2 | 1 | ± | 0 | |
| (−) | 30% | 4 | 3 | 1 | 1 | ± | ± | 0 | 3.22 |
| | 20% | 2 | ± | ± | ± | ± | ± | 0 | |
| | 10% | ± | 0 | 0 | 0 | 0 | 0 | 0 | |
| | 40% | 4 | 4 | 4 | 4 | 4 | 2 | ± | |
| 3 days | 30% | 4 | 4 | 4 | 4 | 4 | 1 | ± | 3.0 |
| | 20% | 4 | 4 | 4 | 4 | 4 | 1 | ± | |
| | 10% | 4 | 4 | 4 | 2 | 1 | ± | 0 | |
| | 40% | | | | 4 | 4 | 4 | 4 | |
| 12 days | 30% | | 4 | 4 | 4 | 4 | 4 | 4 | ≦0.5 |
| | 20% | | 4 | 4 | 4 | 4 | 3 | 2 | |
| | 10% | | 4 | 4 | 3 | 2 | 1 | ± | |
| | 20% | | | | 4 | 3 | 2 | 1 | |
| | 10% | | | 3 | 2 | 2 | 1 | ± | |
| | 5% | 2 | 2 | 1 | 1 | 1 | 1 | ± | |
| 18 days | 2.5% | 1 | 1 | ± | ± | ± | ± | 0 | ≦0.5 |
| | 1.25% | ± | 0 | 0 | 0 | 0 | 0 | 0 | |
| | 0.63% | 0 | 0 | 0 | 0 | 0 | 0 | 0 | |
| | 20% | 4 | 4 | 4 | 4 | 4 | 4 | 4 | |
| | 10% | 4 | 4 | 4 | 4 | 4 | 4 | 4 | |
| | 5% | 4 | 4 | 3 | 3 | 3 | 3 | 3 | ≦0.5 |
| 37 days | 2.5% | 1 | 1 | ± | ± | ± | ± | ± | |
| | 1.25% | ± | ± | 0 | 0 | 0 | 0 | 0 | |
| | 0.63 | ± | 0 | 0 | 0 | 0 | 0 | 0 | |

results are shown in Table 4. The virus infectivity was lost between the 3rd and 12th day after exposure. On the other hand, CF antigenicity was found even on the 18th day although the antigen acquired an anticomplementary effect. From the findings, it was possible that virus was not isolated from the putrid brains of animals even when the animals were truly rabid. During the study period, there were two cases from which no virus was isolated but CF antigen was detected. These animals were strongly suspected of true rabies. Diagnosis by CF test is presently the best among the several diagnostic methods for rabies when a putrid animal brain has to be tested.

5) CF antigenicity of saliva and salivary glands

CF antigenic substance was also found in the saliva and salivary glands, but the antigenicity was inferior to that of the brain.

## DISCUSSION

Comparative results from various methods for diagnosis of rabies are summarized in Table 5. Out of 194 rabies-suspected animals tested, 73 rabid animals, including six dogs whose brains were putrid, were detected by CF test. There were no cases in which a negative reaction was shown by CF test and a positive reaction by any test other than the CF test. Rabiesvirus was detected in 65 cases (89%), encephalitic picture in 62 cases (85%) and Negri bodies in 55 cases (75%).

Table 5. Comparison between the Results Obtained by Various Diagnostic Methods
(Sept. '52 to June '53; Number tested: 194 cases)

| State of specimens | Virus isolation | CF antigenicity | No. of cases | |
|---|---|---|---|---|
| | + | + | 58 | |
| fresh | + | ± | 3 | 67 |
| | − | + | 4 | |
| | − | ± | 2 | |
| | + | + | 4 | |
| putrid | − | + | 2 | 6 |

It is important to know whether or not any false positive cases are included in the CF-tested positive cases. The CF antigens from brain tissues were found in 73 cases in which putrid material from six dogs was included. On the other hand, rabiesvirus was isolated from the brains of 65 cases of which four were in a putrid state. These 65 cases were undoubtedly rabid animals. It was possible that some false positive cases were included in the remaining eight cases which were virus isolation negative and CF antigen positive (see Table 5).

These eight cases consisted of six fresh specimens and of two putrid specimens. In this study, virus isolation was attempted from the salivary glands in some cases. There were two cases which were CF antigen positive and virus isolation positive for salivary glands, in spite of negative virus isolation from the brain tissues. From these findings, it was certain that there might be genuinely rabid animals in which virus isolation from brain tissue was negative. The virus infectivity of brain tissue was lost during a shorter period than was the CF antigenicity (see Table 4). From this finding, we also hesitated in deciding that the two putrid cases, which were CF antigen positive but virus isolation negative, were nonrabid animals. Thus, we could not find certain false positive cases by CF test, although some false positive cases might have existed in cases which we tested.

Diagnosis by CF test as well as by the fluorescent antibody technique is completed within 5 hours after receiving a specimen. These diagnostic methods are superior with respect to the short time required and their high sensitivity to other diagnostic methods. Nevertheless, in principle, the combination of several reliable methods is recommended for the diagnosis of rabies in suspected dogs.

## SUMMARY

An attempt to detect antigenic substance in the brains of rabies-suspected animals was made by the CF test. Standard preparation of CF antigen and the CF test procedure were modified to save time without reducing sensitivity. The diagnostic value of the modified CF test was compared with that of the pathological and virological methods hitherto used.

The results obtained by CF test was equal to the results using virus isolation and were superior to Negri body detection and histopathological observation. The CF test and fluorescent antibody technique as well were superior with respect to the short time required. For these reasons, it was possible to use CF test in place of fluorescent antibody technique for diagnostic purposes. Besides, since CF antigenicity is more stable than virus infectivity, the CF test is suitable for testing the putrid brain specimens of rabies-suspected animals.

## REFERENCES

Ando, K., Ishii, K., Oka, Y., Irisawa, J., Shimada, K. and Kato, T. (1953a). Studies on the immunological diagnosis of animals suspected of rabies. *Jap. Jour. Med. Sci. Biol.*, **6**, 221.

Ando, K., Ishii, K., Oka, Y., Irisawa, J., Shimada, K., Kato, T. and Murakami, H. (1953b). Studies on the immunological diagnosis of animals suspected of rabies (second report). *Jap. Jour. Med. Sci. Biol.*, **6**, 659.

Casals, J. and Palacios, R. (1941). The complement fixation test in the diagnosis of virus infections of the central nervous system. *Jour. Exp. Med.*, **74**, 409.

For Discussion, see page 105.

# Discussion*

DAVENPORT: May I ask Dr. Ishii if he has encountered false positive complement fixation tests where the diagnosis made proved to be in error. I should also like to ask Dr. Lennette if he would comment for our benefit on whether he feels that the fluorescent antibody test is more hindered by having to examine putrid brains than is the complement fixation test. In his opinion, does the complement fixation have an advantage when the material received at the laboratory has been delayed in shipping?

ISHII: There might be some possibilities of making erroneous diagnoses by the CF test just as Dr. Davenport mentioned. I think the most reliable diagnosis can be made by virus isolation from suspected animal brains. However, we have 2 cases in dogs of CF positive in which we isolated the virus not from their brain but from their salivary gland. From this point, it is difficult to say whether the case which showed CF positive without virus isolation is false or positive.

JO: I have a question for Dr. Lennette. What are the kinds of immune serum being used practically for the fluorescent antibody test in your laboratory? If the commercial serum has a disadvantage, how does it differ?

LENNETTE: We use hamster serum. The hamsters are immunized with virus-containing hamster brain so that there is no heterologous, non-specific staining problem to contend with. The animals are hyperimmunized so that the serums, at least by our technique, have quite good neutralizing antibody titers. We have been utilizing this method for so long now that we no longer take the trouble to determine neutralizing antibody levels—we merely immunize the animals and then bleed them and use the serum. I do not know what the secret of our success might be, because others who have employed our method obtain sera which are either very weak in staining capacity or produce non-specific reactions.

---

* This Discussion refers to the report by Ishii.

Commercial serums for fluorescent antibody work are available, and while some have proved to be of excellent quality for us, our experience in general has been that such serums leave much to be desired from several standpoints.

We have examined material which has undergone some deterioration or decomposition during shipment and have obtained good staining with fluorescein-conjugated antiserum. Much of our material comes to the laboratory in glycerol, and if this dehydrating preservative is thoroughly washed out, we have little difficulty with staining. The only major problem that shipment of tissue in glycerol-saline poses is the minute amount of tissue that may be sent; not infrequently such a small fragment becomes emulsified and the examination is thus precluded. If large pieces of tissue are used, there is almost invariably some available for examination.

JO: Have you had experience with sera from other animals? Is the hamster the best animal for preparing immune serum?

LENNETTE: I am sure that immune serum can be prepared in animals other than hamsters and, indeed, some larger species might be preferable from several standpoints. However, we have used hamsters for the preparation of immune serum against so many viruses that we have probably developed a prejudice in favor of this useful beast. Hamster immune sera present the versatility that sera from certain other species do not, i.e., they may be used in a variety of different tests as complement-fixation, neutralization, fluorescent staining, gel diffusion, precipitation, etc.

JO: Does that mean the specificity is also very high?

LENNETTE: Specificity is very high when one uses serum from animals which have been immunized with virus-containing tissues from the same species.

DAVENPORT: I have another question to ask Dr. Lennette. Is it not true, Dr. Lennette, that in your fluorescent antibody staining procedures you usually fractionate the serum on a column, the hamster serum after immunization? If so, I can understand why your laboratory does not have difficulty with these sera when others do—because the man who does the fractionation was trained in Ann Arbor, Michigan.

LENNETTE: That is not quite so, as Dr. Davenport knows. The scientist in question is the one who devised the isothiocyanate technique for conjugation of fluorescein to globulins, and the situation is actually the other way around in that he was not trained by the Michigan people, he trained them.

DAVENPORT: This I deny.

SIKES: I have another response to the question regarding other animal sera used in conjugation. We at C.D.C. also used the hamster back in 1959 and found it to be very good, just as Dr. Lennette has found. And the thing that we searched for was the use of a larger animal, the same way with commercial people, to make large quantities in order to provide large quantities of conjugate throughout a country. There are problems occasionally in using large animals for preparing serum for conjugates. There is an individual animal's variation in response to immunization, such as in burros, horses, mules and goats. We have had success and B.B.L. has had success, Pasteur Institutes have had success, and Suponzo in Argentina has had success making conjugates from these larger animals. But, you cannot count on each animal that you immunize making good conjugatable serum. It will have a high neutralizing antibody titer but not necessarily make a good conjugate. The acid test comes in your evaluating it after conjugation or tagging it yourself. In other words, not every S.N. high titer makes a good conjugate from these larger animals. So it is up to the investigator to immunize several of these animals and then count on maybe one out of five providing him with a good serum, then running this crude serum through DEAE column chromatography and getting a purified, generally 7 S globulin, tagging this and then ending up usually with a good conjugate that would titer about as high as a hamster conjugate. So you can use these other species, and many people do. It is just that it is sort of a trial and error method to get one out of X number to make a good serum.

# Dr. Nomura, additional remarks

I would like to give a short additional presentation of some findings which we have made in a study (Takehara, K., Nomura, Y. and Nakamura, J.) of the modes of infection in mice inoculated with various strains of rabies virus, especially with respect to the development of complement-fixing (CF) antigen and antibody.

The viruses which we used were four types: F (fixed virus), ST (street virus), H (Nishigahara egg high passage virus) and Fl.H (Fury egg high passage virus). These were inoculated intracerebrally in groups of mice, and in the course of time we sacrificed five of the animals to titrate the virus (thick solid line), the CF antigen (thick dotted line) in the brain, the neutralizing antibody (thin solid line) and CF (thin dotted line) antibodies in the serum.

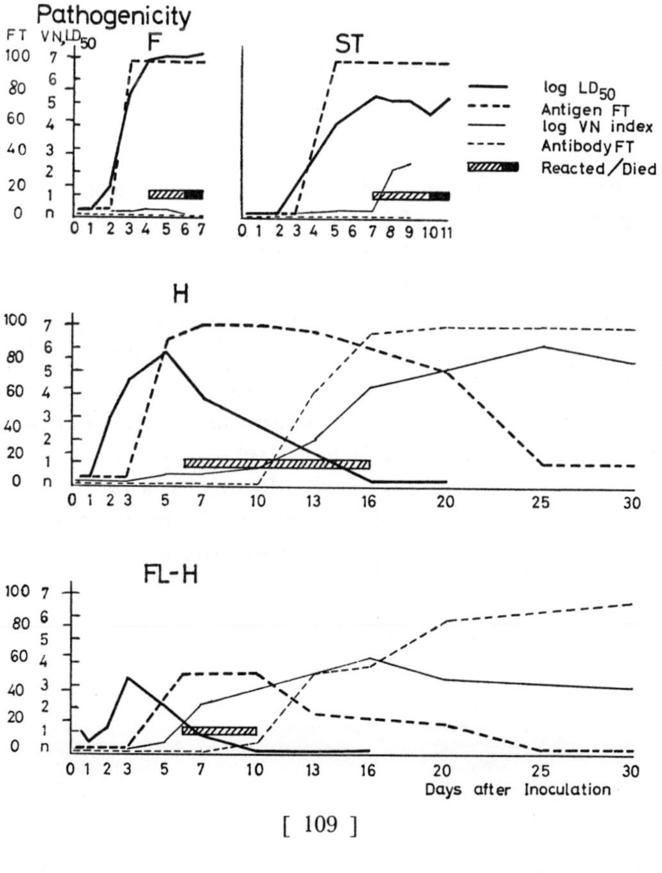

## RESULTS

1) The F infection was the strongest, with all the mice dying within 7 days. During this time, we observed a high degree of virus replication and CF antigen production, but no antibodies were demonstrated.

2) The ST infection was also fatal but with a prolonged course, all animals dying within 11 days, and during this time we saw marked growth of virus and production of CF antigen. The development of neutralizing antibody was demonstrated on the 8th day although no CF antibody was detected in the final sample obtained on the 9th day.

3) The H infection was much milder and although the majority of the animals revealed slight symptoms from day 6 to 16 only a few died (day 13 to 16). The virus reached a peak on the 5th day with a moderately high titer and decreased thereafter and disappeared on day 16. CF antigen showed a steep rise on the 5th day and reached a peak on the 7th with a high titer. Its decrease was rather gradual, a definite titer still maintained on the 20th day. Both antibodies became demonstrable on the 13th day.

4) The Fl.H infection was the weakest and none of the mice died, with only a small portion of them revealing slight, transient abnormality 6 to 10 days after inoculation. The development curves of virus, CF antigen and the two antibodies resembled those in the infection but were obviously lower in height.

As for the CF antigen in the brain, the findings appear worthy of emphasizing that it was demonstrated not only in strongly infected mice with such virulent strains as F and ST but also in weakly infected mice with such attenuated strains as H and Fl.H, and that it persisted in surviving animals for a relatively long time after the virus disappeared. These results should suggest a possibile use of the CF method to demonstrate the antigen in the brain as a specific and sensitive means for the diagnosis of naturally infected animals.

# Pre- and Postexposure Prophylaxis: Present Status and Current Trends

HILARY KOPROWSKI

*The Wistar Institute of Anatomy and Biology, Philadelphia, Pennsylvania 19104*

## INTRODUCTION

Since the late nineteenth century when Pasteur, elaborating on Roux's idea, immunized man against rabies with desiccated rabbit cord, little if any improvement has been made in the preparation of rabies vaccines. In fact, were the original Pasteur vaccine available today, it would perhaps be singled out as the best of the currently used products, provided of course that the live, fixed virus present in the vaccine did not cause rabies in recipients, such as occurred in individuals in South America receiving suckling mouse brain vaccine (Held, 1969).

The "notoriety of badness" associated with the production of rabies vaccine cannot be blamed solely on the vaccine producers. The concept of postexposure immunization, so alien to the principle of prophylaxis through antibody formation, has never been thoroughly analyzed and evaluated, particularly within the context of a modern approach to immunology. Be that as it may, there is no need to play Cassandra at this meeting, since progress in rabies research looks bright at present. Results of scientific investigations conducted during the past decade are providing us with tools for successful treatment of man (Hummeler & Koprowski, 1969).

Rabies vaccines made in the past were objectionable mainly because of their crudeness (Koprowski, 1967). Produced in either animal brain or avian embryo, they contained so much extraneous protein material that it was virtually impossible to purify the rabies antigen bound to the nonspecific carrier, and worse, the nonrabies proteins "competed" with the rabies antigen as antibody inducers, thus effectively inhibiting an adequate antibody response following vaccination. To overcome these difficulties, we turned to rabies virus grown in tissue culture as a source of antigen for experimental vaccine production.

Rabies virus will infect cell cultures derived from tissues of any warm-blooded animal as well as those from some cold-blooded animals. The virus replicates better in some cells than in others; why this is so is not yet clear. In the studies now underway, we are using BHK-21 cells for experimental vaccine production and human diploid cell strains for human vaccine production. Vaccines presently under investigation are produced from extracellular virion material obtained from infected tissue cultures and concentrated and purified by one of three methods (Sokol *et al.*, 1968; Wiktor *et al.*, 1969; Schlumberger *et al.*, 1970):

1) Precipitation by zinc acetate, desalting on Sephadex column, concentration by high-speed centrifugation.
2) Concentration by ultrafiltration through nitrocellulose membrane or
3) Purification by continuous zonal centrifugation.

Using any one of these techniques, virions present in the tissue culture fluids can be concentrated 100- to 200-fold (Schlumberger, 1970). Such concentrates contain less than 10% extraviral impurities consisting mainly of serum albumin in which the virions were maintained during processing (Sokol, 1970). Since the virus does not incorporate cellular protein in its envelope, the remaining contaminants of the preparation are components of the host cell.

We shall now examine some of the properties of experimental vaccines produced from infected extracellular rabies virions.

Of the vaccines listed in Table 1 (Sikes *et al.*, 1970), only HEP-LI contained living virus. In all other preparations, except for SMBP, the virus was inactivated by Beta-propiolactone (BPL) usually after, but sometimes before, processing for concentration and purification of the antigenic material.

The BHK-FC vaccines were produced from medium from BHK-21 tissue cultures infected with the PM strain of virus. In the BHK-FC vaccine, the virions were concentrated by ultrafiltration through nitrocellulose membrane and in FCC by ultrafiltration and high-speed centrifugation. The 200-fold concentration of BHK-FCC vaccine resulted in an infectivity titer of $10^{9.77}$ PFU/m*l* before inactivation. Strangely enough, results from the mouse potency test gave a 10-fold lower antigenic value (AV) than that obtained from the BHK-FC preparation, which was less concentrated as evidenced by $10^8$ PFU/m*l* titer before inactivation. The latter vaccine also showed a higher titer in the complement-fixation test. Whether the infectivity titer before inactivation or the AV obtained from the mouse potency test will correlate with the protective capacity remains to be determined. I am uneasy about attaching great significance to the mouse potency test, not only because of the results obtained with these two vaccines, but also because of experiments in immunization of monkeys.

The next five vaccine batches listed in Table 1 were produced in human diploid cell strain WI-38. The first three batches (HDCS-FCa, FCb and FCc) were produced by ultrafiltration of the infectious tissue culture media, whereas FCA-I vaccine was obtained from FCa after further filtration through a Sephadex G-150 column and adsorption on aluminum hydroxide gel. The HDCS-FCA-II vaccine was concentrated by means of a Diaflow ultrafiltration system and the concentrate mixed with aluminum phosphate. Because of the low initial concentration of rabies virus in the medium of HDCS cells, none of the five vaccines was concentrated enough to be compared directly with the two BHK vaccines. Their infectivity titers before inactivation, potency test AV's, and concentrations of complement-fixing antigen were much lower than those of the BHK vaccine. At present, however, it is possible to obtain a tenfold higher yield of virus in HDCS cultures, and following concentration of the infectious medium, vaccines have been obtained with AV's similar to those obtained with BHK vaccines.

Table 1. Properties of the Experimental Vaccines

| Vaccine | Concentration Factor | Infectivity before Inactivation PFU × Log 10 | NIH-AV | CFU/m*l* |
|---|---|---|---|---|
| SMBP | | | 0.39 | |
| BHK-FC | 40 | 8.0 | 407.0 | 1,024 |
| BHK-FCC | 200 | 9.77 | 49.0 | 512 |
| HDCS-FCa | 100 | 6.43 | 7.3 | 128 |
| HDCS-FCb | 150 | 6.42 | 8.3 | 16 |
| HDCS-FCc | 100 | 6.33 | 3.0 | 32 |
| HDCS-FCA-I | 100 | 6.43 | 1.7 | 160 |
| HDCS-FCA-II | 9 | 7.2 | 2.8 | 32 |
| MK-ZC | 150 | 8.3 | 93.2 | 640 |
| HEP-LI | 120 | 9.4 | 467.0 | 320 |
| HEP-IN | 120 | 9.4 | 81.1 | 320 |

The MK-ZC represents a vaccine produced from PM strain-infected green monkey kidney tissue cultures concentrated and purified by the zinc acetate precipitation method. This vaccine showed high infectivity titer before inactivation and high antigenicity after inactivation. The HEP vaccines were prepared from BHK tissue cultures infected with HEP-Flury strain of rabies rather than with the PM strain, as in all other vaccines. The HEP vaccines were concentrated by the zinc acetate precipitation method, and in HEP-IN, the virus was inactivated by BPL. Although the AV from the mouse potency test dropped following inactivation, these vaccines elicited antibody responses similar to those observed in vaccinated monkeys.

I shall now discuss briefly the possibility of achieving immunization against rabies with viral subunits or other products of virus synthesis instead of with intact, inactivated virion vaccines. The advantage of having a vaccine which contains the coat component of the virus, but which is free of viral nucleic acid and core proteins is obvious, since the presence of core proteins may partially suppress formation of antibodies by coat components, and the release of viral nucleic acid from inactivated vaccine and its subsequent "integration" in the cell genome, with all of its consequences, is at least theoretically possible (Sokol, 1970).

Attempts to produce RNA-free rabies virus coat protein have been successful, and it was possible to identify four protein component (Sokol *et al.*, 1970). One component, the viral nucleocapsid, was isolated after disruption of the virion by sodium dodecyl sulfate and treatment with 2-mercaptoethanol. By combining velocity and equilibrium gradient centrifugation, the two coat proteins and the glycoprotein were separated from the viral RNA and from nucleocapsid proteins; these preparations were found to be both immunogenic and immunosensitive.

It is true that antibody levels induced by these preparations in animals are lower than those observed after vaccination with inactivated rabies virions, but this may be caused by the fact that the coat proteins must reaggregate in order to regain their original immunogenic capacity. This assumption is somewhat supported by results from a study on antigenicity of infectious tissue culture fluids freed from rabies virions by high-speed centrifugation or by zinc acetate precipitation. The results shown in Table 2 (Schlumberger *et al.*, 1970) indicate that it is possible to isolate immunogenic virion-free rabies antigen, which, following precipitation with zinc acetate, can be sedimented by centrifugation. If zinc-acetate precipitation is omitted in the processing of the virion-free fluid, the immunogenic capacity of the preparation is low. Aggregation of the proteinaceous material by zinc acetate probably helps to re-establish its immunogenicity.

Table 2. Protective Activity of Infective Tissue Culture Fluid Component Obtained by Fractionation with Zinc Acetate
(H. D. Schlumberger, T. J. Wiktor and H. Koprowski, *J. Immunol.*, **105**(2), 291, 1970, © The Williams & Wilkins Co., Baltimore, Md., reprinted with permission)

| Fraction | Protective Activity ($ED_{50}$) | | |
|---|---|---|---|
| | Per m*l* | Total | % recovery |
| Unconcentrated tissue culture fluid[a] | 9.5 | 5,700 | 100 |
| Sediment after zinc acetate precipitation, resuspended in EDTA solution (×133[b]) | 260 | 11,700 | 205 |
| Supernatant fluid after zinc acetate precipitation, concentrated by ultrafiltration (×6.3) | 93 | 8,930 | 157 |
| 17,100×G sediment of the virus-depleted preparation (×11) | 154 | 8,383 | 148 |
| 17,100×G supernatant fluid of the virion-depleted preparation (×6.3) | 5 | 538 | 10 |

[a] The unconcentrated tissue culture fluid contained $7\times10^7$ PFU of rabies virus/m*l*
[b] Concentration factor: for explanation see Table 1.

Had I brought my crystal ball with me to Japan, I would predict that nucleic acid and nucleocapsid protein-free material would one day be used for immunization of man against rabies. More extensive and better supported studies, however, must be conducted in order to achieve this goal. In the meantime, we have available the purified concentrated vaccines containing inactivated virions, whose potency must be evaluated in animals more akin to man than a mouse.

*Immunogenicity of tissue culture rabies vaccines in monkeys.*

For the past two years, we have participated in a cooperative project with the National Communicable Diseases Center involving vaccination of rhesus monkeys with the new vaccines and challenge of the vaccinated animals with street virus (Sikes *et al.*, 1970). In the first two trials, we vaccinated monkeys before challenge, in the last trial, after challenge. The results from prechallenge immunization clearly indicated that the monkeys were better protected against challenge by immunization with any one of the tissue culture virion vaccines listed in Table 1 than they were by the control NIH reference vaccine, by duck embryo vaccine or by suckling brain mouse vaccine, the last two vaccines being presently used for vaccination of man in the Western Hemisphere. In general, the better immunogenicity of these vaccines for monkeys correlated with the higher antigenic values obtained in mouse potency tests; on occasion, however, marked discrepancies between the results of the two tests were observed. Immunization with tissue culture vaccine as compared to the commercially available vaccines in general elicited higher antibody levels, and the antibodies appeared in the blood earlier.

The results of postexposure treatment of monkeys with a tissue culture vaccine alone or in combination with immune serum are shown in Table 3. In the face of an 86% mortality ratio among control animals, only one animal died from the group receiving one injection of tissue culture vaccine (BHK-FCC) 6 hours after challenge. Also, simultaneous administration of either homologous or heterologous serum and vaccine yielded the same mortality ratio as that observed in the group receiving vaccine alone. Conversely, when serum administration preceded the vaccine treatment by 8

Table 3. Postexposure Evaluation of Antirabies Serum and Vaccine in Rhesus Monkeys. SN Antibody Titers and Challenge Results

| Postexposure Treatment | Mortality | |
|---|---|---|
| | Days | Ratio (%) |
| Challenge Controls | 17<br>18<br>16<br>22<br>14<br>18 | 6/7 (86%) |
| Vaccine alone on day 1 (BHK-FCC)* | 12 | 1/8 (12%) |
| Vaccine plus homologous serum on day 1 | 10 | 1/8 (12%) |
| Homologous serum alone on day 1 | 69<br>19<br>12<br>28<br>17 | 5/8 (63%) |
| Vaccine plus heterologous serum on day 1 | 11 | 1/8 (12%) |
| Heterologous serum on day 1 and vaccine on day 8 | 17<br>20<br>21 | 3/8 (37%) |
| Heterologous serum alone on day 1 | 40<br>23<br>10<br>21<br>58<br>28<br>12 | 7/8 (88%) |

* Antigenic Value (AV)=49.0

days, the mortality ratio was higher than in the preceding three groups. In contrast to the results obtained with the vaccine, results of postexposure treatment of monkeys with either heterologous or homologous antirabies serum were poor, although monkeys dying in these groups became ill after a longer incubation period than the control animals.

Levels of neutralizing antibody observed in four of the six groups treated after exposure are shown in Table 4. Animals which received treatment with vaccine alone showed no demonstrable antibodies on the third day after challenge, but antibody levels determined on succeeding days were the highest of all groups observed. Monkeys treated with immune sera had antibodies on the third day after challenge, but the level decreased rapidly in the groups receiving serum alone. Animals which received serum and vaccine simultaneously showed a rise in antibody levels on the 8th day after challenge, but the levels were lower than those observed in the groups receiving vaccine alone.

Although animals in groups with low mortality ratios generally showed higher antibody levels than those in groups with higher mortality ratios, an absolute correlation could not be established between the level of neutralizing antibody in an individual animal and protection against death. In the groups receiving either vaccine alone or serum and then vaccine, two animals which died showed higher levels of neutralizing antibody than some of their mates which were protected. Neither could the time of appearance of neutralizing antibodies in sera of animals treated after challenge with street virus be correlated with protection of the animals against challenge. Monkeys which showed no neutralizing antibodies in their sera on the 3rd day after challenge and treatment with vaccine alone fared better than animals which had passively acquired antibodies on the 3rd day after treatment with serum. Thus we must ask several fundamental questions: What is the nature of the immune mechanism which protects an animal against death from rabies? And, is the antibody detected in the neutralization test the "protective" antibody?

*Antibody response versus cell-mediated immunity*

Examination of the nature of the immune mechanism relates to another fundamental problem, that of antibody response versus cell-mediated immunity. Experiments which have thrown some light on this phenomenon involved groups of parabiotic rabbits (Wiktor & Koprowski, 1971). One partner in each group was vac-

Table 4. Postexposure Evaluation of Antirabies Serum and Vaccine in Rhesus Monkeys. SN Antibody Titers and Challenge Results

| Postexposure Treatment | Serum Quantities | | Antibody Level (Days) | | | | | Mortality | |
|---|---|---|---|---|---|---|---|---|---|
| | Recommend. (I.U.) | Actual (I.U.) | 3 | 8 | Death | 31 | 56 | Days | Ratio (%) |
| Vaccine alone on day 1 (BHK-FCC)* | | | <2 | 1750 | | 1400 | 1400 | | |
| | | | <2 | 350 | | 1400 | 1150 | | |
| | | | <2 | 95 | | 480 | 350 | | |
| | | | <2 | 350 | | 1400 | 800 | | |
| | | | <2 | 280 | | 1400 | 1150 | | |
| | | | <2 | 350 | | | | 12 | 1/8 (12%) |
| | | | <2 | 350 | | 1400 | 1150 | | |
| | | | <2 | 480 | | 1750 | 625 | | |
| Vaccine plus homologous serum on day 1 | 72 | 88 | 5 | 15 | | 95 | 45 | | |
| | 92 | 103 | 18 | 95 | 280 | | | 10 | |
| | 108 | 103 | 15 | 95 | | 70 | 70 | | 1/8 (12%) |
| | 84 | 88 | 18 | 230 | | 230 | 95 | | |
| | 88 | 88 | 11 | 33 | | 56 | 70 | | |
| | 80 | 88 | 15 | 95 | | 95 | 160 | | |
| | 80 | 88 | 33 | 95 | | 350 | 230 | | |
| | 72 | 69 | 5 | 70 | | 350 | 480 | | |
| Homologous serum alone on day 1 | 80 | 88 | 30 | 9 | | 7 | <2 | 69 | |
| | 112 | 123 | 18 | 5 | | 2 | 3 | | |
| | 84 | 88 | 13 | 9 | | | | 19 | |
| | 88 | 88 | 16 | 18 | | | | 12 | 5/8 (63%) |
| | 84 | 88 | 22 | 7 | <5 | | | 28 | |
| | 96 | 103 | 26 | 18 | | 11 | 3 | | |
| | 84 | 88 | 12 | 11 | | 3 | <2 | | |
| | 84 | 88 | 12 | 7 | | | | 17 | |
| Heterologous serum on day 1 and vaccine on day 8 | 88 | 119 | 26 | 18 | | 800 | 625 | | |
| | 104 | 139 | 32 | 15 | | 1150 | 800 | | |
| | 80 | 119 | 31 | 11 | | | | 17 | 3/8 (37%) |
| | 93 | 139 | 33 | 9 | 800 | | | 20 | |
| | 88 | 119 | 44 | 15 | | 800 | 280 | | |
| | 124 | 166 | 13 | 9 | | 95 | 70 | | |
| | 84 | 119 | 19 | 9 | 70 | | | 21 | |
| | 88 | 119 | 30 | 7 | | 1150 | 1150 | | |

* Antigenic Value (AV)=49.0

cinated against rabies and at various time intervals after vaccination, the other partner was separated, as shown in Table 5; both were then challenged with virulent virus. As shown in Table 5, the vaccinated animal always survived challenge, but the partner was

Table 5. Results of Parabiosis Experiments

| Separation of rats[a] after vaccination of one partner (days) | Mortality ratio after challenge inoculation[b] | |
|---|---|---|
| | Vaccinated animals | Nonvaccinated partners |
| 3 | 0/6 | 6/6 |
| 7 | 0/6 | 4/6 |
| 10 | 0/6 | 0/6 |
| not separated | 0/6 | 0/6 |

*a* All animals were kept in parabiosis for 7 days prior to vaccination.
*b* Fourteen days after vaccination.

resistant only if challenged while still in the parabiotic state or if separated 10 days after vaccination. Since the non-vaccinated animal is confronted with the entire immunological armament of the vaccinated animal such as immune globulins and antibody-producing cells, one may legitimately question the role of cell-mediated immunity in the protection against rabies. From these results, it is clear that animals which were separated either three or 7 days after vaccination of their partners and challenged 14 days after vaccination did not engender an immune response from cells donated by the vaccinated partner. It is easy to presume that at the time of their separation, only small amounts, if any, of circulating antibody was made available by the vaccinated partner. In contrast, those non-vaccinated animals which survived challenge after being in parabiosis for a longer period of time were probably protected by the "transfusion" of circulating antibody.

These results follow a pattern established by Parish (1970) for reaction of adult rats to immunization with *Salmonella flagellin*. He found that suppression of cell-mediated immunity in the adult animal accompanied a rise in the antibody response. On the other hand, antibody tolerance (nonresistance) was accompanied by a rise in cell-mediated immunity. If the same situation exists in immunization of an animal or human subject against rabies, how are we to evaluate the protection a man receives following vaccination since for obvious reasons, we cannot challenge him with virulent virus?

*Is the neutralizing antibody the "protective" antibody?*

We do not know enough about the nature and properties of rabies immune globulins to answer this question definitely. There are, however, preliminary data which may throw some light on this problem. As shown in Fig. 1, when $10^7$ PFU of rabies virus are mixed with a 1:200 dilution of antirabies rabbit serum incubated for 5~10 minutes, the concentration of the infectious virus drops to $10^{4.6}$ PFU. From then on, the infectivity of the mixture will stay at the same level. If, after incubation for 60 minutes, the virus-antibody mixture is treated with a 1:50 dilution of antirabbit globulin, the resulting precipitate will become noninfectious. These results seem to indicate that virus particles infectious at a concentration of $10^{4.6}$ PFU/m*l* were coated by an antibody, since they were precipitated and rendered noninfectious by an antibody against the rabies antibody. Thus, it appears that the neutralizing antibody cannot render the rabies virus completely noninfectious even though receptors of all virus particles participate in a reaction with rabies antibody.

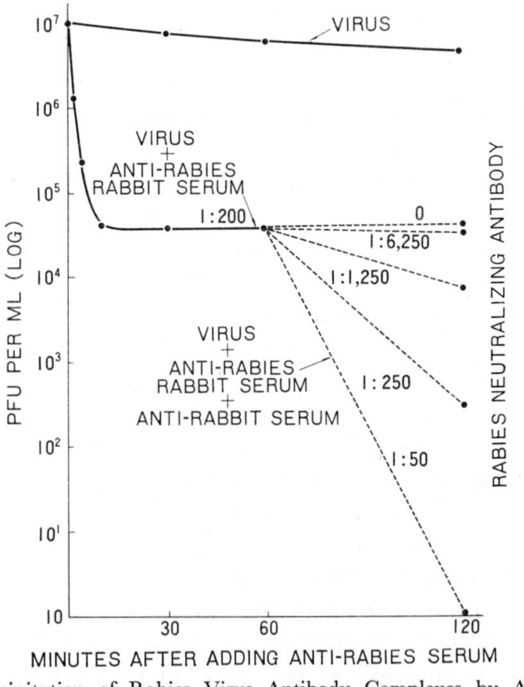


Fig. 1. Precipitation of Rabies Virus Antibody Complexes by Antirabbit Serum

The futility of looking to neutralizing antibody as a measure of protection is best shown in Table 6 which shows levels of neutralizing and "lytic" antibody in the serum of a child who lived 151 days after exposure, and died displaying a titer of 1:12,000 (Wiktor, unpublished data, 1970) of neutralizing antibody. Apparently this level of antibody is unrelated to the final outcome of the disease. The cytotoxic antibody may be the one involved in the death of this child, but it is clear that the neutralizing antibody does not affect the lethal outcome of the infection.

Table 6. Antibody Levels in a Human Case of Rabies

| | Dilution of patient's serum showing positive reaction in test | | | |
|---|---|---|---|---|
| | | | Cytotoxicity against: | |
| Days after exposure | Neutralization | Indirect immunofluo-rescence | Rabies infected Nil-2 cells | "Carrier" culture of MR-8 cells |
| 24 | 10 | 13 | 16 | 12 |
| 30 | 1,024 | 1,024 | 200 | 96 |
| 35 | 2,000 | 256 | 400 | 192 |
| 39 | 6,300 | 2,048 | 1,000 | 192 |
| 63 | N.T.[b] | 16,384 | 400 | 48 |
| 151[a] | 12,000 | 16,384 | 1,250 | 768 |

*a* Time of death
*b* Not tested

*Effect of immune serum on vaccination*

Finally, I shall turn to perhaps the most important problem of post-exposure treatment: that of the combined serum-vaccine treatment. From the results of experiments conducted in monkeys, it became clear that passively-acquired antibody may inhibit the active antibody response engendered by vaccination. Results of experiments bearing directly on this problem are shown in Figs. 2–5 (Wiktor *et al.*, 1971).

Data summarized in Fig. 2 show that the antibody response to vaccine in rabbits which received one dose of immune serum followed a day later by one injection of highly immunogenic vaccine was completely obliterated. Even when the rabbits received three injections of the vaccine rather than one, the immune serum still inhibited the antibody response (Fig. 3). When the rabbits received five injections, the degree of inhibition of the immune response was less than that after three injections, but the level of neutralizing antibody was still lower than after administration of vaccine alone.

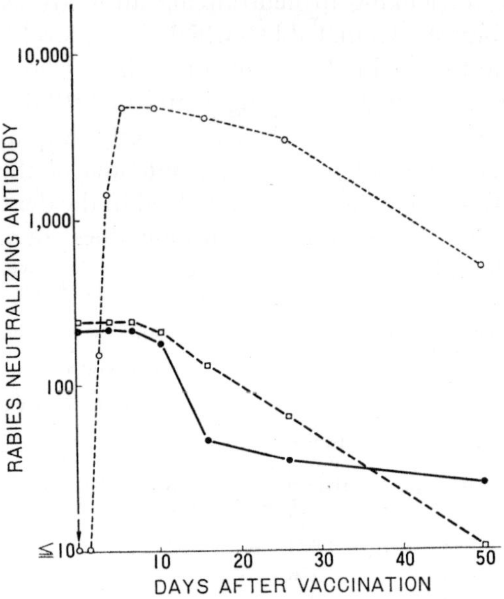


Fig. 2. ○ Vaccine one dose □ Immune serum 100 I.U./kg
● Immune serum and vaccine one dose

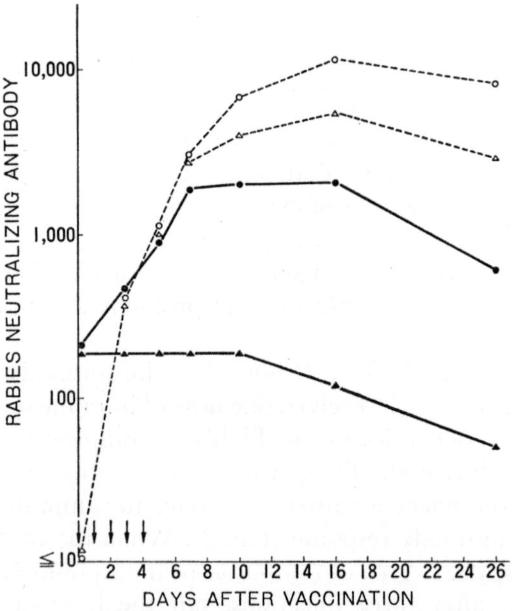


Fig. 3. △ Vaccine three doses ▲ Vaccine three doses and immune serum 50 I.U./kg
○ Vaccine five doses ● Vaccine five doses and immune serum 50 I.U./kg

In another series of experiments, rabbits received one injection of 50 I.U. of immune serum per kg of body weight followed by three injections of immunogenically potent vaccine administered starting either on the 8th day or the 15th day after serum injection. As shown in Fig. 4, serum effectively blocked antibody response to vaccine given 8 days after serum. If, however, the vaccine was given on the 15th day after the serum, then active antibody response to vaccine occurred.

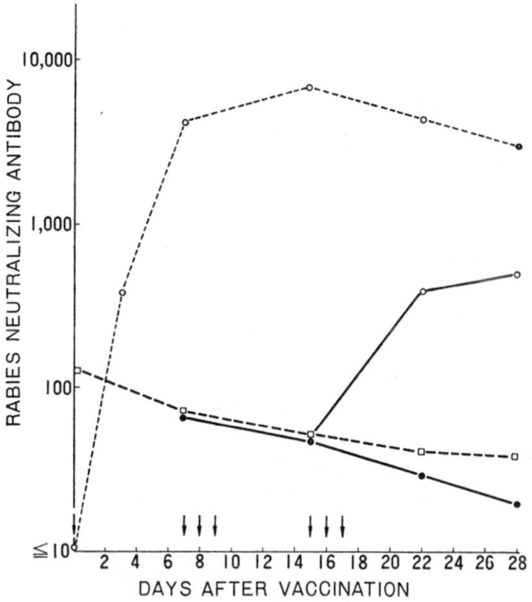


Fig. 4.
○ Vaccine three doses
● Immune serum 50 I.U./kg and three doses of vaccine starting on days 8 or 15
□ Immune serum on day 0

Since it has been claimed that administration of 19S antibody in contrast to 7S antibody does not inhibit antibody response to an antigen, rabbits received an injection of 19S fraction isolated from rabies immune globulin or an injection of immune serum containing chiefly 7S antibody simultaneously with vaccine. The results shown in Fig. 5 indicate that the two types of antibody exhibited a similar inhibitory effect against an active antibody response following vaccination.

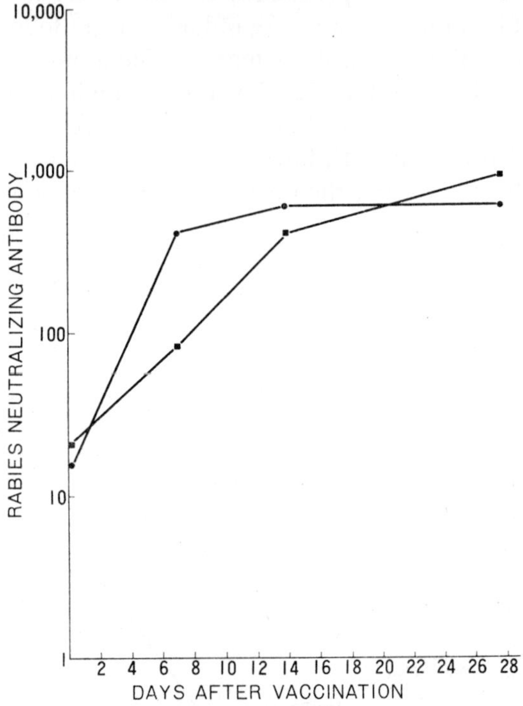


Fig. 5.
■ Vaccine and 19S antibody 5 I.U./kg
● Vaccine and immune serum 4 I.U./kg

These results confirm data obtained several years ago from trials in man (Atanasiu *et al.*, 1967). It was shown then that serum interferes with the active immune response, and as a result, a booster inoculation following the regular schedule of 14 daily injections of vaccine was recommended. At that time, we were dealing with brain tissue vaccines. What happens today when an immunogenically weak duck embryo vaccine is administered in the presence of passively-acquired antibodies is anybody's guess. Treatment failures in human subjects who received immune serum and duck embryo vaccine may be caused by the void in circulating antibody once passive immunity wanes.

Conversely, we have as yet to untangle the thorny problem of antibody which is beneficial to the exposed patient and antibody which is harmful. If lysis of cells which retain rabies-induced antigen occurs *in vivo*, then each batch of immune serum destined for human application should be examined for the presence of the cytotoxic antibody. If present, it should be absorbed from the serum before it can be used in man. Similar control of actively engendered antibodies is impossible to undertake. One has to bear in mind, however, that we cannot predict whether the presence of street virus in the body of the patient at the time when antibody-producing cells are also stimulated by intensive vaccine treatment might not lead to the formation of an antibody that not only cannot completely neutralize street virus particles, but may be of the deadly cytotoxic variety which will destroy cells of a vital part of the central nervous system. We have to admit that we do not know how to cope with this problem; only intensive research into the immunopathology of rabies may open doors to the solution of this problem.

At present caution is the password of antirabies treatment. Do not overtreat. Use the combined treatment of immune serum and vaccine sparingly and after judicious evaluation of each case. When new immunogenically-potent vaccines become available, the whole problem of post-exposure treatment will have to be re-evaluated and redesigned in the light of new facts, ideas and concepts.

## ACKNOWLEDGMENTS

This investigation was supported in part by Public Health Service Research Grant No. R01-AI 02954 from the National Institute of Allergy and Infectious Diseases; Grant No. R22-AI 07988 SSS of the United States-Japan Cooperative Medical Science Program, administered by the National Institute of Allergy and Infectious Diseases; Public Health Service Research Grant No. R01-CA 10028 from the National Cancer Institute; and funds from the World Health Organization.

## REFERENCES

Atanasiu, P., Dean, D. J., Habel, K., Kaplan, M. M., Koprowski, H., Lepine, P. and Serie, C. (1967). *Bull. Wld. Hlth. Org.*, **36**, 361.

Held, J. R. (1969). In: "Proceedings of the Annual Meeting of the Association for Research in Nervous and Mental Disease, Inc.," Vol. 49, edited by L. P. Rowland, Williams & Wilkins, Baltimore, Md., in press.

Hummeler, K. and Koprowski, H. (1969). *Nature*, **221** (5179), 418.

Koprowski, H. (1967). In: "Proceedings of First International Conference on Vaccines Against Viral and Rickettsial Diseases of Man." Pan American Health Organization, 488.

Parish, C. R. (1970). Presented at the Conference on Immunological Tolerance to Microbial Antigens, New York Academy of Sciences.

Schlumberger, H. D., Wiktor, T. J. and Koprowski, H. (1970). *J. Immunol.*, **105** (2), 291.

Sikes, R. K., Cleary, W. F., Koprowski, H., Wiktor, T. J. and Kaplan, M. M. (1970). *Bull. Wld. Hlth. Org.*, in press.

Sokol, F. (1971). Presented at Symposium on "The Future of Viral Vaccines" at the X International Congress for Microbiology, in press.

Sokol, F., Kuwert, E., Wiktor, T. J., Hummeler, K. and Koprowski, H. (1968). *J. Virol.*, **2**, 836.

Sokol, F., Stancek, D. and Koprowski, H. (1971). *J. Virol.*, **7**, 241.

Wiktor, T. J., unpublished data (1970).

Wiktor, T. J., Sokol, F., Kuwert, E. and Koprowski, H. (1969). *Proc. Soc. Exptl. Biol. Med.*, **131**, 799.

Wiktor, T. J., Lerner, R. A. and Koprowski, H. (1971). WHO Bull., in press.

For Discussion, see page 225.

# Postbite Rabies Prophylaxis in Humans with Ultraviolet Ray Inactivated Vaccine

O. Kitamoto, S. Otani, Y. Nagano* and M. Shibuki**

*The Institute of Medical Science, University of Tokyo, Tokyo*

## INTRODUCTION

At the University of Tokyo Institute of Medical Science rabies vaccination was carried out using the Pasteur vaccine up to 1949. The use of this type of vaccine often failed to prevent the onset of rabies and death. Having confirmed that the formol-inactivated vaccine was more effective in protecting mice than the phenol-inactivated vaccine, we vaccinated human subjects with a combination of the formolized and Pasteur vaccines in 1950. No deaths were recorded (Otani *et al.*, 1951).

Rabies virus inactivated by ultraviolet rays was found to be highly immunogenic (Webster & Casals, 1940). We confirmed that the immunizing capacity of the irradiated virus was superior to that of the formol-inactivated virus. We therefore decided to use the irradiated vaccine at the Institute of Medical Science beginning in 1951.

The objective of this report is to present the results of a series of animal experiments conducted with the above-mentioned vaccines and the results of postbite vaccination of humans with the irradiated vaccine.

## MATERIALS AND METHOD

*Virus:* The Denken No. 1 strain of fixed virus was used to prepare the vaccine after 50 passages in guinea pigs by intracerebral route. We removed the brain of the inoculated animal in the agonal stage and prepared a 10% emulsion with phosphate buffered saline at pH 7.2 and centrifuged it at 1,000 rpm for 10 minutes. The $LD_{50}$, as evaluated by intracerebral inoculation of mice, was $10^{-8} \times 0.025$ m*l*.

*Phenol vaccine:* We added 0.5% phenol to the virulent emulsion

* Present address: Kitasato Institute, Shirokane-5, Minatoku, Tokyo

** Present address: Takeda Pharmacy Co., Hikari, Yamaguchi, Japan

and maintained it at 37°C for 48 hours to ensure complete inactivation of the virus. The vaccine was preserved at 4–10°C.

*Formol vaccine:* We added 0.25 formaline (a solution of 37% formaldehyde) to the virus emulsion and maintained it at 1–2°C for 72 hours in order to completely inactivate the virus.

*Ultraviolet ray irradiated vaccine:* A low-pressure mercury vapor lamp was used. The virulent emulsion was delivered in petri dishes in 1 m*l* amounts (thickness of 0.17 mm) and iradiated at a distance of 10 cm for 30 seconds. The inactivation of the virus was complete.

*Test of vaccine potency:* The mice injected with the vaccines received a challenge inoculation by the intracerebral route. The number of injections, the interval between the vaccination and the challenge inoculation, and the inoculum size varied according to the objective of the experiment.

*Evaluation of the protective effect of the vaccine in humans:* Our statistics were derived from only those cases which satisfied the following conditions:

The biting animal was diagnosed as having rabies either by histological examination or by mouse inoculation.

An evident wound made by the bite without the interposition of clothing was confirmed by one of us.

The treatment was initiated before the seventh day.

The patient was observed for at least six months by one of us.

*Laboratory diagnosis of the biting dogs:* This was carried out at the Tokyo Institute of Health by means of histological examination of the brain and virus isolation. The methods of these diagnostic examinations were described by Dr. Shimada at this conference (p. 11).

## RESULTS

*Vaccination of humans with the Pasteur vaccine*

*Protective effect:* Up to 1949, the classic Pasteur vaccine was administered according to the classic regimen. However, laboratory diagnosis of biting animals and long term observation of vaccinated persons were initiated on a regular basis in 1947. Therefore, we analyzed only the results obtained during the period 1947–1949. During these three years, 6,367 persons were vaccinated, of whom 460 were found to have been clearly bitten by dogs proven to be rabid. As shown in Table 1, we had 20 deaths among the 460 cases, a mortality rate of 4.4%.

Table 1. Protective Effect of Pasteur Vaccine

| Site of bite | Period of vaccination | | | | | | | | |
|---|---|---|---|---|---|---|---|---|---|
| | 1947 | | 1948 | | 1949 | | Total | | Percentage mortality |
| | Vaccinees | Death | Vaccinees | Death | Vaccinees | Death | Vaccinees | Death | |
| Head | 16 | 2 | 16 | 4 | 33 | 1 | 65 | 7 | 10.8 |
| Upper extremities | 31 | 1 | 79 | 4 | 149 | 4 | 259 | 9 | 3.5 |
| Lower extremities | 20 | 2 | 43 | 0 | 73 | 2 | 136 | 4 | 3.0 |
| Total | 67 | 5 | 138 | 8 | 255 | 7 | 460 | 20 | 4.4 |
| Percentage mortality | 7.5 | | 5.8 | | 2.7 | | 4.4 | | 4.4 |

*Postvaccinal paralysis:* Examination for postvaccinal paralysis was carried out at three- and six-month intervals after vaccination for all vaccinees, regardless of the condition of the bite. The frequency of this complication clearly differed according to the age of the subjects. A total of 2,835 vaccinees under 14 years of age showed no incidence of paralysis. Among 3,532 subjects over 15 years of age, we confirmed 36 cases of paralysis of which 10 proved to be fatal.

## COMPARISON OF THE FORMOL AND PHENOL VACCINES FOR PROTECTIVE ACTIVITY IN ANIMALS

A virulent emulsion was divided into two parts. One part was used for preparation of the formol vaccine and the other for preparation of the phenol vaccine. With the formol vaccine, we found that three injections of the vaccine every two days gave mice a greater resistance than six daily doses and that one dose was sufficient to protect the animal against the challenge inoculation given two weeks after vaccination.

To compare the effect of the formol vaccine with that of the phenol vaccine, groups of mice received a single dose of 0.5 m*l* of the vaccine by the intraperitoneal route. At intervals varying from one to six weeks after vaccination, a virus dose of 10 $LD_{50}$ was injected intracerebrally. The animals were observed for 30 days. As indicated in Table 2, the survival rate of the treated animals with the formol vaccine tended to be higher than that of the animals which had received the phenol vaccine.

Table 2. Comparison of Protective Activity of Formol- and Phenol-Inactivated Rabies Virus

| Inactivating agent | Interval in weeks between vaccination and challenge | | | | | |
|---|---|---|---|---|---|---|
| | 1 | 2 | 3 | 4 | 5 | 6 |
| Phenol | 6/18*<br>33% | 6/13<br>46% | 9/17<br>53% | 7/14<br>50% | 2/13<br>15% | 5/13<br>38% |
| Formol | 6/17<br>35% | 13/19<br>68% | 7/15<br>47% | 6/15<br>40% | 7/15<br>47% | 12/18<br>67% |

* Survival of mice after challenge

In other series of experiments, we gave mice six daily doses of the vaccine or three doses at two-day intervals. The formol vaccine was also proven to be more protective than the phenol vaccine.

## COMPARISON OF THE ULTRAVIOLET-IRRADIATED AND FORMOL VACCINES FOR PROTECTIVE ACTIVITY IN ANIMALS

Under the conditions of our experiments, ultraviolet-irradiation for 10 seconds completely inactivated the virus. In order to ascertain the optimum dose of the ultraviolet ray, we irradiated the material under the conditions described in "materials and method" for 15, 20 or 30 seconds. Mice were injected with 6 doses of 0.25 *ml* of different dilutions of vaccine at two-day intervals by the intraperitoneal route. Two weeks after the last dose, the mice received an intracerebral challenge inoculation with varying doses of virus. The results recorded in Table 3 indicate that the immunizing capacity of the virus was not greatly affected by a 30-second irradiation. In order to ensure complete inactivation of the virus, the virulent materials were irradiated for 30 seconds in subsequent experiments.

Table 3. Protective Activity of Rabies Virus Irradiated for Varying Time

| Time of irradiation in seconds | Dilution of irradiated viral material | | | | |
|---|---|---|---|---|---|
| | 1:10 | 1:20 | 1:30 | 1:50 | 1:100 |
| 15 | | >5.7 | | 2.2 | |
| 20 | >5.7* | | >3.8 | | |
| | | >5.4 | | <1.2 | |
| | | >5.7 | | 4.6 | <2.4 |
| 30 | >5.6 | | | | |
| | >5.6 | | 4.3 | | |
| | | 4.5 | | 1.9 | |
| | | 5.1 | | 4.5 | |

* Log $LD_{50}$ of challenge virus survived

Table 4. Comparison of Protective Activity of Formol- and Ultraviolet Ray-inactivated Rabies Virus

| Inactivating agent | Dilution of inactivated viral material | | | |
|---|---|---|---|---|
| | 1:20 | 1:30 | 1:50 | |
| Formol | 2.0* | 2.7 | 1.4 | <1.4 |
| Ultraviolet rays | 3.5 | 5.1 | 3.2 | 1.3 |

* Log $LD_{50}$ of challenge virus survived

For comparison between formolized virus and irradiated virus in protecting activity, a virulent emulsion was divided into two parts and inactivated by formol and by irradiation. The vaccination and the challenge were carried out as in the preceding experiment. The results are recorded in Table 4. The rabies virus inactivated by ultraviolet rays protected animals better than the virus inactivated by formol.

## VACCINATION OF HUMANS BITTEN BY RABID ANIMALS WITH ULTRAVIOLET-INACTIVATED VACCINE

From April, 1951, bitten persons were vaccinated with the irradiated vaccine. They were given daily subcutaneous doses of 1.0 m*l* of the vaccine and daily intracutaneous doses of 0.2 m*l*. The vaccination was continued for 7 to 15 days. During the period from July 1951 to December 1954, 4,718 persons were vaccinated. The results obtained during this time have already been published, but only partially (Nagano *et al.*, 1954a, b).

*Protective effect:* The cases which satisfied all the aforementioned conditions numbered only 448 (Table 5). Of these, 26 persons had been bitten on the head, 296 on the upper extremities and 126 on the lower extremities. After six months of observation, we could find no deaths among these persons.

*Postvaccinal paralysis:* Of the 4,718 subjects vaccinated, 2,014 subjects under 14 years of age did not show postvaccinal paralysis.

Table 5. Protective Effect of Pasteur Vaccine and U.V. Irradiated Vaccine in Postbite Treatment of Human Subjects

| Vaccine | Period of vaccination | Site of bite | Vaccinees | Death | Percentage mortality |
|---|---|---|---|---|---|
| Pasteur | From April 1947 to December 1949 | Head | 65 | 7 | 10.8 |
| | | Upper extremities | 259 | 9 | 3.5 |
| | | Lower extremities | 136 | 4 | 3.0 |
| | | Total | 460 | 20 | 4.4 |
| U.V. irradiated | From July 1951 to December 1954 | Head | 26 | 0 | 0 |
| | | Upper extremities | 296 | 0 | 0 |
| | | Lower extremities | 126 | 0 | 0 |
| | | Total | 448 | 0 | 0 |

Of 2,704 subjects over 15 years of age, three showed nervous symptoms. The following is the clinical data for these cases of complications:

*Case 1:* M.W., farmer aged 30. Anamnesis: Malaria and trauma in the upper right extremity in New Guinea during the war.
Bite: Bitten on the lower left extremity. The biting dog was proven to be rabid.
Day 1: Vaccination begun.
Day 5: Marked induration at the site of the vaccination. Vaccination ceased. Malaise.
Day 8: Fever of 39°C and chills. Fever persisted for the following three days. Intense headache.
Day 11: Restlessness. Facial convulsions. Trifacial neuralgia. Lumbar movement disorder. Abdominal paresthesia. Administration of corticosteroid.
Day 45: Complete recovery.

*Case 2:* A. K., student aged 18. Anamnesis: Nothing in particular.
Bite: Bitten on the left hand. The biting dog proven to be rabid.
Day 1: Vaccination begun.
Day 11: Fever of 38–40°C. Vaccination ceased. Fever dropped. Motor paresis in the lower extremities. Analgesia in the abdomen and lower extremities. Anuria. Constipation. Administration of corticosteroid.
Day 21: The results of an examination of cerebrospinal fluid showed signs of meningitis.
Day 24: Able to walk. Spontaneous urination.
Day 32: Complete recovery.

*Case 3:* S. Y., factory worker, aged 26. Anamnesis: Nothing in particular.
Bite: Bitten through clothing on the upper right extremity by a dog proven to be rabid.
Day 1–7: Intracutaneous vaccination.
Day 50: Sight disorder in the right eye. Examination of fundus oculi showed nothing in particular.
Day 90: Sight regained.

## DISCUSSION AND CONCLUSION

We wish to repeatedly stress that for the evaluation of the protective effect of an antirabies vaccine in postbite treatment, it is absolutely necessary to consider only those cases in which the biting animal was definitely proven to be rabid. Furthermore, one must choose only those cases in which the wound is clearly confirmed by physicians and the vaccinated subjects must be observed for at least six months. The results presented in this paper were obtained with cases satisfying these conditions.

The results summarized in Table 5 strongly suggest that the protective effect of the ultraviolet-irradiated vaccine is superior to that of the Pasteur vaccine.

The Pasteur vaccine caused neuroparalytic complications in 1.0 % of persons over 15 years of age with a fatality rate of 28%.

The irradiated vaccine caused milder nervous complications in 0.1% of the subjects over 15 years of age. Among these cases, there were no deaths (Table 6).

Table 6. Neuroparalytic Complications Caused by Pasteur Vaccine and U.V. Irradiated Vaccine

| Vaccine | Age of vaccinees | | | | |
|---|---|---|---|---|---|
| | ≤14 years | | ≥15 years | | |
| | Vaccinees | Neuroparalytic complications | Vaccinees | Neuroparalytic complications | Death |
| Pasteur | 2835 | 0 | 3532 | 36 | 10 |
| U.V. irradiated | 2014 | 0 | 2704 | 3 | 0 |

## REFERENCES

Nagano, Y., Shibuki, M., Kitamoto, O. and Otani, S. (1954a). *Rev. d'Immunol.*, **18**, 339.

Nagano, Y., Shibuki, M., Kitamoto, O. and Otani, S. (1954b). *Nihon Iji Shimpo,*, No. 1559, 1038.

Otani, S., Shibuki, M. and Kato, T. (1951). *Tokyo Iji Shinsi*, **68**, 21.

Webster, L. T. and Casals, J. (1940). *Science*, **92**, 610.

For Discussion, see page 225.

## Additional Remarks

Y. NAGANO: To obtain significant statistics, the authors have chosen only people actually bitten by dogs proven to be rabid. The fatality rate was 20 out of 460 or 4.4% with the Pasteur vaccine and zero out of 448 with the U.V. vaccine. But these two vaccines were not used in the same period. The Pasteur vaccine was utilized until 1949, and the U.V. vaccine has been used since 1951. The statistics for the Pasteur vaccine were taken from 1947 to 1949. The fatality rate declined year after year during this three-year period: it was 7.5% in 1947, 5.8% in 1948, and 2.7% in 1949.

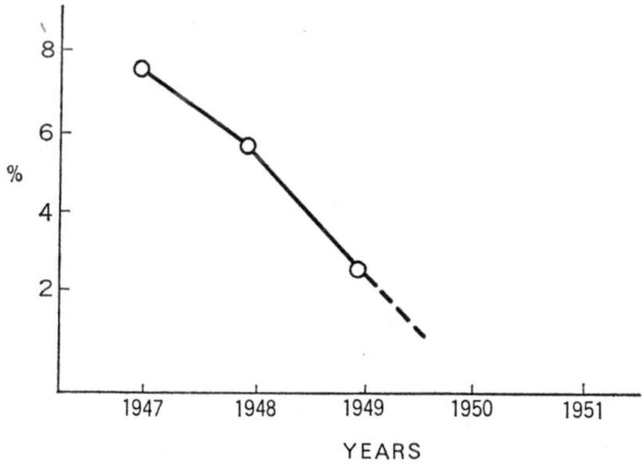


If we extend the curve in this figure, we get zero in 1951. We may have obtained a zero fatality rate by continuing to use the Pasteur vaccine. Through these three years the rabies epidemic continued, and the vaccine was prepared using the same procedure and administered on the same schedule. It is possible that there was some unknown factor which contributed to the decline in the fatality rate. Alternatively, this decline might be due simply to a fluctuation in the effect of the vaccine.

## Additional Remarks

# Efficacy of Rabies Inactivated Vaccine

YOSHITOSHI NOMURA AND JUNJI NAKAMURA

*Nippon Institute for Biological Science, Tachikawa, Tokyo*

## SUMMARY

When mice and guinea pigs were inoculated by the peripheral route with such rabies viruses as the L, M, and H of Nishigahara strain and the Fl and Fl•H of Flury strain at varying levels of passage in chick embryos, most of them acquired immunity against rabies, without showing any evidence of cerebral infection. This immunity was essentially comparable in effectiveness with that established by a single inoculation with inactivated vaccine.

Animals which responded to the intracerebral inoculation of the same viruses, manifesting clinical symptoms and allowing the virus to multiply in the brain, were proved to have acquired a stronger immunity. It was, however, difficult to distinguish this immunity either qualitatively or quantitatively from that obtained by multiple inoculations with inactivated vaccine.

## INTRODUCTION

Koprowski *et al.* (Koprowski & Cox, 1947; 1948; Koprowski & Black, 1950; Koprowski *et al.*, 1957) developed the chick embryo-adapted Flury strain of rabies virus. Following Koprowski *et al.*, (1952), immunity conferred in experimental dogs by vaccination with the low egg passage (LEP) virus of this strain lasted at least 2 years, and the survival rate against the challenge street virus given at this period was obviously greater in these animals (88%) than in control dogs (58%) which had been immunized with a phenol inactivated vaccine. When Koprowski *et al.* (1955) vaccinated experimental calves with the high egg passage (HEP) virus, the smallest dose (3 m*l*) applied produced as satisfactory antibody response and good protection against the challenge as larger doses (up to 15 m*l*). Although these findings appear to lead to the assumption that the vaccine virus might possibly be propagated in the body of inoculated animals themselves, as discussed by Koprowski *et al.* (1955) it has not yet been confirmed.

Could it be generally expected in animals receiving the live rabies virus vaccine peripherally that an immunity would be produced as a result of actual infection (growth of the virus)? If so, how does this immunity differ from that established by inoculation with inactivated rabies vaccine? To give clues to these questions, experiments were carried out with mice and guinea pigs to study aspects of infection and immunity following inoculations and comparing them with living and killed rabies viruses. This paper deals with the results obtained from these experiments.

## MATERIALS AND METHODS

Mice: Commercial mice of the dd strain produced at the Fuchu Experimental Animal Laboratory were used. Of these, 4-week-old mice were used for the experiment proper and 3-week-old mice for the titration of virus and the neutralization test.

Guinea pigs: Hartley guinea pigs 5∼6 weeks old, weighing 250∼300 g, were used. They were produced on the Funabashi Farm. Equal numbers of males and females were mixed together for each experiment.

Live viruses used for vaccination: The viruses used included the Nishigahara chick-embryo strain originated from the Nishigahara fixed-virus strain F (Pasteur fixed-virus origin), adapted by Takamatsu *et al.* (Takamatsu & Oshima, 1959; Takamatsu *et al.*, 1959) to chick embryos and including viruses at low passage level L (24∼26 passages in eggs), intermediate passage level M (158∼165 passages in eggs), and high passage level H (291∼295 passages in eggs). The Flury chick-embryo-adapted strain was supplied by courtesy of Dr. Akira Kondo of the National Institute of Health, Ministry of Health and Welfare, and included viruses at intermediate passage level Fl (126∼128 passages in eggs) and high passage level Fl•H (237∼243 passages in eggs). As viral material, the infected chick embryo body was used in the case of L, and the chick embryo brain in the case of M, H, Fl, and Fl•H.

Inactivated viruses used for vaccination: Three viruses of L, Fl•H and F were inactivated by ultraviolet ray irradiation (UV•L, UV•Fl•H and UV•F). The viral materials used were first, those that were used for live viruses in the case of L and Fl•H, and second, infected goat brain in the case of F.

Each material was made to 20% emulsion in distilled water and centrifuged. The resulting supernatant was exposed to ultraviolet rays in an apparatus of rotating ampoule system especially devised in the authors' laboratory. After irradiation, each virus was inoculated into chick embryos or mice to confirm that the infectivity of the virus had been completely inactivated.

Challenge virus: Goat brain infected with the above-mentioned highly virulent Nishigahara strain of fixed virus F (1,868~1,869 rabbit passages) was made into an emulsion in distilled water and centrifuged. The resulting supernatant was used as a challenge virus.

Titration of viruses: The titration of the F and L viruses was conducted with mice, that of the M, H, and Fl•H viruses with 7-day-old embryonated eggs, and that of the Fl virus either with mice or with 7-day-old embryonated eggs.

For the assay in mice, each material was made to tenfold dilutions with physiological saline (pH 7.6) to which 10% skim milk had been added. A group of 3 or 4 mice was inoculated intracerebrally with 0.03 m*l* of each dilution and held under observation for 2 weeks. The $LD_{50}$ was calculated from the mortality rate by Behrens's method.

The titration of viruses with 7-day-old embryonated eggs was carried out by the method already described by the authors (Nakamura *et al.*, 1959). Each material was diluted tenfold to form a broth at pH 7.6. Six to 7 eggs were inoculated with 0.2 m*l* of each dilution by the allantoic route and incubated for 6 or 7 days at 36°C in the case of the M and H viruses, or inoculated by the yolk sac route and incubated for 9 days at 36°C in the case of the Fl and Fl•H viruses. All the eggs were then opened to examine specific hemorrhagic changes appearing in the brain of the embryos and to demonstrate the presence of complement-fixation antigen in the brain. The $ID_{50}$ was calculated from the results obtained.

Serum neutralization test: Serum samples were collected from guinea pigs and frozen immediately at −20°C for storage. Before testing, they were thawed and heated at 56°C for 30 minutes. The fixed virus F was used throughout. As a diluent, 2% normal horse serum heated at 60°C for 30 minutes in distilled water was employed.

The method adopted for the neutralization test was essentially the same as the standard method of WHO (1957). Either the virus or the serum was serially diluted and three or four mice were allotted for each test mixture.

## EXPERIMENTAL DESIGN AND RESULTS

*Features of infection and immunity provoked by intracerebral or intraperitoneal inoculation of live attenuated or killed viruses in mice.*

The following experiment was carried out with L, M, H, Fl, and Fl•H live viruses and with UV•L and UV•F inactivated viruses. Four-week-old mice were divided into 2 groups of about 30 each. The virus to be tested was serially diluted by a factor of 5 or 10 and inoculated into the first group by the intracerebral route (IC) and into the second group by the intraperitoneal route (IP). After 2 weeks of observation, surviving mice in each group were divided into

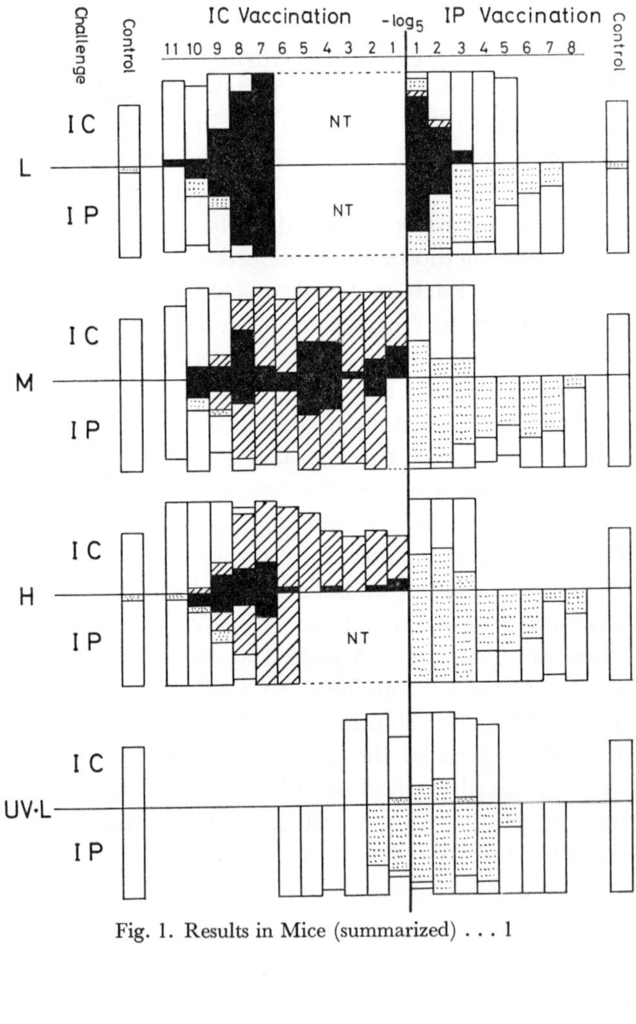


Fig. 1. Results in Mice (summarized) . . . 1

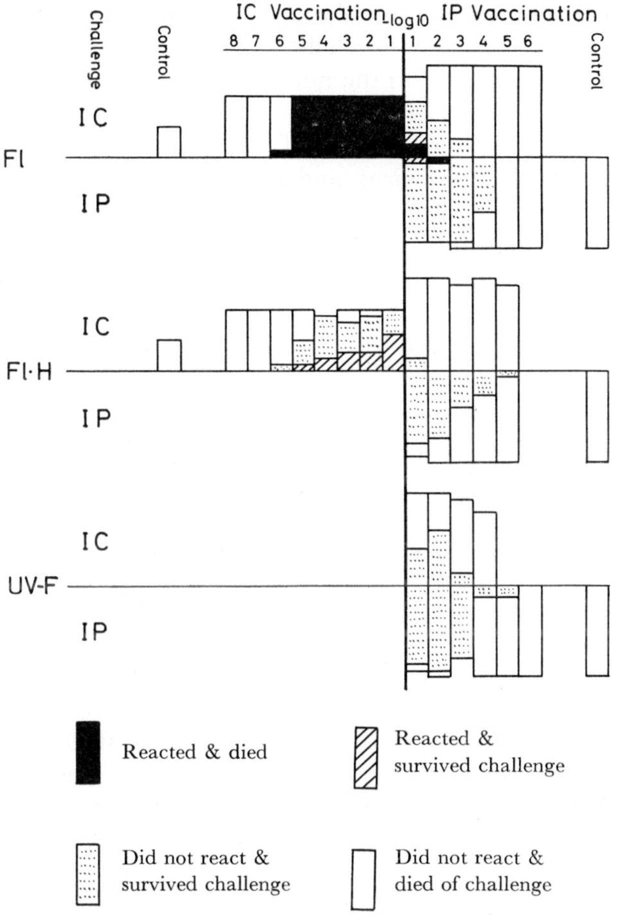


Fig. 2. Results in Mice (summarized) . . . 2

2 subgroups, one of which was then challenged with 1,000 IC-$LD_{50}$ (0.03 m*l*) of the F virus by the IC route (IC challenge) and the other with 20 IP-$LD_{50}$ (0.3 m*l*) by the IP route (IP challenge). They were further observed for 2 weeks.

In this manner, 13 experiments were carried out. The results obtained from them are summarized in Figs. 1 and 2.

In these figures, the results obtained from each of the vaccination viruses (L, M, H, UV•L, Fl, Fl•H, and UV•F) are given separately in each section. Each section presents the collective results of vaccination and challenge with symbols (solid spot, oblique line, dot, and blank spot as explained in the footnote of the figures), and is classified by the route of inoculation, the dilution ($-\log_5$ or $-\log_{10}$) of vaccine, and the route of challenge. The area occupied by each diagram is proportional to the number of mice.

The L virus was still rather strongly pathogenic for mice. When vaccinated with this virus by the IC route, mice were infected even at a high dilution of the virus, and all of them died after manifesting clinical symptoms. When inoculated by the IP route, however, only the lower dilutions induced clinical infection leading to the animals' death. Mice exempt from clinical infection died, with very few exceptions, of the IC challenge but were resistant to the IP challenge even when they had been treated previously with considerably high dilutions of the virus.

When mice were vaccinated with the M virus by the IC route, they contracted infection and presented clinical signs even with higher dilutions of the virus. Death occurred, however, irregularly and infrequently, regardless of the dilution of the virus inoculated. When the average death rate was calculated in the aggregate covering all the dilutions of the virus, it was 27% (63/234) among mice involved in clinical infection. Mice which had recovered from clinical infection withstood the IC challenge without exception. No clinical infection was observed among mice vaccinated with the M virus by the IP route. Immunity against the IC challenge was established only in a few of the mice vaccinated with lower dilutions of the virus. Immunity against the IP challenge was produced in mice, including even those vaccinated with higher dilutions of the virus. This pattern of immunity was similar to that presented by the L virus.

In the two experiments on the IC and IP vaccination, both with the M virus, attempts were made to recover the virus from the brains of some of the mice vaccinated. For this purpose 5 animals were randomly selected from each series of virus dilutions in the IC inoculation group and were sacrificed on the 10th day. Three of the 10 animals from the series of the lowest virus dilution ($5^{-1}$) in the IP inoculation group were sacrificed on the 7th, 10th and 13th days, respectively. As a result, the virus was recovered from mice inoculated intracerebrally with dilutions of virus up to $5^{-10}$. The value of $ID_{50}$ calculated from the rate of virus isolation was $5^{-8.9}$, which agreed with that calculated from the rate of clinical reaction. On the other hand, no virus was isolated from any of the IP inoculated mice tested.

The patterns of infection and immunity exhibited by the H virus were essentially similar to those exhibited by the M virus, although the death rate among IC vaccinated mice was obviously lower with the former than with the latter. Thus the mean death rate calculated through all the dilutions of the H virus inoculated was 19% (28/150) among the mice involved in clinical infection.

When the UV-inactivated L virus was applied by the IC route, one of the 11 mice receiving the lowest dilution $5^{-1}$ resisted the subsequent challenge by the IC route. The result against the IP challenge was slightly superior, but the resistant animals were found only in the first two series treated with the lower dilutions of the virus. However, when the same inactivated virus was applied by the IP route, the immunizing effect was markedly increased against both routes of challenge. Such an increase in immunizing effect in the IP vaccinated animals cannot be interpreted merely as the result of the tenfold increase in the amount of antigen. The difference in the route of inoculation also seems to have had considerable influence upon results. It may also be important to note that the immunity against the IP challenge was similar in both the group of IP vaccinations using the inactivated virus and the group using the living L virus, not only in respect to patterns but also in their quantitative aspects.

The immunizing effect of the IP vaccination with UV•F virus (tenfold serial dilutions) was remarkably stronger than that with the UV•L. It was demonstrated in this case that even a single vaccination with lower dilutions could confer immunity against the IC challenge to a reasonable proportion of the vaccinated mice.

No essential difference in the patterns of infection and immunity in mice has been found between the two chick embryo-adapted virus strains, the Flury strain and the Nishigahara strain. So far as pathogenicity is concerned, the Fl virus is located between the L and the M viruses. The IC vaccination with the Fl virus killed mice even at a considerably high dilution of virus. The IP vaccination with the same virus killed a few at the lowest dilution. The Fl•H virus was proved to be more attenuated than the H virus. It did not kill mice even when applied to them by the IC route. From summarized data the chick embryo-passage viruses used in the present study may be arranged in the following decreasing order of pathogenicity for mice: L, Fl, M, H, and Fl•H.

Although infection was readily established when a very small amount of any of these viruses had been inoculated into mice by the IC route, it varied in intensity with the pathogenicity of the respective virus. Those infected with the L or Fl virus manifested clinical symptoms and died, without exception. Those involved in infection with the M or H virus showed moderate or mild clinical symptoms, without exception, but few of them died and most of them recovered. Those infected by inoculation with the Fl•H virus either recovered after showing a slight response or took a subclinical course, presenting no fatal cases at all. The mice involved in infection, clinical or subclinical, were generally proved to have acquired strong immunity. Even those infected subclinically with the most highly attenuated Fl•H virus withstood the IC challenge.

In the case of IP inoculation, however, only such less attenuated viruses as the L and Fl could induce infection in a few of the mice inoculated, which usually resulted in death. Such viruses as the M, H, and Fl•H generally failed to induce infection when inoculated into mice by the peripheral route. The immunity produced in them was so weak that it could not withstand the IC challenge, although it withstood the IP challenge. It was of apparently the same strength as an immunity established by a single IP injection with an inactivated virus.

*Features of infection and immunity provoked by intracerebral or intraperitoneal inoculation of live attenuated or killed viruses in guinea pigs.*

An experiment was carried out with 8 groups of Hartley guinea pigs 5∼6 weeks of age. Four of the 8 groups served as live virus vaccination groups and were inoculated with the M virus by the IC route, with the Fl•H virus by the IC route, with the Fl virus by the IP route, and with the Fl•H virus by the IP route, respectively. The remaining 4 groups served as inactivated-virus vaccination groups and were injected with 1 dose of UV•Fl•H, 1 dose of UV•F, 3 doses of UV•F with intervals of 3 days, and 5 doses of UV•F with the same intervals by the IP route. The doses of virus used for inoculation are shown in Figs. 3 and 4.

In the live virus vaccination groups, some guinea pigs were sacrificed 4∼5 days after inoculation and examined to determine if the demonstrated virus in the brain confirmed the establishment of infection. The remaining guinea pigs underwent clinical examination (body temperature and nervous symptoms) twice a day for 28 days after inoculation. They were challenged with the F virus by the IC or IP route after blood samples were collected for an antibody survey. Of the inactivated-virus vaccination groups, the single-dose groups were bled and challenged by either route 21 days after injection, and the three- and five-dose groups 18 and 14 days, respectively, after the last dose had been administered. The amounts of virus used for challenge by the IC route ranged from $10^{3.2}$ to $10^{3.7}$ IC-$LD_{50}$ and for the IP route, from $10^{1.2}$ to $10^{2.1}$ IP-$LD_{50}$.

The results obtained are summarized in Figs. 3 and 4.

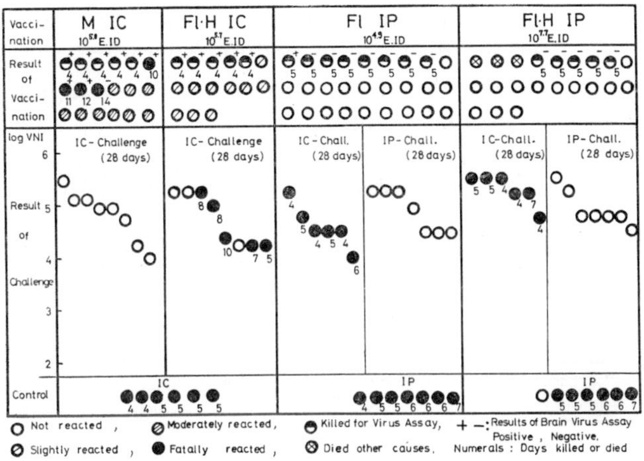


Fig. 3. Results in Guinea Pigs A: Living Virus

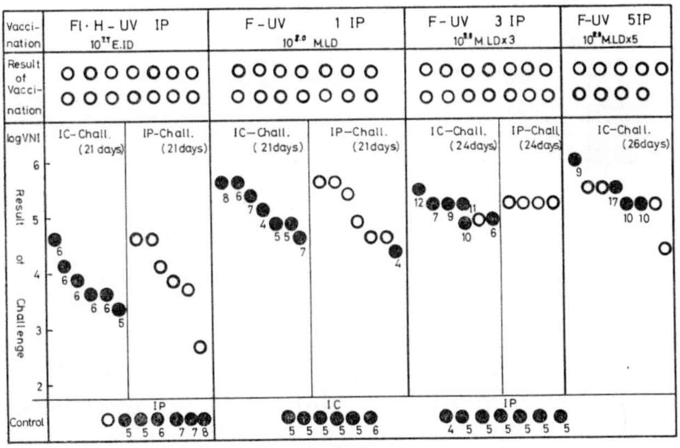


○ Not reacted, ● Fatally reacted,
Numerals: Days died

Fig. 4. Results in Guinea Pigs B: Killed Virus

The 18 guinea pigs of group 1, inoculated with the M virus by the IC route, exhibited fevers higher than 40°C and anorexia after an incubation period of 3 or 4 days, without exception. Accompanying continued fever, such clinical symptoms as staggering gait, unilateral or bilateral hind-leg paralysis, and nervous excitement (moderate) appeared successively. As nervous symptoms progressed, somewhat severe signs were presented, including unilateral or bilateral foreleg paralysis. Of the 18 animals, five were sacrificed on the 4th day for virus recovery. Clinical reactions were particularly severe in 4 (31%) of the remaining 13, showing higher body temperature (41°C), cervical paralysis, and general weakness leading to recumbency. Then, with a sudden decrease in body temperature, these animals died 7~11 days after the appearance of the first symptoms. In the other 9 animals, normal body temperature returned after a febrile stage lasting for 6~11 days, the other symptoms vanished a little later and recovery took place eventually, although growth was noticeably retarded. Figure 5 gives the clinical pictures of an animal which died after manifesting severe symptoms and another animal which recovered after presenting a milder response.

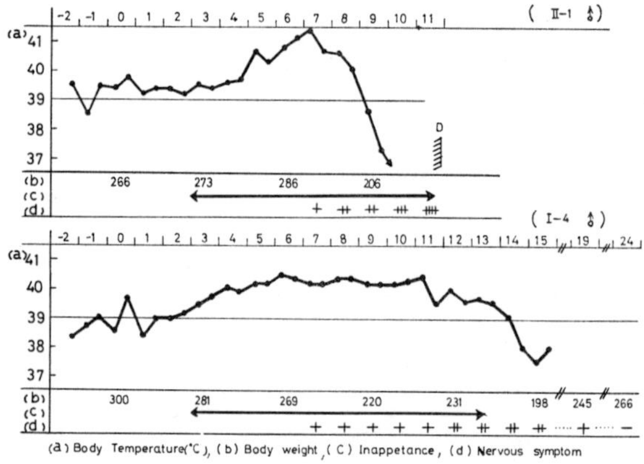


Fig. 5. Clinical Response in a Guinea Pig Inoculated Intracerebrally with M

Virus was recovered from the brain in all of the 5 sacrificed animals, and the establishment of 100% infection was thus demonstrated. Eight surviving animals were challenged with the F virus by the IC route 28 days later, but all of them withstood the challenge without showing any reaction at all.

The 15 guinea pigs of group 2, inoculated with the Fl•H virus by the IC route, exhibited a milder fever (39.5~40.0°C) than those in group 1 and anorexia. None of them presented such nervous symptoms as observed in group 1, nor did any take a fatal course. Nevertheless, virus was isolated from the brain of all 5 animals sacrificed on the 4th day of inoculation. Thus the establishment of 100% infection was also demonstrated in this group. Figure 6 gives the clinical picture of one of the guinea pigs of group 2.

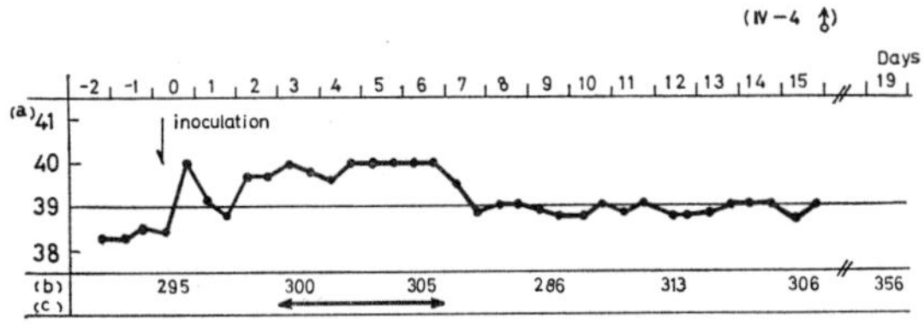


Fig. 6. Clinical Response in a Guinea Pig Inoculated Intracerebrally with Fl•H

(a) Body temperature (°C), (b) Body weight, (c) Inappetance

All the 6 untreated guinea pigs set as controls remained normal all the time during the period of the present experiment.

Although the production of neutralizing antibodies was as satisfactory in group 2 as in group 1, five of 8 animals of group 2 died when challenged by the IC route. These results suggest that the immunity produced in guinea pigs following the growth of a highly attenuated rabies virus in the brain will not always be strong enough to protect the animals from a fatal infection caused by subsequent IC challenge with a highly virulent virus.

No clinical symptoms were manifested by the guinea pigs of groups 3 and 4 inoculated with the Fl and Fl•H viruses by the IP route. Five animals were sacrificed in each of these groups 5 days after inoculation and examined for the presence of virus in the brain. The result was negative in all of them, except one animal of group 4 in which the result was equivocal since one of 7 eggs inoculated was weakly positive in complement fixation test although negative in lesions. From the results mentioned above it is highly probable that no infection of the central nervous system occurred in either of the 2 groups.

The guinea pigs of groups 3 and 4 were divided into two subgroups 28 days after virus inoculation. These were then bled and challenged with the F virus by the IC for one group and IP route for the other. The neutralizing antibody titer was at essentially the same level in these two groups as in groups 1 and 2. Nevertheless, all the animals in the subgroups of IC challenge died, while those of the subgroups of IP challenge withstood the challenge 100%.

Groups 5 and 6, which had received a single dose of the inactivated viruses of UV•Fl•H and UV•F, respectively, were each also divided into 2 subgroups and challenged by the IC and IP routes. In both groups, animals challenged by the IC route died with no exception, while survival of those challenged by the IP route was total or almost total. These features are comparable with those shown by the two groups 3 and 4 which had been treated with the living Fl and Fl•H viruses through the same IP route.

The guinea pigs of groups 7 and 8 were injected with the UV•F virus 3 and 5 times, respectively, at 3-day-intervals by the IP route. One of the 7 animals in group 7 and four of the 8 animals in group 8 withstood the IC challenge. The results obtained from group 8 were almost comparable with those from group 2 in which the cerebral infection had been induced by IC inoculation with the live Fl•H virus.

So far as the data were available, there was no noticeable relationship recognized between the neutralization titer of the serum (determined with a fixed dilution 1:3) and the establishment of immunity against the IC challenge.

*Duration of immunity acquired in guinea pigs by infection with live attenuated viruses or repeated injections with inactivated vaccine.*

Two similarly designed experiments were carried out as follows. Experimental guinea pigs were divided into 3 groups. Group 1 was inoculated with the M virus by the IC route, group 2 with the Fl•H

| Vaccination Virus, Route & Dose | Number of G.pig | | | | Result of Challenge (IC)$^{\$}$ | | | | |
|---|---|---|---|---|---|---|---|---|---|
| | Vaccinated | Virus positive / tested | Reacted (incub.) | Died (course) | 1 m | 2 m | 4 m | 6 m | 12 m |
| M-IC $10^{4.9}$ $EID_{50}$ | 12 | · | 10 (6~7d) | 5 (9~18d) | · | · | · | · | ○○○○ ○○○ |
| Fl·H-IC $10^{5.2}$ $EID_{50}$ | 41 | 10/10 | 3 (71~101d)* | 0 | ○○○○ ○○● (10) | ○○○○ ○○○ | ○○○○ ○○ | · | ○●●● ●● (4~10) |
| F·UV-5 IP $5\times10^{7.8}$ $MLD_{50}$ | 33 | · | 0 | 0 | ○○○○ ●●● (7~8) | ○○○○ ○●●● (6~8) | ○○○○ ○● (7) | ○○● (6) | ○○○○ ● (6) |
| Control | · | · | · | · | ●●●● ● (4~6) | ●●●● (6) | ●●● (6) | ●●● (6) | ●●● (5~7) |
| Challenge dose $MLD_{50}$ | · | · | · | · | $10^{2.2}$ | $10^{3.0}$ | $10^{2.5}$ | $10^{2.5}$ | $10^{3.5}$ |

* $\left(\frac{\text{Incubation • Course}}{\text{Termination}}\right)$ V (brain virus)
CF (brain CF Ag.)
ME (meningoencephalitis)

$\left(\frac{71 \cdot 1}{K}\right)$ V− CF− $\left(\frac{75 \cdot 1}{K}\right)$ V− CF− ME+ $\left(\frac{101 \cdot 5}{K}\right)$ V− CF− ME+

○, Survived; ● Died (days)

Fig. 7. Duration of Immunity in Guinea Pigs Vaccinated with Living and Killed-virus Vaccines (I)

virus by the IC route, and group 3 with the UV•F virus 5 times at 3-day-intervals by the IP route. A portion of animals in group 2 were sacrificed 4 days after inoculation for assay of the virus in the brain. To estimate the comparative duration of immunity between groups 2 and 3, surviving animals in each group were subjected to the IC challenge at varying intervals during a period of 12 months in the first experiment and 21 months in the second. All the surviving animals in group 1 were challenged at the final challenge. Some normal animals served as controls at every challenge. Figures 7 and 8 show the results obtained from the two experiments.

| Vaccination Virus Route & Dose | Number of G·pig: Vaccinated | Virus positive/tested | Reacted (incub) | Died (Course) | Result of Challenge(IC) § 15d | 1m | 3m | 9m | 15m | 21m |
|---|---|---|---|---|---|---|---|---|---|---|
| M - IC $10^{4.1}$ $EID_{50}$ | 15 | • | 15 (6~7d) | 6 (4~11d) | • | • | • | • | • | ○○●● ● (4) |
| Fl·H - IC $10^{5.1}$ $EID_{50}$ | 50 | 7/7 | 6 ※ (6~88d) | 2 (4~6d) | ○○○○ ○○ | ○○○○ ●●● (7~11) | ○○○○ ○○● (6) | ○○○○ ● (10) | ○●● (5~7) | ○○●● ●● (5~6) |
| F-UV-5IP $5\times10^{7.3}$ $MLD_{50}$ | 40 | • | 0 | 0 | ○○○○ ○●● (8~12) | ○○○○ ○○○ | ○○○○ ○○○ | ○○○○ ● (6) | ○○○○ | ●●●● ● (4~9) |
| Control | • | • | • | • | ●●● (5~6) | ●●● (5~6) | ●●● (6) | ●●● (5~7) | ●●● (5~6) | ●●● (4~5) |
| Challenge dose $MLD_{50}$ | • | • | • | • | $10^{3.0}$ | $10^{2.5}$ | $10^{2.5}$ | $10^{3.3}$ | $10^{2.5}$ | $10^{2.5}$ |

| * Incubation • Course / Termination | 6 • 4 / S | 9 • 6 / S | 11 • 2 / S | 11 • 4 / D | 88 • 6 / S | 88 • 6 / D |
|---|---|---|---|---|---|---|

§ ○, Survived; ●, Died (days)

Fig. 8. Duration of Immunity in Guinea Pigs Vaccinated with Living and Killed-virus Vaccines

Almost the same tendency was observed in both experiments. In the two groups inoculated with live viruses by the IC route, the appearance of clinical symptoms and the demonstration of virus indicated the establishment of infection at 100%, but the duration of immunity was not as long as expected. Particularly in group 2, inoculated with the Fl•H virus and involved in relatively mild infection, a portion of the animals started to succumb to the challenge a short time after inoculation, and more than 66% died of infection at the final challenge in both experiments. In group 1, inoculated with the M virus and involved in severer infection, three of the 5 animals died of infection when challenged 21 months after inoculation in the second experiment. In group 3, injected with 5 doses of inactivated vaccine by the IP route, the results after challenges conducted during the course before the final one were almost comparable with those in group 2, and the results at the final challenge were apparently better in the first experiment but worse in the second. The results noted above indicate that no essential difference exists between the persistence of an immunity developed as a result of mild cerebral infection with a highly attenuated virus, and that produced by repeated peripheral injections with an inactivated virus.

Finally, it should be mentioned that out of the many guinea pigs in group 2 which had been kept under long term observation after inoculation with the Fl•H virus, 3 in the first and 2 in the second experiments developed nervous symptoms such as paralysis of the hind quarters, torticollis and sudden general paralysis 71 to 104 days after inoculation, and were dead or sacrificed in a few days. Of the 3 animals in the first experiment, all were subjected to bacterial examinations and assays for rabiesvirus and complement-fixation antigen in the brain, and 2 were investigated histologically. All the bacterial and viral assays had negative results. However, the two animals examined histologically revealed an outstanding picture of nonpurulent encephalomyelitis. In addition to inflammatory changes, lesions were characterized by atrophy and diminution in neurons, combined with a mild reparative gliosis. No such fresh circulatory disturbance as congestion, hemorrhage or edema could be observed, suggesting the chronicity of the lesions. There were no changes suggestive of the allergic encephalomyelitis.

Among the many animals in the control group and group 3 which had been vaccinated with the inactivated virus, there was found no case at all during the long periods of observation which showed symptoms similar to those in the above-mentioned paralytic cases in group 2. Accordingly, it is possible that the paralytic cases that occurred in group 2 may have been related to the IC inoculation with the Fl•H virus given so many days before.

## DISCUSSION

On the field application of the HEP vaccine of Flury strain (Fl•H) to cattle in Brazil, Carneiro *et al.* (1955) found that the rate of immunized animals tended to be proportionate to the dose of vaccine injected. Schwab *et al.* (1954) and many other investigators (Fox *et al.*, 1957a; Atanasiu *et al.*, 1956; Atanasiu *et al.*, 1957; Fox *et al.*, 1957b; Scharpless *et al.*, 1957; Ruegsegger *et al.*, 1961; Tierker & Sikes, 1967) could not present any evidence for the growth of the same virus in the body when applied to man. All of these investigators presumed that the inoculated virus might act in cattle and man in essentially the same manner as the inactivated vaccine. Their conception seems to be supported by the following conclusions obtained from the results of the present experiments in which the egg adapted viruses of the two rabies strains at varying levels of attenuation were inoculated intraperitoneally into mice and guinea pigs. With any of these viruses, there existed little possibility of conferring immunity to those animals, primarily because the establishment of infection carried no risk of fatality. The sufficiently attenuated viruses were presumably no more infectious by this route, but induced an immunity which was difficult to differentiate from that induced by injection of the inactivated virus, either in respect to the amount of virus required for immunization or the strength of immunity that followed.

As an important warning in relation with the use of a live rabies vaccine, Potel (1958) reported the development of clinical cases with nervous symptoms among experimental dogs vaccinated with the LEP virus of Flury strain. In the present study, fatal infection not infrequently occurred among mice inoculated intraperitoneally with lower dilutions of the Fl virus that belonged to the same Flury strain as, and was at a more advanced stage of the egg passage than, the LEP virus.

The general conception that the persistence of immunity induced as a result of infection with an active virus might be much longer than that produced by the use of an inactivated vaccine was not verified with rabies virus in guinea pigs in this study. Five repeated injections with the properly prepared inactivated vaccine conferred in this animal an immunity, the persistence of which was determined by the intracerebral inoculation with the virulent fixed virus and was almost comparable with that following cerebral injection with the live Fl•H virus. The immunity was extinguished in most of the immunized animals in both groups in 21 months.

## ACKNOWLEDGMENTS

We wish to express our hearty thanks to Mr. Satoshi Hirai and Mrs. Toshiko Miura for technical assistance given to this investigation and Dr. Masanori Tajima, chief of the pathological laboratory at the Institute, for help in the histopathological examination of the guinea pigs.

## REFERENCES

Atanasiu, P., Bahmanyar, M., Baltazard, M., Fox, J. P., Habel, K., Kaplan, M. M., Kissling, R. E., Komarov, A., Koprowski, H., Leppine, P., Gallardo, F. Perez, and Schaeffer, M. (1956). Rabies neutralizing antibody response to different schedule of serum and vaccine inoculations in non-exposed persons. *Bull. Wld. Hlth. Org.*, **14**, 593–611.

Atanasiu, P., Bahmanyar, M., Baltazard, M., Fox, J. P., Habel, K., Kaplan, M. M., Kissling, R. E., Komarov, A., Koprowski, J., Leppine, P., Gallardo, F. Perez, and Schaeffer. M. (1957). Rabies neutralizing antibody response to different schedule of serum and vaccine inoculations in non-exposed persons. Part II. *Bull. Wld. Hlth. Org.*, **17**, 911–932.

Carneiro, V., Black, J. and Koprowski, H. (1955). Rabies in cattle. V. Immunization of cattle in Brazil against exposure to street virus of vampire bat origin. *J. Amer Vet. Med Assoc* , **127**, 366–369

Expert Committee on rabies (1957). Third Report. Wld. Hlth. Org. tecnh. Rep. Ser. No. 121.

Fox, J. P., Conwell, D. P. and Gerhardt, P. (1957a). Antirabies vaccination of man with HEP Flury virus. *Vet. Med.*, **52**, 81–85.

Fox, J. P., Koprowski, H., Conwell, D. P. and Gelfand, H. M. (1957b). Study of antirabies immunization of man. Observations with HEP Flury and other vaccines, with and without hyperimmune serum, in primary and recall immunizations. *Bull. Wld. Hlth. Org.*, **17**, 869–904.

Koprowski, H. and Cox, H. R. (1947). Studies on rabies infection in developing chick embryo. *J. Bact.*, **54**, 74–76.

Koprowski, H. and Cox, H. R. (1948). Studies on chick embryo adapted rabies virus. I. Culture characteristics and pathogenicity. *J. Immunol.*, **60**, 533–553.

Koprowski, H. and Black, J. (1950). Studies on chick embryo adapted rabies virus. II. Pathogenicity for dogs and use of egg-adapted strains for vaccination purpose. *ibid.*, **64**, 185–196.

Koprowski, H., Black, J. and Doris, J. N. (1957). Studies on chick-embryo-adapted rabies virus. VI. Further changes in pathogenic properties following prolonged cultivation in the developing chick embryo. *ibid.*, **72**, 94–106.

Koprowski, H. and Black, J. (1952). Studies on chick embryo adapted rabies virus. III. Duration of immunity in vaccinated dogs. *Proc. Soc. Exp. Biol. & Med.*, **80**, 410–415.

Koprowski, H., Black, J. and Johnson, W. P. (1955). Rabies in cattle. IV. Vaccination of cattle with high-egg-passage, chicken embryo-adapted rabies virus. *J. Amer. Vet. Med. Assoc.*, **127**, 363–366.

Nakamura, J., Takehara, K., Nomura, Y. and Kishi, S. (1959). Studies on the complement-fixation in rabies. WHO/Rabies/124 (Expert committee on rabies): 1–24.

Potel, K. (1958). Das histologische Verhalten des Zentralnervensystems bei Hunden nach Impfung mit einer eiadaptierten Lebendvakzine (Flury-Vakzine) gegen Tollwut. *Arch. Exp. Vet.-med.*, **12**, 612–626.

Ruegsegger, J. M., Black, J. and Scharpless, G. R. (1961). Primary antirabies immunization of man with HEP Flury virus vaccine. *Am. J. Publ. Hlth.*, **51**, 706–716.

Scharpless, G. R., Black, J. and Cox, H. R. (1957). Preliminary observations in primary antirabies immunization of man with different types of high-egg-passage Flury virus. *Bull. Wld. Hlth. Org.*, **17**, 905–910.

Schwab, M. P., Fox, J. P., Conwell, D. P. and Robinson, T. A. (1954). Avianized rabies virus vaccination in man. *Bull. Wld. Hlth. Org.*, **10**, 823–835.

Takamatsu, Y. and Oshima, Y. (1959). Studies on the production of the Nishigahara egg-strain of rabies fixed virus. I. Propagation of virus in embryonated eggs. *NIBS Bull. Biol. Res.*, **IV**, 11–21.

Takamatsu, Y., Oshima, Y. and Takehara, K. (1959). Studies on the production of the Nishigahara egg-strain of rabies fixed virus. II. Experiments on passage of virus in chick embryos. *ibid.*, **IV**, 22–68.

Tierker, E. S. and Sikes, R. K. (1967). Preexposure prophylaxis against rabies. Comparisons of regimens. *J. Am. Med. Ass.*, **201**, 911–914.

For Discussion, see page 225.

# Rabies Postvaccinal Encephalomyelitis

## Considered from Clinical, Neuropathological and Epidemiological Standpoints with Reference to Postvaccinal Nervous System Complications against Japanese Encephalitis and Smallpox

HIROTSUGU SHIRAKI

*Institute of Brain Research, Faculty of Medicine, University of Tokyo, Tokyo*

## INTRODUCTION

Although the clinical, pathological and epidemiological features of rabies postvaccinal encephalomyelitis in the Japanese have already been discussed in detail (Uchimura *et al.*, 1955; Uchimura & Shiraki, 1957; Uchimura *et al.*, 1958; Shiraki & Otani, 1959; Shiraki *et al.*, 1962; Shiraki, 1968a, 1968b) and no rabies has been encountered in Japan for more than 10 years, the key points from our studies will briefly be recalled here. There are several reasons for this:

1. Since some types of antirabies vaccines which are still being used in other parts of the world contain a certain amount of animal neural tissue, there still exists a possibility that rabies postvaccinal encephalomyelitis can occur.
2. As found in our careful follow-up survey of rabies postvaccinal encephalomyelitis on every individual inoculated, we believe that the incidence of the disease in other parts of the world may be much higher than one might expect.
3. A central nervous system type of vaccine, such as the Japanese encephalitis vaccine, still contains a small amount of neural tissue, and thus, there is a possibility that certain neuropsychiatric complications similar to those of rabies postvaccinal encephalomyelitis can occur.
4. The pathological features of rabies postvaccinal encephalomyelitis closely resemble those of acute multiple sclerosis, certain phases of chronic multiple sclerosis and allied disorders, postvaccinal encephalomyelitis for smallpox, postinfectious encephalomyelitis of certain viral origins and experimental "allergic" encephalomyeli-

tis. The former can still contribute to an understanding of the etiopathogenesis of the latter disease groups.

5. In spite of extensive studies on experimental "allergic" encephalomyelitis, definite conclusions as to an "allergic" etiopathogenesis of the latter disease groups have not yet been reached. A slow viral infection, such as measles virus infection, being the developmental mechanism of multiple sclerosis, on the other hand, has recently been suspected.

6. Both theories, however, still remain a matter of conjecture, and I therefore believe that we should return to the essential features of rabies postvaccinal encephalomyelitis and start again.

## MATERIALS

The materials with which I am dealing here comprise the following: 11 autopsy cases of rabies postvaccinal encephalomyelitis in the Japanese as well as a large series of clinical observations on the disease from 1947 to 1957 in the Tokyo area; clinical data of antirabic complications particularly in Thai children; one autopsy case of the spinal form of rabies postvaccinal encephalomyelitis in an Austrian male; autopsy cases of postvaccinal encephalomyelitis for smallpox, chicken pox encephalitis and experimental "allergic" encephalomyelitis; acute multiple sclerosis and classic type of chronic multiple sclerosis in Japanese and Caucasians; one autopsy case of demyelinating encephalitis due to repeated inoculation of desiccated neural tissue of calf in an Austrian male; physical and neuropsychiatric impairment due to vaccination against Japanese encephalitis as well as one autopsy case of postvaccinal polyneuritis against Japanese encephalitis.

## RABIES POSTVACCINAL ENCEPHALOMYELITIS AND RELATED DISORDERS

### *Clinicopathological features of spinal form of rabies postvaccinal encephalomyelitis*

The clinicopathological features of rabies postvaccinal encephalomyelitis encountered during the period from 1947 to 1957 in the Tokyo area can be classified into two main forms, i.e., spinal and cerebral.

The *spinal form* (*early form*) of the disease was characterized clinically by the initial onset of systemic reactions such as persistent fever of a spiking character during or immediately after the vaccination, a relatively rapid improvement in various involvements of the spinal cord occasionally, though fatal termination under an ascending paralysis, a rare incidence of severe sequelae, and an incubation period usually of about fifteen days (Fig. 1). This form of antirabic complications is, as a rule, observed in the European and American cases as well (Fig. 1).

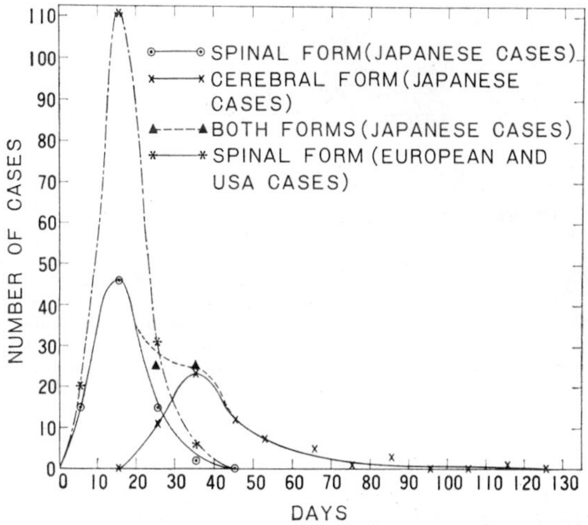


Fig. 1. Latent Period of Rabies Postvaccinal Encephalomyelitis. Latent period means the number of days from the first inoculation to the onset of the central nervous system involvements. The data from Japan consist of 141 cases, while those from Europe and USA include 168 cases reported in the references. In the former, attenuated live vaccine was used.

Autopsy examinations in the most acute cases as a rule revealed multiple, tiny perivascular demyelinated foci in a coalescence predominantly in the upper portion of the spinal cord, chiefly in its white matter and less in the grey matter, and with pronounced inflammatory cell cuffs perivascularly (Fig. 2A). A higher magnification clearly indicated a perivascular multicentricity of the foci, while a large number of the so-called epithelioid cells proliferated in both dilated perivascular space of the central venule and periadventitial demyelinated area as well (Fig. 2B). Axis cylinders within the demyelinated areas were comparatively well preserved, however (Fig. 2C). In the more protracted cases, a coalescent tendency of the perivascular foci became pronounced, while a perivascular multicentricity of the foci still remained at the edge of the coalescent lesions

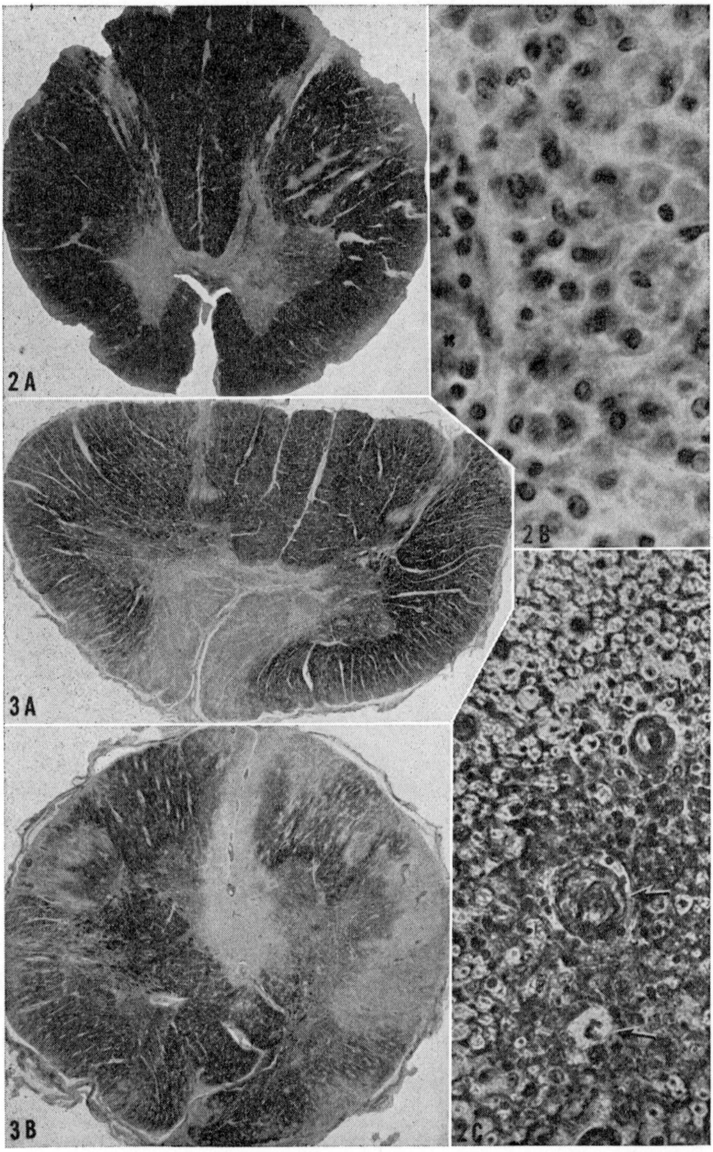


Fig. 2. Spinal Form of Rabies Postvaccinal Encephalomyelitis in the Japanese. 22-year-old female; Calmette vaccine 2cc × 10, subcutaneously; 16 days from first inoculation to death; negative rabies in dog.

A. Cervical cord. Multiple, tiny perivascular demyelinated foci are disseminated in the unilateral lateral tract, marginal areas are more or less demyelinated, and myeloarchitecture of the grey matter is bilaterally and confluentially disintegrated as well.

(Figs. 3A, B). Although the main localization of the foci was restricted mainly to the caudal-most medulla oblongata and upper cervical cord continuously involving both anterior and posterior nerve rootlets (Figs. 3A, B), a fair number of the tiny perivascular foci were widespread in the subcortical white matter of the cerebrum (Figs. 4A, D, E). In addition, the exceedingly confluent cortical lesions in which nerve cells and axis cylinders were completely preserved were widespread in the different gyri (Figs. 4A, B, C).

Autopsy cases of the spinal form of rabies postvaccinal encephalomyelitis have been reported not only in Japanese but also in Caucasians. For example, Jellinger and Seitelberger (1963) has reported a case in which the spinal cord disclosed multiple, tiny demyelinated foci of a perivascular multicentricity in a coalescence, predominantly in its white matter (Fig. 5A). Coarse spongy tissue disruption where swollened axonal structures were aggregated was an unusual feature in the present example (Figs. 5A, B, C). Questions still remain as to whether those may indicate an essential disease process, a result of acute circulatory disturbance or unknown metabolic error.

*Relationship of the spinal form of rabies postvaccinal encephalomyelitis to experimental "allergic" encephalomyelitis and postvaccinal or postinfectious encephalomyelitis*

So far, the characteristics of the foci of the spinal form of rabies postvaccinal encephalomyelitis in relation to their pathomorphology, localization and distribution patterns are essentially the same as

---

B. Highly magnified demyelinated focus in A. Mononuclear cells ("epithelioid cells") proliferate in the demyelinated parenchyma. *Crosses* indicate the lumen of the central vein.

C. Similar area to B. Two perivascular foci in a coalescence consist of a proliferation of the darkly-stained "epithelioid cells," while axis cylinders are comparatively preserved. *Arrows* indicate the two central vessels. (A; Sugamo myelin. B; H.E. C; Bielschowsky.)

Fig. 3. Spinal Form of Rabies Postvaccinal Encephalomyelitis in the Japanese. 58-year-old female; inactivated carbol vaccine 0.2cc × 3, intracutaneously into upper arm; 47 days from first inoculation to death; no information on rabies in dog.

A. Upper cervical cord. Severe demyelination is symmetrical, bilaterally restricted to the anterior tract and adjacent grey matter.

B. Caudal-most medulla oblongata. Demyelinated foci in a coalescence are particularly pronounced in the regions closely related to the subarachnoid space, posterior median fissure and central canal. An exceedingly large number of the tiny perivascular foci develop as well. (A & B; Woelcke myelin.)

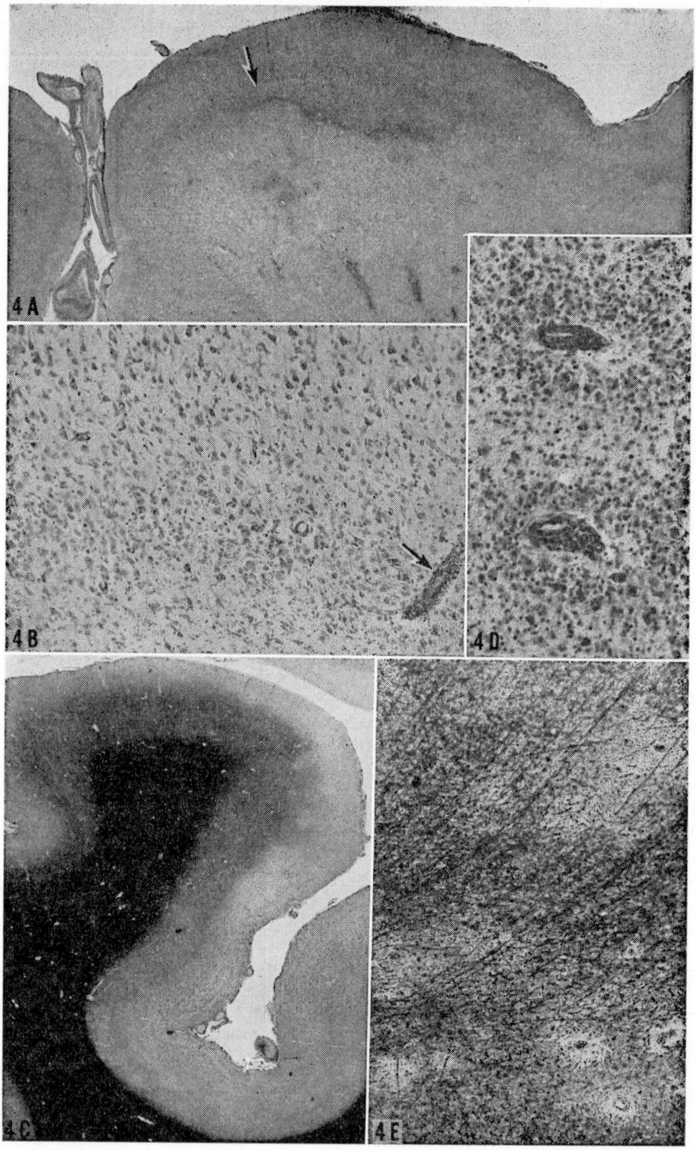


Fig. 4. Spinal Form of Rabies Postvaccinal Encephalomyelitis in the Japanese (Same case as in Fig. 3).

A. Insulotemporal gyri. Marginal cellular activity develops in the deeper cortical layers and is widespread, while leptomeningitis is visible as well. Multiple, tiny perivascular foci are pronounced in the subcortical white matter as well.

B. Magnified area indicated by *arrow* in A. Band-like cellular proliferation in

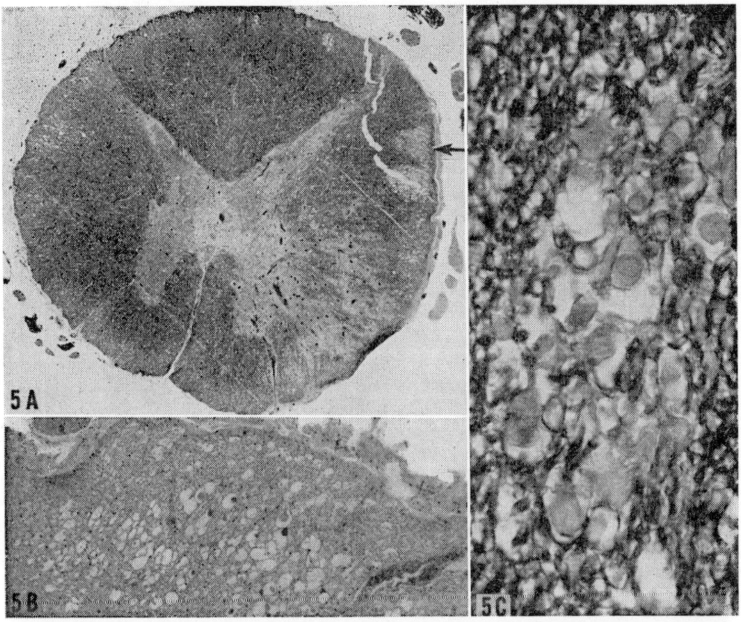


Fig. 5. Spinal Form of Rabies Postvaccinal Encephalomyelitis in a Caucasian. 50-year-old Austrian male; Hempt vaccine 6x; 26 days from first inoculation to death; no information on rabies in dog.

A. Spinal cord. Multiple, perivascular demyelinated foci in a coalescence are predominant in the unilateral lateroventral tract and grey matter. Different-sized, coarse spongy foci are disseminated at the marginal white matters.

B. Magnified area indicated by *arrow* in A. Coarse spongy tissue disruption consists of a vacuolar formation and spheroid bodies. ×70.

C. Magnified area similar to B. Faintly-stained axonal swellings aggregate and are separated from the normal myelin sheaths by an enlarged space formation. ×513. (A & C; Woelcke myelin. B; H.E.)

---

the deeper cortical layer consists of the activated astrocytes and phagocytic cells, while nerve cells within the focus are completely preserved. *Arrow* indicates the perivascular lymphocytic cell cuffs.

C. Similar area to A. Lower border of the band-like demyelination in the cortex corresponds to the marginal cellular activity in A.

D. Two tiny perivascular foci in the subcortical white matter in A highly magnified. The former consist of the central vessels infiltrated with the lymphocytes, periadventitial narrow tissue loosening and proliferated cellular marginal zone.

E. Tiny foci in A and D develop a demyelination and tend to coalesce. (A, B & D; Thionine. C & E; Woelcke myelin.)

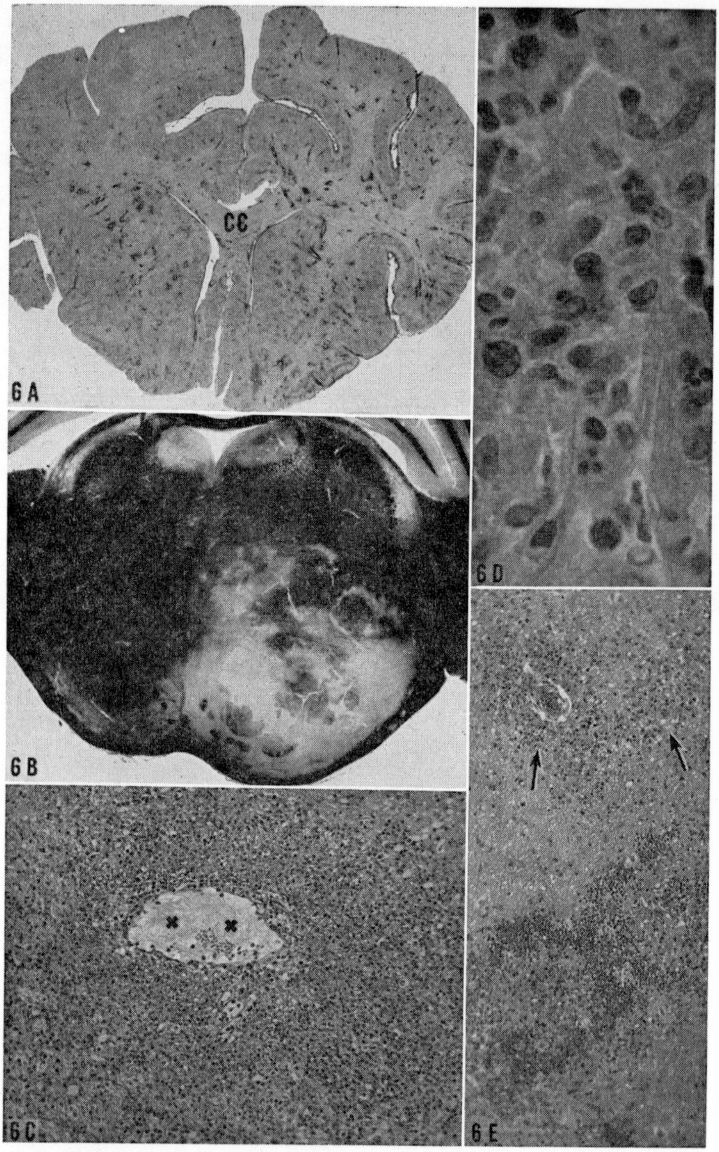


Fig. 6. Experimental "Allergic" Encephalomyelitis with Adjuvant Method.
A. (Dog; rabbit brain, 0.2cc lx, intracerebrally; 23 days' duration) Frontal-cut cerebral hemispheres through the rostral part of the corpus callosum (CC). An exceedingly large number of the tiny perivascular foci are visible not only in the white matter but also in the cortices and subcortical grey matters.
B. (Monkey; rabbit brain, 0.1cc lx, intramuscularly; 25 days' duration) Pons. An exceedingly large, confluent demyelinated focus is restricted mainly to the unilateral basis where an edematous swelling developed.

those of experimental "allergic" encephalomyelitis, postvaccinal encephalomyelitis or postinfectious encephalomyelitis of certain viral origins.

For example, in the *experimental "allergic" encephalomyelitis with Freund's adjuvant method* (Murofushi, 1958) multiple, tiny, perivascular demyelinated foci predominantly in the white matter of the cerebrum and spinal cord were essentially similar to those of the spinal form of rabies postvaccinal encephalomyelitis (Fig. 6A). Besides, a higher magnification clearly indicated that those foci consisted of the central venule and periadventitial proliferation of the "epithelioid cells" (Figs. 6C, D, E) similar to those in rabies postvaccinal encephalomyelitis mentioned above (Fig. 2B). Occasionally, those foci tended to coalesce, and developed a large confluent, demyelinated focus (Fig. 6B), while the blood-brain barrier in those foci was, as a rule, disintegrated. Consequently, erythrocytes, plasmic fluids or fibrinous materials migrated to the parenchyma which became necrotic or was edematously swollen (Figs. 6B, E).

This was the same as with the multiple perivascular demyelinated foci mainly in the cerebral white matter in *postvaccinal encephalitis against smallpox* (Figs. 7A, B) as well as the multiple, perivenous, coalescent demyelinated foci in the pontine basis in the case of *chicken pox encephalitis* (Fig. 8).

*Clinicopathological features of the cerebral form of rabies postvaccinal encephalomyelitis*

In the *cerebral form* (*delayed form*) of rabies postvaccinal encephalomyelitis, on the other hand, the onset of the illness, accompanied by general systemic reactions, occurred several weeks to a few months (about thirty-five days in a majority of the cases) after the antirabic vaccination. This form was never observed in Europeans or Americans (Fig. 1). The patients in this form remained only slightly

---

C. (Monkey; 20% rabbit spinal cord, lx, subcutaneously; 26 days' duration) Cerebral white matter. A conspicuously large number of both "epithelioid cells" and inflammatory cells migrate in the periadventitial parenchyma. *Crosses* indicate the engorged central venule. ×100.
D. (Monkey; mice brain, lx, subcutaneously; 35 days' durations) Highly magnified, focus similar to C. A. majority of the cellular elements comprise "epithelioid cells," while a smaller number of them, the polymorphonuclear leukocytes. Compare with Fig. 2B. ×900.
E. (Same case as in D) Cerebral white matter. Similar foci to C (*arrows*) are of a looser nature, while two ring hemorrhages are visible in the lower part. ×115. (A; Thionine. B; Sugamo myelin. C–E; H.E.)

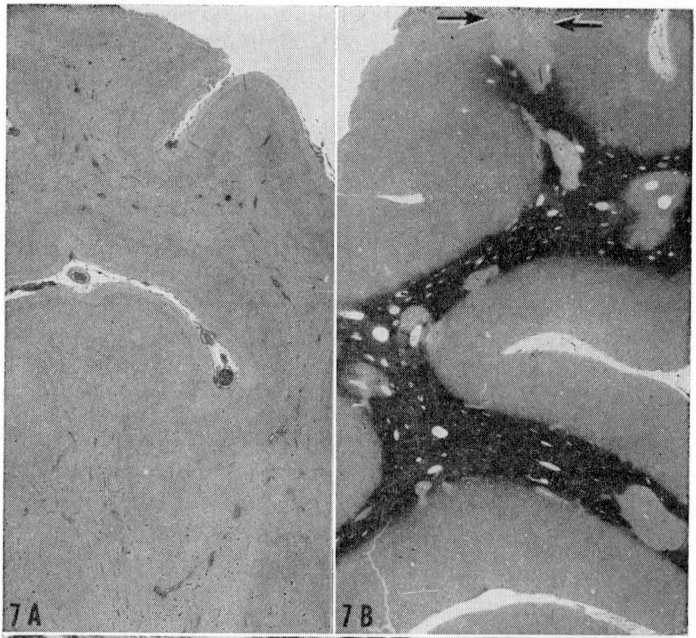


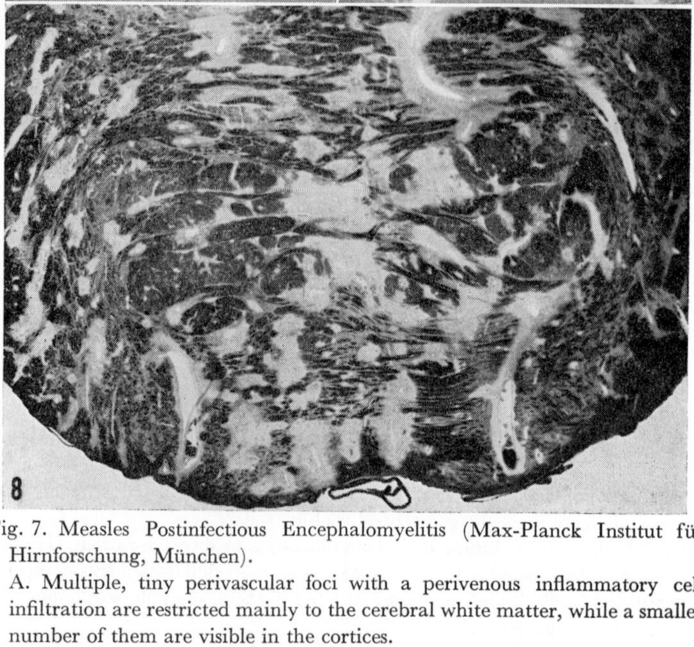


Fig. 7. Measles Postinfectious Encephalomyelitis (Max-Planck Institut für Hirnforschung, München).

A. Multiple, tiny perivascular foci with a perivenous inflammatory cell infiltration are restricted mainly to the cerebral white matter, while a smaller number of them are visible in the cortices.

B. Similar demyelinated foci in a coalescence are multiple in the cerebral white matter. *Arrows* indicate the focus continuously involving the cortical myeloarchitecture. (A; Thionine. B; Spielmeyer myelin.)

febrile (approximately 37°C) throughout the entire course, while at the acute stage, the neurological disturbances, such as impaired visual acuity, and motor and sensory disturbances as well as psychic impairments characterized by disturbed consciousness and Korsakow's syndrome, developed without exception. Pleocytosis and increased protein in the cerebrospinal fluid were, as a rule, observed. Subsequently, the above-mentioned impairments tended to show gradual improvement, representing neurasthenia-like symptoms transitionally, and finally, neuropsychiatric sequelae including personality changes not infrequently left behind.

At the comparatively acute stage, the exceedingly confluent demyelinated foci were found mainly in the white matter of both hemispheres adjacent to the lateral ventricles (Fig. 9A), while a cellular increase was particularly dominant at the edge of the demyelinated foci where perivenous inflammatory cell cuffs were disseminated (Fig. 9B). Similar demyelinated foci which became edematously swollen and developed multiple petechiae and well-preserved nerve cells occurred not infrequently in the optic chiasm, brain stem and spinal cord, representing a somewhat close spatial relationship to the cerebrospinal fluid spaces (Figs. 10A, B).

In the protracted cases, on the other hand, the lesions closely related to the lateral ventricles became confluent, were sharply demarcated, and developed a conspicuous gliosis, while a perivascular multicentricity of the foci still remained at the periphery of the confluent foci (Figs. 11A, B, 13D). In the others, a sharply-defined, confluent demyelinated focus developed in the white matter of the temporal gyri, continuously involving the basal ganglions, optic tract, hypothalamus and other areas (Figs. 12A, 13A), while an intense gliosis as well as a proliferation of the mesenchymal fibers developed not only in the demyelinated foci but also in the adjacent non-demyelinated white matter (Figs. 12B, 14). Similar demyelinated foci were sporadically seen in the optic nerve and chiasm (Fig. 13B), brain stem (Figs. 13C, 15) and spinal cord (Fig. 13D).

---

Fig. 8. Chicken Pox Postinfectious Encephalomyelitis (Max-Planck Institut für Hirnforschung, München).
Pontine basis. Irregular-shaped, different-sized demyelinated foci develop perivenously and tend to coalesce. (Spielmeyer myelin.)

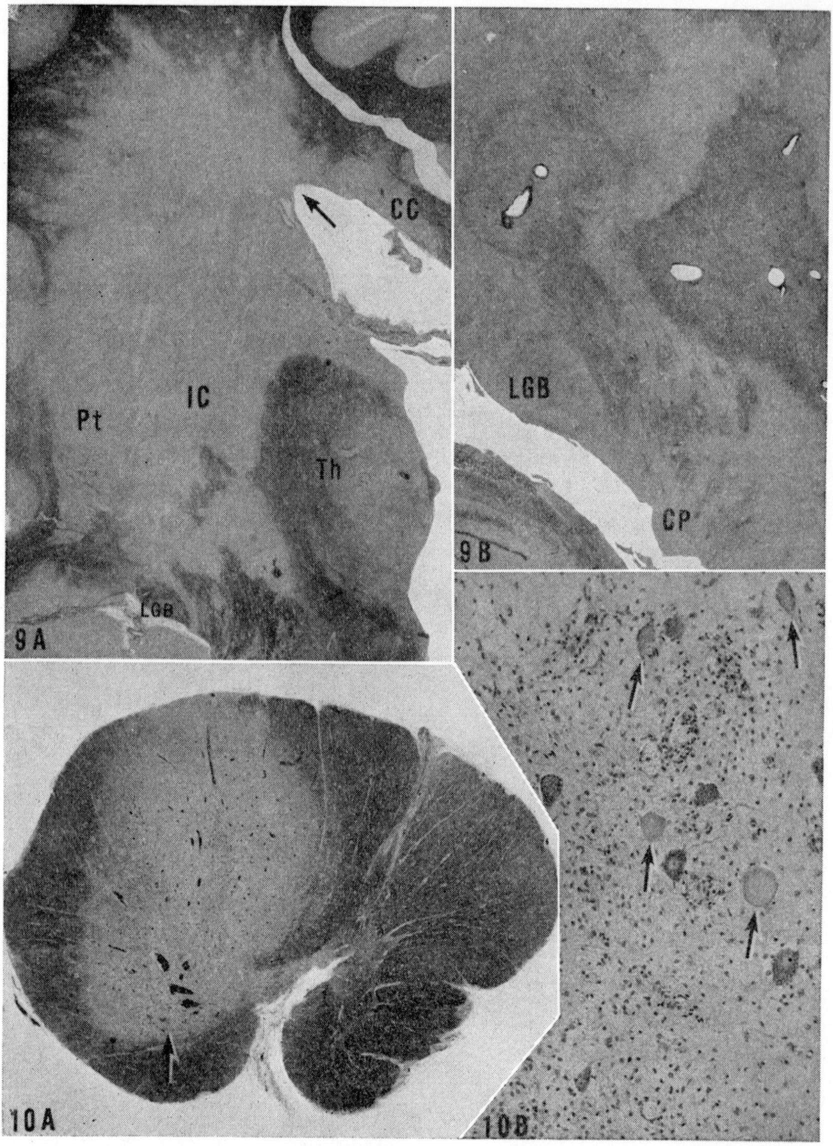


Fig. 9. Cerebral Form of Rabies Postvaccinal Encephalomyelitis in the Japanese (41-year-old male; Calmette vaccine 2cc × 17, subcutaneously; 90 days from first inoculation to death; negative rabies in dog).

A. Frontal-cut diencephalon through the lateral geniculate body (LGB). Exceedingly large, confluent demyelinated foci involve the corpus callosum (CC), centrum semiovale, internal capsule (IC), putamen (Pt), marginal area of the thalamic nuclei (Th) and other areas. Multiple, tiny demyelinated foci at the periphery of the former are of a perivascular nature. *Arrow* indicates the "Steiner's Wetterwinkel."

B. Lower magnified area in A. LGB; lateral geniculate body. CP; cerebral peduncle. Cellular activity is particularly pronounced at the edge of the confluent foci in which perivenous inflammatory cell cuffs are pronounced. (A; Woelcke myelin. B; Thionine.)

Fig. 10. Cerebral Form of Rabies Postvaccinal Encephalmyelitis in the Japanese (48-year-old female; Calmette vaccine 2cc × 18, subcutaneously; 83 days from first inoculation to death; no information on rabies in dog).

A. Cervical cord. An exceedingly large, confluent demyelinated lesion develops unilaterally involving both white and grey matter where veins are engorged and hemorrhagic foci are disseminated. The site of the lesion is edematously swollen, while multiple, tiny perivascular demyelinated foci are closely adjacent to the former.

B. Magnified demyelinated anterior horn indicated by *arrow* in A. Although gliomesenchymal cells proliferate intensely in the parenchyma, pyramidal cells are well preserved. Certain of them develop an axonal alteration, however (*arrows*). ×115. (A; Woelcke myelin. B; Thionine.)

⇨

Fig. 11. Cerebral Form of Rabies Postvaccinal Encephalomyelitis in the Japanese (27-year-old male; Calmette vaccine 2cc × 18, subcutaneously; 129 days from first inoculation to death due to a coincidental complication; no information on rabies in dog).

A. Confluent demyelinated lesion develops in the regions adjacent to the anterior horn of the lateral ventricle, such as the caudate nucleus (CN), internal capsule (IC), anterior commissure (AC), putamen (Pt) and elsewhere.

B. Frontal-cut occipital gyri through the caudal-most part of the corpus callosum (CC). Both coalescent and tiny perivascular demyelinated foci are disseminated in the white matter adjacent to the dilated posterior horn of the lateral ventricle (*crosses*) as well as in the deeper white matter. (A & B; Woelcke myelin.)

Fig. 12. Cerebral Form of Rabies Postvaccinal Encephalomyelitis in the Japanese (35 year-old, Male; Calmette vaccine 2cc × 18, subcutaneously, 168 days from first inoculation to death; negative rabies in dog).

A. An exceedingly large, confluent, sharply-defined demyelinated lesion involves the temporal white matter, myeloarchitecture of the hippocampal, fusiform and insular gyri, external capsule, claustrum, putamen (Pt), globus pallidus, optic tract (*arrow with cross*), and a part of the cerebral peduncle and internal capsule (IC). *Arrows* indicate the similar small focus in the dorsal part of the thalamic nuclei.

B. Frontal-cut hemisphere through the tuber cinereum (TC). A moderate to intense gliosis is widespread in the temporal white matter, external capsule, subcortical white matter of the insular cortex, ventral part of the globus pallidus (GP), and optic tract (*arrow*) and adjacent white matter. Gliosis is seen at the "Steiner's Wetterwinkel" as well. A slight gliosis in the temporal white matter is more widespread than demyelination. Pt; putamen. CN; caudate nucleus. (A; Woelcke myelin. B; Holzer.)

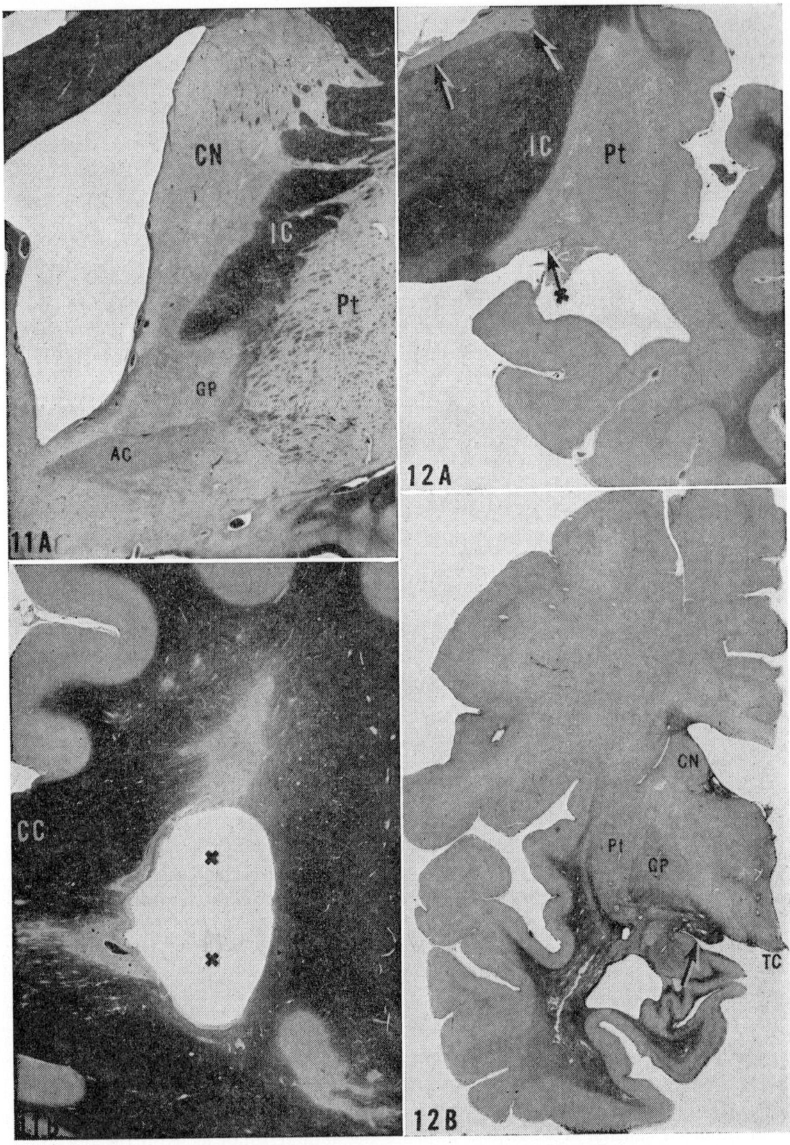
CN
IC
Pt
GP
AC
11A
12A
CC
12B
TC

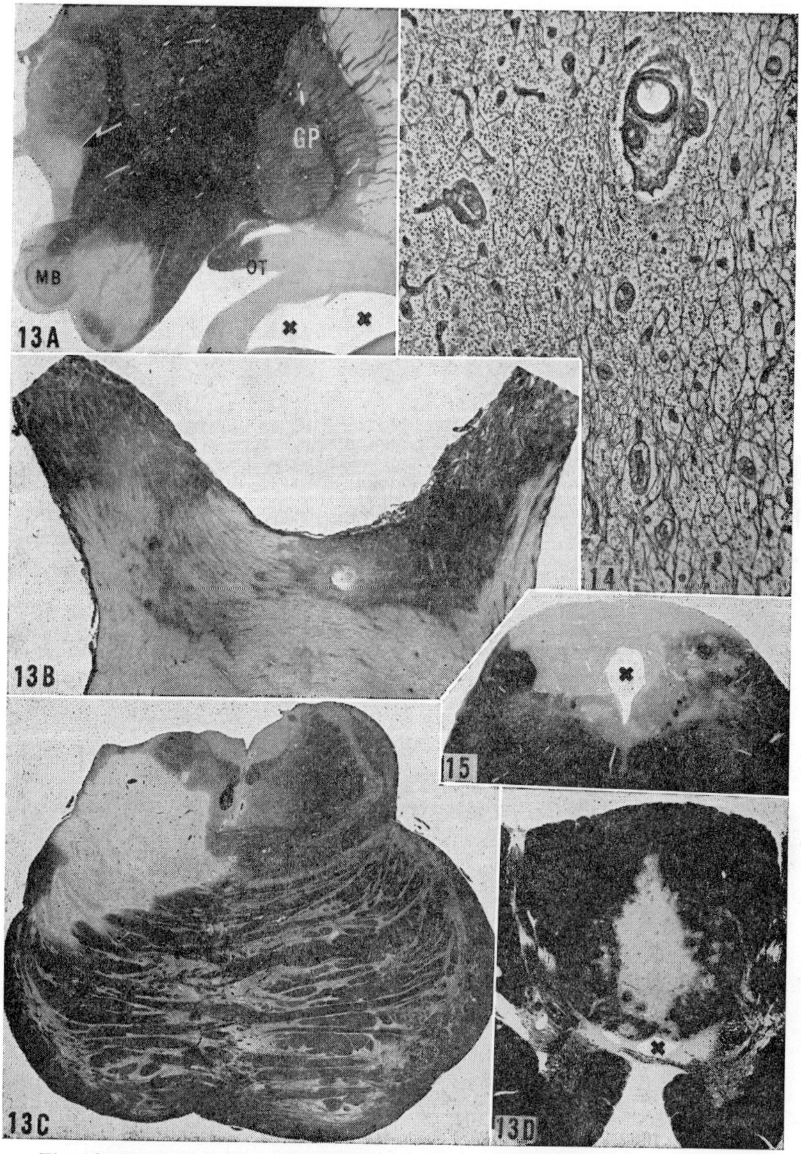


Fig. 13. Cerebral Form of Rabies Postvaccinal Encephalomyelitis in the Japanese (Same case as in Fig. 12).

A. Frontal-cut diencephalon through the mamillary body (MB). Sharply-defined, demyelinated foci are visible in the cerebral peduncle, third ventricular wall and thalmamic nuclei (*arrow*). Confluent demyelination occurs around the inferior horn of the lateral ventricle (*crosses*) continuously involving the uncus, ventral part of the lenticular nucleus and lateral part of the optic tract (OT). GP; globus pallidus.

*Relationship of cerebral form of rabies postvaccinal encephalomyelitis to acute multiple sclerosis and classic type of chronic multiple sclerosis*

As a consequence, these features of the distribution and localization of those foci in the cerebral form of rabies postvaccinal encephalomyelitis cannot be differentiated from those of *acute multiple sclerosis* (Figs. 16A, B, C; Maeda *et al.*, 1962; Fig. 17; Totsuka *et al.*, 1970) or certain phases of *classic chronic multiple sclerosis* which are frequently encountered in Caucasians (Figs. 21A, B) and have recently been encountered in Japanese as well (Figs. 18A, B; Takahata, 1970; Figs. 19A, B; Yonezawa, 1970; Figs. 20A, B, C; Matsuyama, 1970).

*Relationship of rabies postvaccinal encephalomyelitis to other demyelinating encephalomyelitides of unknown origin*

Briefly, considering the pathomorphology of both spinal and cerebral forms of rabies postvaccinal encephalomyelitis, a close connection can be established between the group of experimental "allergic" encephalomyelitis, postvaccinal or postinfectious encephalomyelitis, and the group of acute disseminated encephalomyelitis or acute multiple sclerosis as well as certain phases of chronic multiple sclerosis and allied disease groups (Fig. 22).

---

B. Optic chiasm. Severe scar formation develops confluentially in the bilateral optic nerves and chiasm, while tiny foci with an intense gliosis are disseminated in the adjacent areas as well.

C. Pons. Sharply-demarcated, confluent demyelinated focus develops unilaterally in the tegmentum and partially in the basis.

D. Cervical cord. A single confluent demyelinated lesion develops almost symmetrical bilaterally in the deeper part of the Goll's tract. Tiny perivascular foci are disseminated at the edge of the former. *Cross* indicates the central canal. (A & C; Woelcke myelin. B; Holzer. D; Sugamo myelin.)

Fig. 14. Cerebral Form of Rabies Postvaccinal Encephalomyelitis in the Japanese.

(69-year-old male; Calmette vaccine 2cc × 18, subcutaneously; 145 days from first inoculation to death; negative rabies in dog).

Demyelinated cerebral white matter. Vascular sclerosis and proliferation of the mesenchymal fibers are conspicuous. (Perdrau.)

Fig. 15. Cerebral Form of Rabies Postvaccinal Encephalomyelitis in the Japanese

(14-year-old male, Calmette vaccine 2cc × 18?, subcutaneously; 170 days from first inoculation to death; no information on rabies in dog). Midbrain. Both confluent and patchy demyelinated foci are pronounced in the areas around the Sylvian aqueduct (*cross*). (Sugamo myelin.)

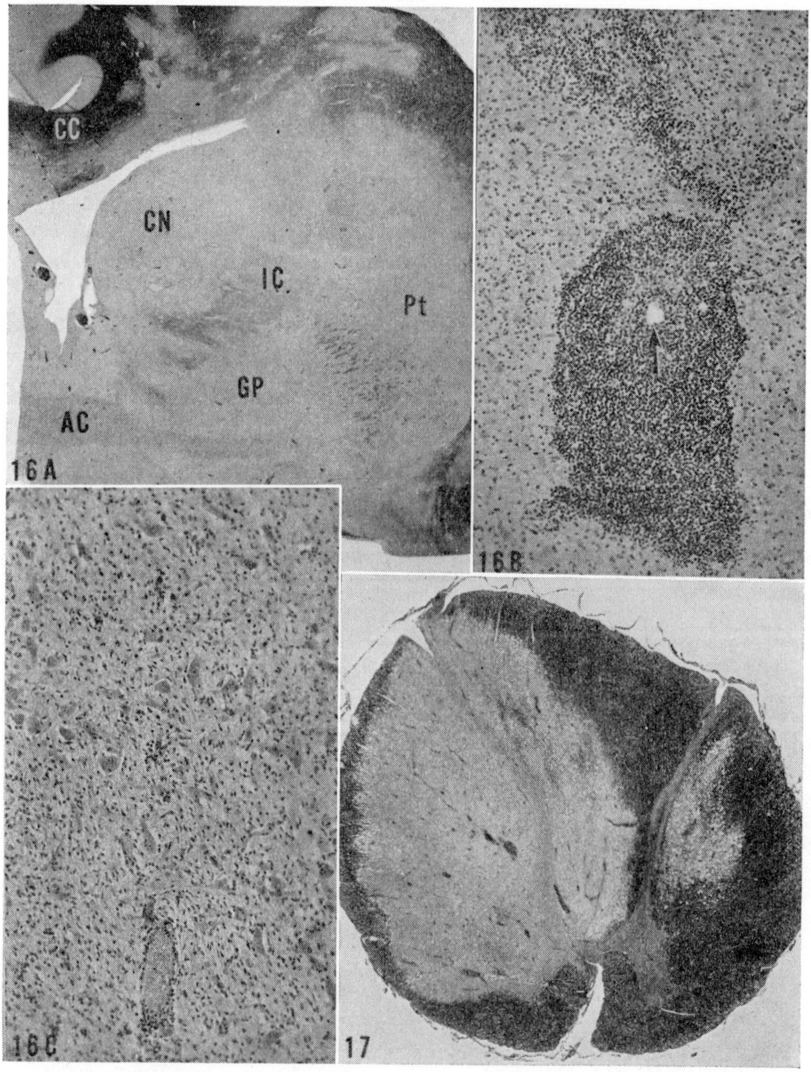
CC
CN
IC
Pt
GP
AC
16A
16B
16C
17

⇦

Fig. 16. Acute Multiple Sclerosis or Acute Demyelinating Encephalitis in the Japanese (25-year-old male; 31 days' duration; unknown cause; monophasic).

A. An exceedingly large, confluent demyelination involves the corpus callosum (CC), caudate nucleus (CN), putamen (Pt), globus pallidus (GP), internal capsule (IC) and anterior commissure (AC). Tiny perivascular foci in a coalescence are disseminated at the marginal area of the former. ×2.7.

B. Globus pallidus in A. Conspicuously dilated perivenous spaces are infiltrated with a large number of the inflammatory cells. *Arrow* indicates the lumen of the central venule. ×97.

C. Substantia innominata in the demyelinated area in A. Activated rod cells and astrocytes proliferate intensely, while nerve cells are completely preserved. ×97. (A; Woelcke myelin. B & C; Thionine.)

Fig. 17. Acute Multiple Sclerosis in the Japanese (37-year-old male; 8 days' duration; unknown cause; monophasic).

Upper thoracic cord. Two coalescent demyelinated foci with a pronounced marginal spongy tissue disruption develop in the white matter and are particularly marked on the left side, which is edematously swollen. Myeloarchitecture of the grey matter on the same side is disintegrated as well. ×8.7. (Woelcke myelin.)

⇨

Fig. 18. Classic Type of Chronic Multiple Sclerosis in the Japanese (31-year-old male; 7 years' duration with multiple relapses).

A. Frontal-cut hemispheres through the tuber cinereum (TC). Sharply-defined, completely-demyelinated foci in a coalescence are multiple in the bilateral cerebral white matters continuously involving both cortices and subcortical grey matter. "Steiner's Wetterwinkel" and septum pellucidum are bilaterally demyelinated, while anterior horn of the lateral ventricle is symmetrically bilaterally dilated. Optic tract (*arrows*) is bilaterally demyelinated and particularly pronounced in the central portion. ×1.2.

B. Demyelinated occipital white matter. Inflammatory cells infiltrate in the dilated perivenous spaces. ×87. (A; Woelcke myelin. B; H.E.)

Fig. 19. Classic Type of Chronic Multiple Sclerosis in the Japanese (22-year-old female; approximately 4 years' duration with multiple relapses).

A. Demyelinated cerebral white matter. Axis cylinders are comparatively preserved, while hypertrophic astrocytes are faintly stained. ×440.

B. Pons. Sharply-demarcated, confluent demyelinated foci in which a preexistent myeloarchitecture is still visible, develop in both tegmentum and basis, and tend to coalesce. Whole structure of the pons is completely preserved, which never occurs in an atrophic process. ×3.0. (A; Bodian. B; Woelcke myelin.)

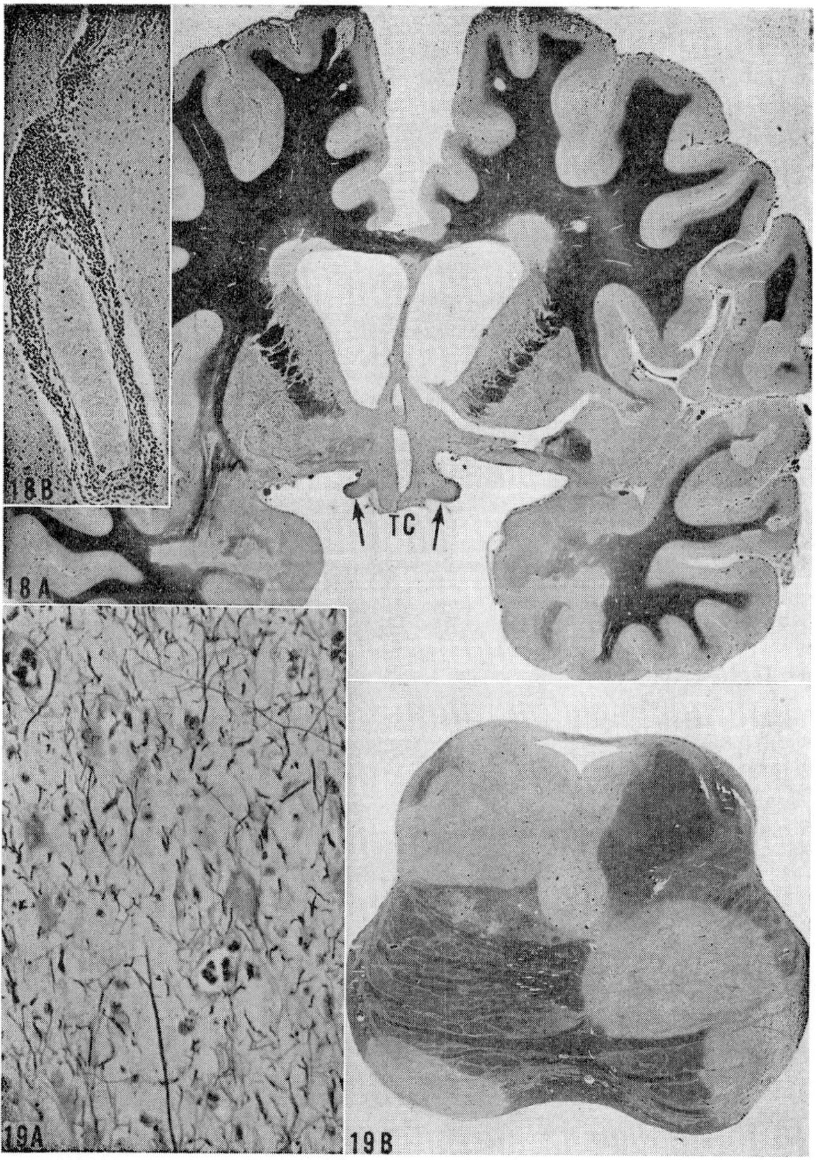
18B
TC
18A
19A
19B

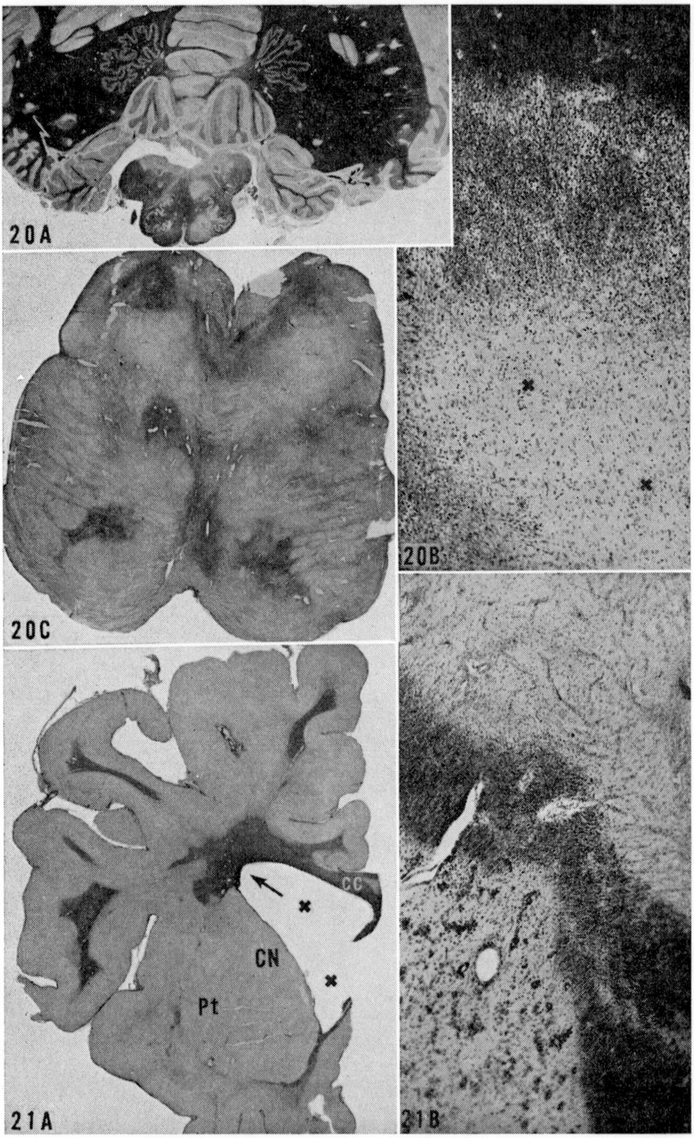


Fig. 20. Classic Type of Chronic Multiple Sclerosis in the Japanese (37-year-old female; 6 years and 7 months' duration with multiple relapses).

A. Mid-medulla oblongata and cerebellum. Sharply-defined, different-sized demyelinated foci are disseminated in the bilateral cerebellar white matters and medulla oblongata as well. ×1.2.

B. Magnified lesion of the cerebellar white matter indicated by *arrow* in A. Shadow plaque is pronounced at the margin of the completely demyelinated central portion (*crosses*). ×96.

However, the question till remains as to a firm relationship of rabies postvaccinal encephalomyelitis to chronic multiple sclerosis, because the latter, as a rule, develops a fluctuating clinical course, discloses both old and recent foci of a polyphasic character (Figs. 20C, 21A, B) or typical shadow plaques (Figs. 20A, B), while rabies postvaccinal encephalomyelitis is essentially of a monophasic character as far as demonstrated by the careful follow-up of surviving patients during the past 10 years, and develops no typical shadow plaques.

*Etiopathogenesis of rabies postvaccinal encephalomyelitis from clinical, pathological and epidemiological viewpoints*

The causative or trigger agent for the development of rabies postvaccinal encephalomyelitis, in our opinion, could not be attributed to the attenuated rabies virus in the vaccine preparations employed, nor to any virulent rabies virus, but to the spinal cord or brain substances contained in the vaccines. The reasons can be summarized as follows:

1. Cerebral damage in cases of rabies postvaccinal encephalomyelitis essentially differed from those of genuine rabies.
2. The possibility that the vaccination varied the course or characteristics of genuine rabies in humans can be ruled out insofar as antirabic complications occurred even in the absence of rabies in biting dogs.
3. Rabies postvaccinal encephalomyelitis occurred even after complete inactivation of the rabies vaccine by physicochemical means.
4. There existed a positive correlation between the incidence of the vaccine accidents and the total amount of the desiccated neural

---

C. Pons. A moderate to intense gliosis develops in the multiple plaques of both tegmentum and basis. ×3.0. (A & B; Woelcke myelin. C; Holzer.)

Fig. 21. Classic Type of Chronic Multiple Sclerosis in Caucasians.

A. (Neurological Institute, Columbia University, New York) Multiple plaques with an intense gliosis are disseminated in the cerebral white matter, while mostly pronounced at the "Steiner's Wetterwinkel" (*arrow*) and corpus callosum (CC). Anterior horn of the lateral ventricle is dilated (*crosses*). CN; caudate nucleus. Pt; putamen.

B. (Max-Planck Institut für Hirnforschung, München) Occipital white matter. Two plaques are closely adjacent. One without a mobilization of the fat granule cells in the upper part indicates an advanced nature, while another with a perivascular accumulation of the fat granule cells in the lower part, a more recent nature. (A; Holzer. B; Sudan III.)

tissues contained in the vaccines. For example, the incidence of rabies postvaccinal encephalomyelitis in the combined use of both attenuated live and inactivated vaccines containing the highest amount of the desiccated neural tissues, i.e., 100~150mg, was highest (0.88%), while that in the small amount of the inactivated vaccine containing the smallest amount of neural tissues, i.e., 5~10mg, was lowest (0.08%). However, the incidence of the disease and the amount of the desiccated neural tissues in other vaccinations ran parallel between them (Table 1).

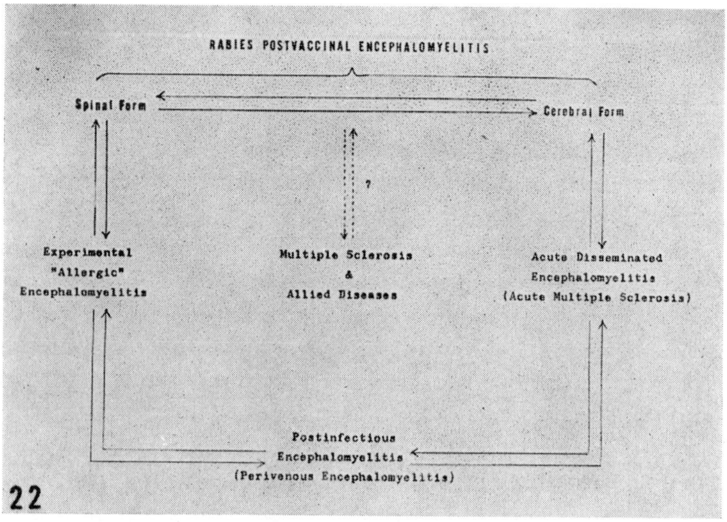


Fig. 22. Relationship of Rabies Postvaccinal Encephalomyelitis to Other Demyelinating Encephalomyelitides (See text).
The reasons for a questionable connection between rabies postvaccinal encephalomyelitis and multiple sclerosis and allied disorders are as follows: both recent and old lesions are concurrently encountered in the same CNS of multiple sclerosis and allied disorders according to a longstanding, fluctuating clinical course (Figs. 20C and 21A, B), while lesions of rabies postvaccinal encephalomyelitis are essentially of a monophasic nature; typical shadow plaques in multiple sclerosis (Figs. 20A, B) are not seen in rabies postvaccinal encephalomyelitis.

5. The lesions of experimental "allergic" encephalomyelitis by inoculation with brain "antigen" alone are practically identical to those of rabies postvaccinal encephalomyelitis.

6. Brain damages in the autopsy case reported by Jellinger *et al.*, 1958, were the same as those of rabies postvaccinal encephalomyelitis.

Table 1. Clinical Form Incidence of Rabies Postvaccinal Encephalomyelitis with the Use of Various Antirabic Vaccines in Tokyo Area and Total Amount of Desiccated Neural Tissue in Vaccines (Institute of Infectious Diseases, Tokyo University: Data from 1947–1957)

| Type of vaccine (Years) | Number of persons inoculated | Number of patients | Clinical form | | Incidence (%) | Total amount of desiccated neural tissue in vaccine (mg) |
|---|---|---|---|---|---|---|
| Attenuated live (1947–50) | 6,367 | 36 | Spinal | 17 | 0.57 | 80–120 |
| | | | Cerebral | 19 | | |
| Attenuated live & inactivated (1950–51) | 1,703 | 15 | Spinal | 9 | | |
| | | | Cerebral | 6 | 0.88 | 100–150 |
| Inactivated | | | | | | |
| Large amount (1951–57) | 970 | 3 | Spinal | 2 | 0.30 | 70–100 |
| | | | Cerebral | 1 | | |
| Small amount (1950–57) | 3,869 | 3 | Spinal | 3 | 0.08 | 5–10 |
| | | | Cerebral | 0 | | |
| Total | 12,909 (1947–57) | 57 | Spinal | 31 | 0.44 | 64–95 |
| | | | Cerebral | 26 | (0.67)* | |

* Symbol indicates the incidence of the disease among individuals above 13 years of age

A 51-year-old Austrian male who had hemiparkinsonism since his 47th year was inoculated seven times, each time with 0.02 grams of sterile, dry-frozen neural tissues of calf during one and one-half years in a therapeutic trial for Parkinsonism by a private practitioner. The inoculated material was prepared from the cerebral cortices, thalamus, hypothalamus, cerebrospinal fluid and placenta of calf. He developed no particular complications with inoculation, while temporary improvement of rigidity and tremor was observed. Twenty-two days later, following the seventh inoculation, he developed a right hemiparesis, involving slight convergent weakness of right ocular bulb, right facial palsy, right hemispasticity, left hemirigidity, right hyperreflexia and pathological reflexes, right abdominal areflexia, weakness of all limbs predominantly on the right side, tremor of the left hand, organic psychotic impairments and diffuse slow waves of EEG on left hemisphere. No abnormality of cerebrospinal fluid was observed. The above-mentioned impairments progressed subsequently and he expired of an acute circulatory disturbance. The total duration of the illness ranged ten weeks after the onset of the encephalitic syndrome.

The confluent demyelinated foci were found in the white matter closely adjacent to the ventricular walls of the left hemispheres (Fig. 23A), while a cellular marginal activity was particularly dominant at the edge of those foci where axonal structures were well-preserved, though focal swellings were more or less conspicuous, and lymphocytic perivascular cell cuffs were also visible (Figs. 23B, C). Besides, a perivascular multicentricity of the tiny foci was particularly pronounced at the edge of the confluent lesions or in isolation in the parenchyma (Figs. 23A, D).

So far, the patterns of those foci in the present example were exactly the same as those in certain cases of rabies postvaccinal encephalomyelitis or acute multiple sclerosis, thereby being attributed exclusively to the repeated inoculations with the animal brain substances.

According to the data of our survey, rabies postvaccinal encephalomyelitis in Japanese occurred in 57 among 12,909 individuals inoculated, 0.44% average (Table 1). Whereas no accidents were seen in 4,452 children below 13 years of age (Table 2), the incidence of rabies postvaccinal encephalomyelitis above 13 years of age ultimately reached 0.67%, the highest ever reported in the world (Table 1).

Meanwhile, as far as we have checked western literature, we

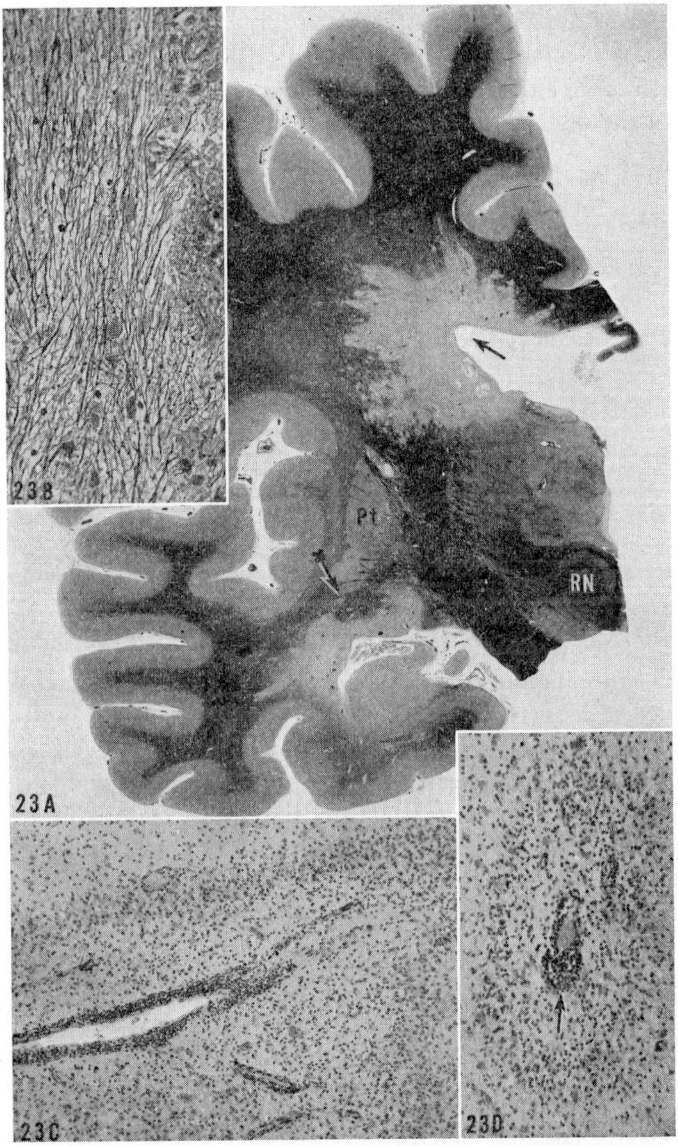


Fig. 23. Demyelinating Encephalitis Due to Repeated Inoculations of Desiccated Neural Tissue of Calf in a Caucasian (See text).

A. Frontal-cut left hemisphere through the red nucleus (RN). Two confluent, sharply-defined demyelinated lesions are visible in the white matter at the "Steiner's Wetterwinkel" (*arrow*) and a part of the dorsal thalamic nuclei as well as in the white matter and hippocampal gyri adjacent to the inferior horn of the lateral ventricle. Perivascular, tiny demyelinated foci in a coalescene are multiple at the margin of the former. Pt; putamen. ×1.7.

never came across cases of the cerebral form (delayed form) of rabies postvaccinal encephalomyelitis, except in the Japanese (Fig. 1). Results were the same in our Thailand survey, where no cerebral form of the disease was observed among Thai people.

Table 2. Age Distribution in Rabies Postvaccinal Encephalomyelitis in Japan (Institute of Infectious Diseases, Tokyo University: Data from 1947–1957)

| Age | Number of inoculated individuals | Number of patients | |
|---|---|---|---|
| | | Spinal form | Cerebral form |
| 1–12 | 4,452 | 0 | 0 |
| 13–20 | 2,351 | 6 | 5 |
| 21–30 | 2,064 | 8 | 7 |
| 31–40 | 1,506 | 9 | 6 |
| 41–50 | 1,307 | 5 | 4 |
| 51–60 | 734 | 2 | 3 |
| 61–70 | 426 | 1 | 1 |
| 71–80 | 69 | 0 | 0 |
| Total | 12,909 | 31 | 26 |

The efforts to clarify the origin of these two prominent characteristics, the highest incidence of the disease in Japanese, and existence of its cerebral form only in Japanese, analyzing possible factors such as the mode of vaccinal preparations, viral strains employed for the preparation of vaccines and mode and site of the inoculation, have failed to yield any significant reasonable solution. A question as to whether the spinal and cerebral forms of rabies postvaccinal encephalomyelitis could have a close relationship to the animal spinal cord or animal brain contained in the vaccine preparations still remained unsolved, because the spinal form of rabies postvaccinal encephalomyelitis occurred more often in cases of the brain-type vaccine from guinea pig, and vice versa (Table 3).

B. Magnified demyelinated corpus callosum in A. Axis cylinders are comparatively preserved, while spheroid bodies and hypertrophic astrocytes are disseminated. ×100.

C. Periphery of the confluent demyelinated focus in A. Marginal cellular activity consisting of the granule cells and activated astrocytes is pronounced, while perivenous inflammatory cell cuffs are disseminated within the lesion. ×86.

D. Magnified perivascular, tiny demyelinated focus indicated by *arrow with cross* in A. The former consists of the central venule infiltrated with the lymphocytes (*arrow*), periadventitial narrow tissue loosing and marginal cellular mobilization. ×100. (A; Woelcke myelin. B; Bodian. C & D; Thionine.)

Table 3. Relationship of Animal Organs Used in Manufacture of Vaccine to Clinical Form of Rabies Postvaccinal Encephalomyelitis in Japan (Institute of Infectious Diseases, Tokyo University: Data from 1947–1957)

| Type of vaccine | Organ of animal used in vaccine | Clinical form | Number of patients |
|---|---|---|---|
| Attenuated live | Rabbit spinal cord | Spinal | 17 |
| | | Cerebral | 19 |
| Ultracentrifuged and | Guinea pig brain | Spinal | 5 |
| Ultraviolet-irradiated | | Cerebral | 1 |

Thus, at present we are unable to obtain any immediate explanation for those, beyond racial differences. In this connection, the fact that among Thai children below 14 years of age severe reactions of either meningitic or of spinal form, some terminating fatally, were occasionally observed may be significant (Table 4). At any rate, no cases with severe sequelae of rabies postvaccinal encephalomyelitis in the Japanese have ever existed among the children below 13 years of age as noted above.

Table 4. Clinical Features of Antirabies Vaccinal Complications in Thai Children below Age 14 (Department of Pediatrics, Medical Faculty of Chulalongkorn University, Bangkok, 1957–1959)

| Age & Sex | Rabies in dog | Number of injections | Incubation period in days[a] | Total clinical course in days[b] | Prognosis |
|---|---|---|---|---|---|
| Meningoencephalomyelitic form | | | | | |
| 5M | ? | 14X | 18 | 23 | Expired |
| 7M | + | 14X | 13 | 21 | Incompletely recovered |
| 12M | ? | 13X | 10 | 15 | Unknown |
| Meningitic form | | | | | |
| 12M | ? | 14X | 17 | 23 | Recovered |
| 6M | — | 12X | 12 | 17 | Recovered |
| 13M | — | 14X | 4 | 10 | Recovered |
| 12F | — | 14X | 14 | 23 | Recovered |
| 13M | — | 14X | 17 | 35 | Recovered |
| 9M | — | 14X | 14 | 23 | Recovered |
| 6M | 0 | 14X | 14 | 22 | Recovered |

Note: — No information; 0 Negative; + Positive; ? Suspicious

*a* Incubation period means from first inoculation to onset of illness.

*b* Total clinical course means from onset of illness to discharge from hospital.

## NEUROPSYCHIATRIC COMPLICATIONS FOLLOWING VACCINATION AGAINST JAPANESE ENCEPHALITIS

These important data mentioned above constituted ground for the decision to use Japanese encephalitis vaccine containing a minimal amount of mouse brain or spinal cord substances, despite an intensive chemicophysical purification, (2–5$\gamma$/cc of protein N in the new type vaccine and 20$\gamma$/cc of total N in the old type vaccine), for the immunization of children or younger individuals in Japan.

A full-scale survey of postvaccinal complications took place on some forty thousand individuals within a month following prophylactic immunization against Japanese encephalitis, either with the old or new type vaccine preparations (Okinaka *et al.*, 1967). The survey failed to reveal the presence of any individuals developing clear-cut neuropsychiatric disturbances (Tables 5, 6).

In 1965 and 1967, requests were sent to major medical institutions throughout the country for reports on cases of neuropsychiatric impairments developing within a month following vaccination against Japanese encephalitis as well. The results thus obtained on such a series of thirty cases were carefully analyzed in detail from the neuropsychiatric viewpoint and could be summarized in Table 7.

Table 5. Full Survey of Physical Reactions Following Vaccination against Japanese Encephalitis in Three Prefectures of Japan, 1965 (Okinaka *et al.*, 1967)

| Subject | Number inoculated | Number of individuals with physical reactions | Percentage |
|---|---|---|---|
| New Type of Vaccine | | | |
| Elementary school | 7,313 | 105 | 1.4 |
| Middle school | 6,367 | 45 | 0.7 |
| High school | 4,721 | 26 | 0.6 |
| Nonschool children & adults | 2,995 | 104 | 3.5 |
| Total | 21,396 | 280 | 1.3 |
| Old Type of Vaccine | | | |
| Elementary school | 6,320 | 38 | 0.6 |
| Middle school | 5,129 | 93 | 1.1 |
| High school | 2,873 | 64 | 2.2 |
| Nonschool children & adults | 2,666 | 138 | 5.2 |
| Total | 16,988 | 333 | 1.9 |

Table 6. Contents of Physical Reactions Following Vaccination against Japanese Encephalitis in Three Prefectures of Japan, 1965 (Okinaka *et al.*, 1967)

| | New Type of Vaccine | | Old Type of Vaccine | |
|---|---|---|---|---|
| | School individuals | Nonschool children & adults | School individuals | Nonschool children & adults |
| Headache | 75 | 14 | 81 | 31 |
| Fatigue | 8 | 26 | 8 | 29 |
| Fever | 55 | 29 | 52 | 35 |
| Fever & fatigue | 0 | 8 | 0 | 0 |
| Headache & fatigue | 0 | 10 | 0 | 0 |
| Headache & fever | 2 | 0 | 2 | 0 |
| Fever & vomiting | 1 | 1 | 0 | 0 |
| Headache, fever & vomiting | 1 | 0 | 0 | 0 |
| Local reddish swelling | 10 | 8 | 34 | 28 |
| Abdominal pain | 3 | 0 | 0 | 1 |
| Diarrhea | 0 | 0 | 0 | 3 |
| Vomiting | 1 | 0 | 0 | 0 |
| Nausea | 1 | 1 | 3 | 0 |
| Palpitation | 0 | 1 | 0 | 0 |
| Buzzing | 0 | 1 | 0 | 0 |
| Loss of appetite | 1 | 0 | 1 | 0 |
| Neuropsychiatric Impairments | 0 | 0 | 0 | 0 |

Of these categories of various complications, the forms of categories (4) and (5) in Table 7 seem to be of prime importance as postvaccinal hazards from prophylactic immunization against Japanese encephalitis, relating to the above-mentioned rabies postvaccinal encephalomyelitis. As indicated in Table 8, of particular note is that both of the two cases of the demyelinating encephalitic form ranged in age from seven to fourteen years, both belonged to children, and the involvements were possibly restricted to the optic nerve, brain stem or spinal cord but not to the cerebrum. In two cases of the polyneuritic form among five patients, on the other hand, the age distribution was three years and four months and four years, respectively (Table 9).

In addition, the author has had an opportunity to examine one autopsy case of the polyneuritic form of the disease. A three-year-old girl was vaccinated against Japanese encephalitis on May 17, 1961. Fifteen days later, she developed paralytic paraplegia and pain of toe, and on the next day, that was succeeded by ascending paralysis to the upper limbs, urinary incontinence, complete tetraplegia,

Table 7. Sporadic Cases with Neurological Impairments Following Vaccination against *Encephalitis Japonica*, 1965 (Okinaka *et al.*, 1967)

| Form of complication | Number of cases | Incubation period | Age |
|---|---|---|---|
| (1) Meningoencephalomyelitis | 6 | 1–9 days | 1–44 years |
| (2) Encephalopathy | 3 | 2–19 days | 1 year & 6 months–7 years |
| (3) Convulsive Seizure | 10 | 2 hours–4 days | 5 months–9 years & 9 months |
| (4) Demyelinating Encephalitis | 2 | 9 & 19 days | 7 & 14 years |
| (5) Polyneuritis | 5 | 1–28 days | 3 years & 4 months–33 years |
| (6) Miscellaneous Neurological Complications | 4 | 30 minutes–8 days | 5–51 years |

Table 8. Two Cases of Demyelinating Encephalomyelitis Following Vaccination against *Encephalitis Japonica* (Okinaka *et al.*, 1967)

| | |
|---|---|
| Age | 7 years & 14 years |
| Sex | Males |
| Incubation period | 9 & 19 days |
| Site & mode of inoculation | 1.0cc, subcutaneously |
| CSF | cell count 253/3, Pandy $3^+$ |
| Neurological impairments | fever, impaired gait, bilateral Babinski, elevated knee & Achilles jerkes, urinary incontinence, impaired sensations below umbilical region, retrobulbar neuritis, impaired visual acuity, central constriction of visual field, optic atrophy, 1-abducence paralysis |
| Prognosis | death & progressive |

Table 9. Five Cases of Polyneuritis Following Vaccination against Japanese Encephalitis (Okinaka *et al.*, 1967)

| | |
|---|---|
| Age | 3 years & 4 months, 16 years, 33 years |
| Sex | 3 males, 2 females |
| Site & mode of inoculation | 0.1–1.0 cc, subcutaneously |
| CSF | cell count 0–6/3, Pandy $2^+$–$3^+$, protein 140 mg/d$l$ |
| Neurological impairments | fever, motor weakness of lower limbs, motor weakness of upper limbs, tetraplegia, impaired gait, unstable gait, hyporeflexia, convulsion, dysarthria, dysphagia |
| Virus isolation | negative |
| Prognosis | death 1, complete recovery 1, incomplete recovery 3 |
| Miscellaneous | Guillain-Barré, abdominal pain, fatigue, pain & swelling of joints |

impaired sensations of the upper limbs, impaired speech and areflexias. Consciousness remained clear, while cerebrospinal fluid developed the findings of pressure 190/150mm$H_2O$, cell count 4/3 and Pandy $\pm$. On the third day of the illness, pain of the lower limbs was observed, while voluntary movement of the upper limbs was slightly improved and facial palsy was observed on the right side. She expired twenty-two days after the vaccination and eight days after the onset of the polyneuritic involvement.

The most conspicuous alterations were found in both posterior and anterior nerve rootlets from the fifth cervical cord to the cauda equina. They consisted of swelling, vacuolation, fragmentation or edematous disruption in the axonal structures, while the latter

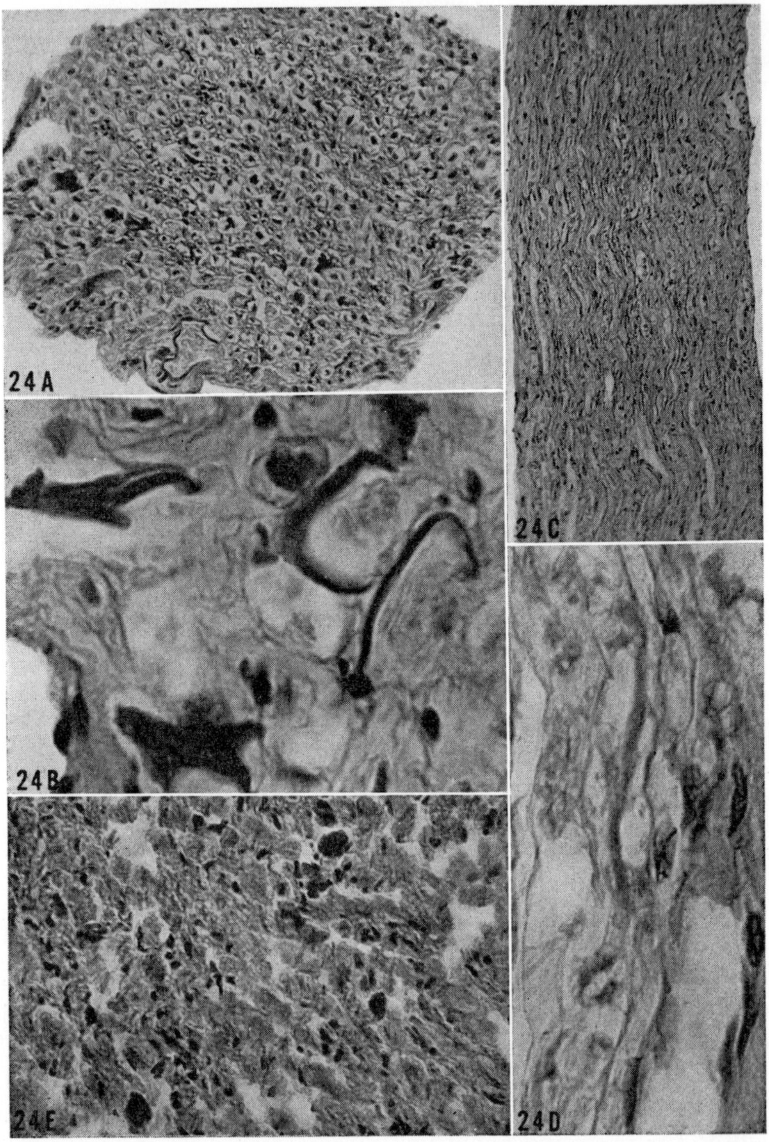


Fig. 24. Polyneuritis following Vaccination against Japanese Encephalitis in the Japanese (See text).
A. Posterior nerve rootlet at the level of the 5th cervical cord. Certain of the axis cylinders are swollen, metamorphosed and deeply hematoxophilic, while others are conspicuously edematous. ×360.
B. Magnified posterior nerve rootlet at the level of the 2nd thoracic cord. Similar to A, while Schwann's cell nuclei become darkly shrunken. ×1130.
C. Anterior nerve rootlet at the level of the 4th lumbar cord. Almost all axis

occasionally became deeply hematoxophilic. Myelin sheaths were more or less disintegrated as well, while Schwann's cell nuclei became darkly shrunken. No perivascular cell cuffs nor granule cells were mobilized, however (Figs. 24A~E). Vagus nerve rootlets at the level of the midmedulla oblongata were degenerated in a similar way. Pyramidal cells of the grey matter at different levels of the spinal cord were partially degenerated and a few of them developed tiny intracytoplasmic bodies. A few spheroid bodies were visible particularly at the medioventral part of the anterior horn of the fifth cervical and second lumbar cords. Diapedetic hemorrhages were disseminated in the spinal grey matter. Coarse spongy tissue disruption occurred bilaterally in the tegmentum of the pons as well.

So far, the present example was clinicopathologically considered to be a polyneuritic process due to vaccination against Japanese encephalitis, though clear-cut perivascular inflammatory cell cuffs were not identified.

## CEREBRAL COMPLICATIONS FOLLOWING VACCINATION AGAINST SMALLPOX IN INFANTS

The same can be said as to certain cases of postvaccinal encephalomyelitis against smallpox (Shiraki, 1968e).

For example, a four-month-old girl was vaccinated against smallpox on October 2, 1965, and that was succeeded by a cold-like syndrome. Four days later, she developed a high fever (41°–42°C), convulsions, impaired consciousness, stiffness of all limbs and neck-stiffness. The findings of cerebrospinal fluid were as follows: pressure 190/−6m*l*/120mm$H_2O$, cell count 349/3 (neutrophiles/lymphocytes = 170/179), total protein 2TS, Nonne 1+ and Pandy 2+. The serum test for Japanese encephalitis, Echo and coxachie were all negative. Subsequently, the high fever persisted, and she finally expired eleven days after the vaccination and eight days after the onset of the cerebral involvements. Virus isolation as well as fluorescent antibody technique for identification of smallpox virus antigen

---

cylinders are edematously swollen and faintly stained. ×120.

D. Magnified area in C. Similar to C, while certain of them are vacuolarly disrupted. ×950.

E. Cauda equina. A great majority of the axis cylinders are edematously swollen and faintly stained, while a less number of them are deeply hematoxophilic. Schwann's cell nuclei became darkly shrunken. ×440. (A–E; H.E.)

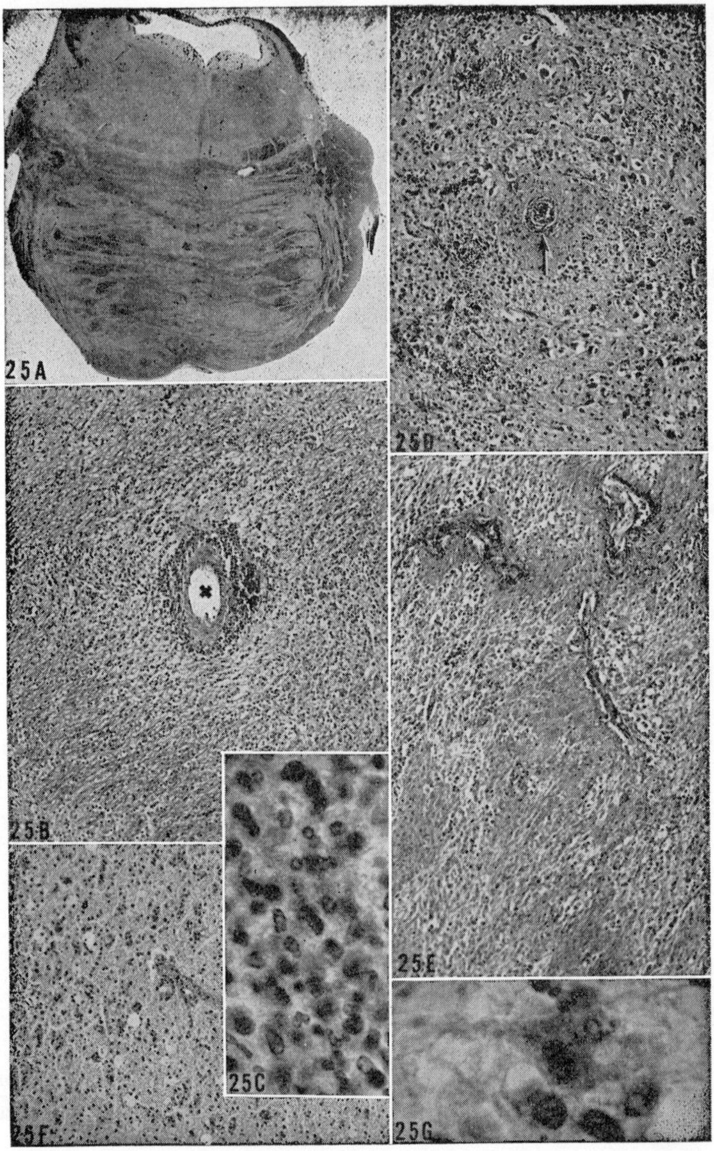


Fig. 25. Postvaccinal Meningoencephalitis for Small Pox in the Japanese (See text).

A. Pons. An exceedingly large number of the isolated or coalescent, tiny demyelinated foci, the details of the distribution of which are illustrated schematically in Figs. 26A and B, are widespread in both tegmentum and basis. Their true features, however, are not conspicuous at this power of magnification since myelination is not yet completed in the 4-month-old patient. ×3.0.

from the postmortem fresh brain tissues were not successful. The brain weighed 790 grams.

The lesions of the central nervous system were, in brief, characterized by a severely disturbed blood-brain barrier as well as pathomorphological complexes peculiar to those of experimental "allergic" encephalomyelitis or of the spinal form of rabies postvaccinal encephalomyelitis which is accompanied by perivascular inflammatory cell cuffs. Those two main foci were predominant in the brain stem, pulvinar thalami and uppermost cervical cord; above all, they were prominent in their tegmental regions. For example, in the pontine area, multiple foci were disseminated in both tegmentum and basis (Fig. 25A), while a higher magnification indicated that the unit focus consisted of the engorged central venule infiltrated with a smaller number of the inflammatory cells, periadventitial migration of the erythroplasmofibrinous materials and conspicuous proliferation of the "epithelioid cells" accompanied by the demyelination with comparatively well-preserved axis cylinders and nerve cells (Figs. 25B, C). In addition, plasmofibrinous migration as well as erythrocytic infiltration in the parenchyma were particularly pronounced in the brain stem and pulvinar thalami (Figs. 25D, E). Consequently, a majority of the remaining nerve cells degenerated ischemically (Figs. 25F, G). The schematic distribution patterns of those foci in both the pontine region and pulvinar thalami are illustrated in Figs. 26A and B. The white matter of the cerebrum, on the other hand, was far less involved and a slight cellular increase and perivascular cell cuffs were observed only in the areas adjacent

---

B. Lower magnified unit focus in the basis in A. The former is round and consists of the central vessel infiltrated with the inflammatory cells (*cross*), periadventitial narrow tissue loosening and marginal proliferation of the "epithelioid cells." ×82.

C. Highly magnified latter area in B. A majority of the cellular elements comprise the "epithelioid cells" and activated rod cells. Compare with Figs. 2B and 6D. ×570.

D. Tegmentum in A. Multiple hemorrhages occur, while periadventitial plasmofibrinous migration around the central vessel (*arrow*) is visible as well. Ischemic-shrunken nerve cells are still preserved. ×96.

E. Pulvinar thalami. PAS-positive fibrinous transudations are exceedingly pronounced in the perivascular spaces and periadventitial parenchyma and tend to coalesce. Cellular mobilization consisting mainly of the "epithelioid cells" develops outside of the latter. ×82. F. "Epithelioid cells" proliferate loosely in the parenchyma where nerve cells are still preserved, while a majority of them develop an ischemic change and neuronophagia. ×82. G. A magnified ischemic nerve cell with a neuronophagia in F. Parenchyma becomes sieve-like and disrupted. ×900. (A & B; Luxol fastblue with cresyl-violet. C, D, F & G; H.E. E; PAS.)

to the ventricular walls. A slight-to-moderate inflammatory cell infiltration of a focal nature occurred in the subarachnoid space of the cerebrum, the cortices of which developed an acute edematous alteration.

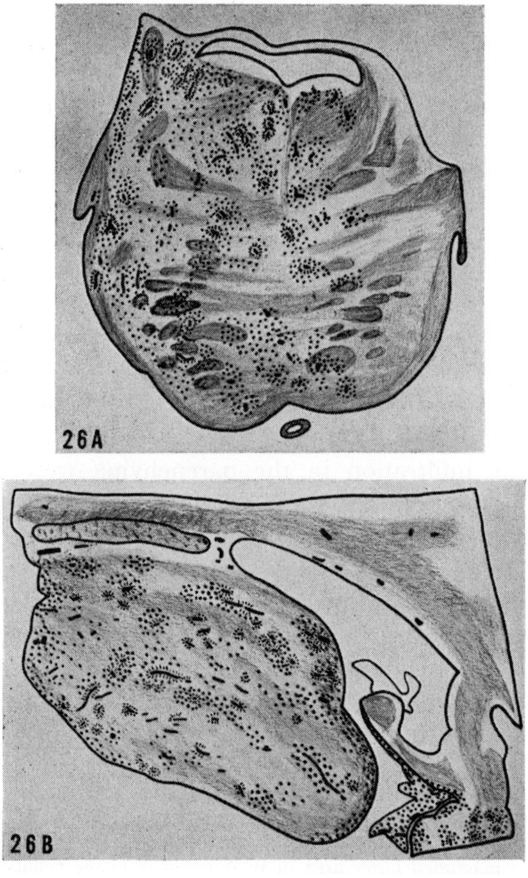


Fig. 26. Schematic Distribution Pattern of Foci in Postvaccinal Meningoencephalitis for Small Pox in the Japanese (Same case as in Fig. 25).
A. Same section as in Fig. 25A. See text.
B. Same section as in Figs. 25E to G. See text. ~; perivascular inflammatory cell cuffs of venules ⁘; periadventitial plasmofibrinous transudation in the former ∴; unit foci as indicated in Fig. 25B and C.

This notable selective localization of the foci in the present example may be interpreted as follows: inasmuch as myelination of the nervous system of babies within six months of age is believed to be virtually complete in those areas, particularly in their tegmental regions, a definite demyelinating process accompanied by the severely impaired blood-brain barrier did occur selectively in those regions and comprised the main cause of death.

## SUMMARY AND CONCLUSION

Mainly from the neuropathological viewpoint, there has been established a close connection of both spinal and cerebral forms of rabies postvaccinal encephalomyelitis with various groups of demyelinating encephalomyelitides of unknown origin, such as acute multiple sclerosis, postvaccinal or postinfectious encephalomyelitis and a certain phase of multiple sclerosis and allied disorders. The question remains as to whether or not a firm connection of the former of a monophasic nature with chronic multiple sclerosis of a polyphasic character can be established.

For various reasons, the causative agent for the developmental mechanism of rabies postvaccinal encephalomyelitis in man could be attributed to the repeated inoculations of humans with animal CNS tissue contained vaccines, and this may contribute to an understanding of the etiopathogenesis of demyelinating encephalomyelitides of unknown origin.

Two main characteristics of rabies postvaccinal encephalomyelitis in the Japanese, i.e., highest incidence of the disease and existence only of its cerebral form, have been emphasized. Reasonable explanations for those, however, except for racial differences, were not forthcoming. No antirabic complications were observed among Japanese children below thirteen years of age. This fact constituted a ground on which vaccination against Japanese encephalitis was performed on the children and younger individuals in Japan.

A full-scale survey on postvaccinal complications against Japanese encephalitis failed to reveal any neuropsychiatric impairments, while sporadic cases of both demyelinating and polyneuritic forms of the disease together with an autopsy case of the latter disclosed a certain relationship of a minimal amount of the animal neural tissues contained in the vaccines to the development of neurological complications.

An autopsy case of the postvaccinal encephalitis against smallpox has been discussed as in the former case.

As a consequence, among postvaccinal complications against both Japanese encephalitis and smallpox, children occasionally developed neuropsychiatric impairments. This observation may be contrasted to the fact that in children below thirteen years of age, rabies postvaccinal encephalomyelitis never occurred.

Thus far, for an essential understanding of the etiopathogenesis of nervous system complications against various vaccinations, it is keenly felt that the interaction of exogeneous causative agents and endogeneous factors of individuals and races should be carefully considered in particular, ontogenesis of nervous system. In other words, two main factors, i.e., quality and quantity of exogeneous agents, as well as stage or grade of development or maturation of both peripheral and central nervous system of different age groups, should simultaneously and seriously be considered here.

## REFERENCES

Jellinger, K. and Seitelberger, F. (1958). Akute tödliche Entmarkungsencephalitis nach wiederholten Hirntrockenzellen-Injektionen. *Klin. Wschr.*, **36**, 437–441.

Jellinger, K. and Seitelberger, F. (1963). Zur Frage der zentralnervösen Komplikation nach Wutshutzimpfung. *Deutsch. Z. Nervenheilk.*, **184**, 508–536.

Maeda, S., Kondo, S., Mukai, A., Hamada, S. and Ishii, T. (1962). An autopsy case of acute demyelinating encephalitis with unilateral diencephalic lesions. *Psychiat. et Neurol. Jap.*, **64**, 1199–1215.

Matsuyama, H. (1970). Atlas of multiple sclerosis. *Jap. J. Clin. Med.*, **28**, 2282–2285.

Murofushi, K. (1958). The studies on experimental demyelinating encephalomyelitis. *Psychiat. et Neurol. Jap.*, **60**, 37–74.

Okinaka, S., Toyokura, Y., Tsukagoshi, H., Kuroiwa, Y., Araki, T., Arima, M., Otani, S., Tsubaki, H., Shiraki, H., Takatsu, T., Narabayashi, H. and Yoshimura, S. (1967). Physical reactions following vaccination against Japanese B encephalitis, with special reference to neurological complications. *Adv. Neurol. Sci.*, **11**, 410–424.

Takahata, N. (1970). Atlas of multiple sclerosis. *Jap. J. Clin. Med.*, **28**, 2285–2287.

Totsuka, S., Higasayama, I., Yazaki, M., Matsumoto, Y. and Nagao, K. (1970). Two autopsy cases of acute disseminated encephalomyelitis. *Adv. Neurol. Sci.*, **14**, 358–366.

Shiraki, H. (1968a). Neurological disorders in Thailand, especially related to rabies. Medical problems in southeast Asia, Symposium series IV, p. 53–69, Center for Southeast Asian Study, Kyoto Univ.

Shiraki, H. (1968b). The comparative study of rabies postvaccinal encephalomyelitis and demyelinating encephalomyelitis of unknown origin, with special reference to the Japanese cases. Central Nervous System, edited by O. T. Bailey and D. E. Smith, p. 87–123, Williams & Wilkins, Baltimore.

Shiraki, H. (1968c). Neuropathology of postvaccinal encephalitis for smallpox. *Jap. J. Infect. Dis.*, **41**, 11.

Shiraki, H. and Otani, S. (1959). Clinical and pathological features of rabies postvaccinal encephalomyelitis in man. Relationship to multiple sclerosis and to experimental "allergic" encephalomyelitis in animal. "Allergic" Encephalomyelitis, edited by M. W. Kies and E. C. Alvord, p. 58–129, C. C. Thomas, Springfield, Illn.

Shiraki, H., Otani, S., Tamthai, B., Chamuni, A., Chitanondh, H. and Charuchinda, S. (1962). Rabies postvaccinal encephalomyelitis and genuine rabies in human beings. *World Neurol.*, **3**, 125–148.

Uchimura, Y., and Shiraki, H. (1957). A contribution to the classification and the pathogenesis of demyelinating encephalomyelitis. With special reference to the central nervous system lesions caused by preventive inoculation against rabies. *J. Neuropath. & Exper. Neurol.*, **16**, 139–203.

Uchimura, Y., Shiraki, H. and Haruhara, Ch. (1955). Zur Histopathologie und Pathogenese der Entmarkungsencephalomyelitiden mit besondere Berücksichtigung der Entmarkungsprozesse der Lyssaschutzimpfung. *Psychiat. et Neurol. Jap.*, **56**, 503–535.

Uchimura, Y., Shiraki, H. and Haruhara, Ch. (1958). Klinik der postvaccinalen Encephalitis nach Tollwutimpfung und ihres Folgezustandes. *Nervenarzt*, **29**, 303–37.

Yonezawa, T. (1970). Atlas of multiple sclerosis. *Jap. J. Cli. Med.*, **28**, 2288–2291.

For Discussion, see page 225.

# Rabies Immune Globulin of Human Origin

Preparation and Dose Determination in Nonexposed Volunteers

V. J. Cabasso,* J. C. Loofbourow,** R. E. Roby* and W. Anuskiewicz*

**Microbiology Research Section, Cutter Laboratories, Berkeley, California 94710*
***Office of Occupational Medicine, Cowell Student Health Center, University of California, Davis, California 95616*

## INTRODUCTION

The use of rabies immune serum or globulin of equine origin, in combination with rabies vaccine, has been routine for many years in postexposure immunization of man (WHO, 1966).

The first recorded preparation of rabies immune serum was reported in 1889 by Babes and Lepp (1889). Between that date and the 1930s a number of reports were published on the use of rabies immune serum or serum concentrates in the prevention of experimental rabies in animals or in the postexposure treatment of man. A comprehensive review of these reports was made by Habel (1945). Results of the early experiments ranged from complete protection against a rabies challenge to no protection at all, but the numbers of animals included in those experiments were small, and they were not adequately controlled. Later experiments in small animals and monkeys were better controlled and, together with results obtained in man, gave suggestive evidence of the value of rabies immune serum.

In a systematic study of rabies immune serum of rabbit origin used in mice, guinea pigs and monkeys, Habel found that serum prophylaxis alone gave better protection in postinfection treatment than vaccine alone, and that protection was enhanced when serum treatment was combined with a course of vaccine administration (Habel, 1945). These observations in animals were later confirmed and extended by Koprowski and coworkers (Koprowski *et al.*, 1950; Koprowski & Cox, 1951; Koprowski & Black, 1954).

The usefulness of rabies immune serum in postexposure treatment of man was dramatically demonstrated in a group of persons bitten by a rabid wolf in Iran, (Baltazard *et al.*, 1955; Habel & Koprowski, 1955), and was later confirmed in the USSR with rabies immune globulin (Selimov *et al.*, 1959).

In Iran, of 17 persons with severe head wounds, 5 received two injections of serum the first and fifth days, and phenolized rabies vaccine for 21 days; 7 received one serum injection and a 21-day course of vaccine; 5 received only the course of vaccine. In addition, a 6-year-old boy suffering from a crushed parietal bone and torn dura mater was given 6 serum injections and vaccine for 21 days. Rabies antibody was detected as early as the second day in all those receiving serum and vaccine, and the antibody remained detectable throughout the observation period. In contrast, antibody became detectable only after 19 days in the vaccine-only group. Of the 18 subjects, 1 of the 7 who received one serum dose and vaccine and 3 of the 5 who received vaccine alone, a total of 4, died of rabies. The most striking survival was that of the 6-year-old boy.

A series of studies coordinated by WHO was subsequently undertaken to determine the optimal conditions under which rabies immune serum of equine origin and rabies vaccine can be used in man (Atanasiu *et al.*, 1956, 1957, 1961, 1967). These studies, carried out in adult humans previously not exposed to rabies and with no history of rabies vaccination, indicated that serum can interfere with the active immunity induced by the vaccine. They further demonstrated that this interference can be overcome by booster doses of vaccine 10 and 20 days after the end of the usual 12– to 14–dose series. But Habel (1966) has recently indicated that a more effective regimen consists of booster doses of vaccine at 20 days, 2 months and 6 months after the initial series.

Preformed rabies antibody of equine origin was also found useful in the local treatment of bite wounds. In the studies on this mode of treatment, the antibody was applied in the form of immune serum, or of its liquid or powdered globulin (Kaplan *et al.*, 1962; Dean *et al.*, 1963; Kaplan & Paccaud, 1963; Dean, 1966). The favorable results obtained in experimental animals culminated in a recommendation by the WHO Expert Committee on Rabies (1966) that the topical use of preformed rabies antibody be considered in all exposures, particularly severe exposures.

The demonstrated utility in man of rabies immune serum of equine origin has not been realized without penalty: a high incidence of serum sickness and the risk of anaphylaxis accompany its use.

Only a preparation of human origin would prevent this side-effect from occurring in man, while preserving the benefit of preformed rabies antibody. Hosty *et al.* (1959) and Anderson and Sgouris (1965) reported their preliminary efforts to prepare rabies immune serum or globulin of human origin. More recently, Winkler *et al.* (1969) described the preparation of three lots of rabies immune globulin of human origin. Even though these lots were subpotent, they served to demonstrate the feasibility of this approach.

Homologous globulin preparations would have the obvious advantage of ending the risk of anaphylaxis or serum sickness. However, the question arises whether the longer lasting homologous passive antibody might not interfere even more than equine globulin with the active immunity induced by the vaccine. Comparing the effect of equivalent dosage of homologous (guinea pig) and heterologous (donkey) rabies immune sera in guinea pigs, Archer and Dierks (1968) found that the former could delay or suppress active immunization when a rabies vaccine of avian origin was used. Delay or suppression did not take place, however, when a vaccine of higher potency was employed.

It is evident that additional studies are needed on the preparation of rabies immune globulin of human origin, and on the conditions of its use in human immunization. This report summarizes our studies in this area.

## MATERIALS AND METHODS

*Rabies immune plasma: source, collection and fractionation*

Rabies immune plasma was obtained from healthy, volunteer adult donors who, because of actual past exposure to rabid animals, had received one or more courses of rabies vaccine—Semple, duck embryo or chicken embryo type—or who, because of the nature of their occupations as veterinarians, veterinary students or animal handlers, underwent routine preexposure immunization against rabies and received periodic boosters of rabies vaccine.

Sample bleedings from potential donors were first tested for rabies neutralizing antibody, and only those with titers deemed high enough to yield an immune globulin preparation of acceptable rabies antibody titer when pooled were asked to donate plasma. Blood was withdrawn by plasmapheresis in accredited blood banks at intervals not shorter than one week. The plasma units were stored frozen until they were tested individually for rabies antibody titer and pooled for fractionation of the IgG.

Fractionation of pooled plasma was carried out by methods 6 and 9 of Cohn *et al.* (1946) and Oncley *et al.* (1949). The 16.5% ($\pm$2.5%) IgG solution obtained was sterile filtered, and the final product was aseptically dispensed in glass vials in 5 m*l* volumes. Biological and chemical control tests were carried out in accordance with the Public Health Service Regulations, Biological Product Title 42, Part 73, Revised June 1969. When all tests were completed, and found to meet the requirements set forth in the Regulations, the assigned potency of the lot was imprinted on the label of the final container in terms of international units per m*l* (IU/m*l*).

*Serum neutralization test (SNT)*

Individual plasma units, prefractionation plasma pools and finished IgG preparations were tested for rabies neutralizing antibody according to the procedure recommended by the Division of Biologics Standards (DBS), National Institutes of Health, Bethesda, Maryland, for the potency testing of Antirabies Serum (Equine Origin). Plasma samples, but not IgG samples, were inactivated at 56°C for 30 minutes before dilution.

The animals used were Swiss Webster mice of the same sex, weighing 10–14 grams. The challenge virus was the CVS strain of rabies virus obtained from DBS. Stock virus was prepared from infected mouse brains and stored at −60°C or below in glass sealed ampoules.

One of the rabies immune preparations used as reference was DBS Reference No. 2. This was in the form of a measured amount of dried globulin which, when reconstituted with 5 m*l* distilled water, was considered to contain 2 IU/m*l* of rabies antibody. The IU is defined as the amount of antibody present in 4 mg. of this particular dried reference globulin. The other preparation was a House Reference Serum made by us in rabbits.

The SNT proper was carried out by preparing 1) equal parts of 2-fold dilutions of the House Reference, each mixed with approximately 200 $LD_{50}$/0.03 m*l* of CVS virus, to monitor the reproducibility of the test system; 2) equal parts of 2-fold dilutions of the DBS Reference and CVS virus as above, to establish the denominator required for computation of the potency of the test plasma or globulin; 3) equal parts of 2-fold dilutions of test plasma or globulin and CVS virus, and 4) 10-fold dilutions of the CVS virus suspension used in above mixtures to determine the number of mouse lethal dose-50 ($LD_{50}$) used in each test.

Incubation of the plasma, or globulin-virus mixtures, was at 37°C for 90 minutes. Mixtures were held in crushed ice until injected. Each dilution was injected intracerebrally into 6 mice, each animal receiving 0.03 m*l*. The mice were observed for paralysis or death for 14 days, after which time virus or antibody titers were calculated by the Spearman-Kärber method (Spearman, 1908; Kärber, 1931).

In 34 consecutive tests carried out as described, the number of virus $LD_{50s}$ used in each varied between 22 and 220. The majority (21 tests) ranged from 47 to 100, the mean value was 91 and the median 100 $LD_{50}$. In the same 34 tests, the serum neutralizing dose-50 ($SN_{50}$) of the House Reference Serum ranged from 1:89 to ≥1:316.

The majority of $SN_{50}$ titers (26 tests) were between 1:100 and 1:200, and their geometric mean was 1:163.

*Clinical study*

A study intended to investigate the optimal dose of Rabies Immune Globulin (Human) (RIGH), i.e., the dose which would result in minimal or no interference with the active immunity induced by rabies vaccine, was conducted at the Cowell Student Health Center and Hospital, University of California at Davis. The study population consisted of consenting young adult volunteers from the School of Veterinary Medicine, 20 to 30 years of age, of either sex, and in good health. Only individuals with no prior history of rabies immunization, who would ordinarily receive preexposure rabies prophylaxis were admitted to the study. They were randomly distributed among the five experimental groups to be described.

The lot of RIGH employed in this investigation was experimental lot no. PR 2316 to be described under Experiments and Results. This lot had a rabies antibody potency of 550 IU/m*l*.

The vaccine used was a recently released lot (no. 3EE97B) of Rabies Vaccine, Duck Embryo Origin (DEV), graciously donated for the study by Dr. F. Bruce Peck, Jr., Eli Lilly and Company, Indianapolis, Indiana. It had a potency ratio of 1.17 against DBS Reference Vaccine No. 175 and, at the time it was administered, was 12–13 months away from the expiration date.

## EXPERIMENTS AND RESULTS

*Lots of RIGH prepared*

Following the procedures described earlier, we prepared two consecutive lots of RIGH, nos. PR 2316 and PR 2342. The first was derived from a pool of about 14 liters of plasma, and the second from 50 liters of plasma. Laboratory test results of the two lots are summarized in Table 1.

Table 1. Rabies Immune Globulin (Human) (RIGH)-Cutter
Laboratory Test Results on Two Experimental Lots

| | Lot No. | |
|---|---|---|
| | PR 2316 | PR 2342 |
| Date prepared | 5-12-69 | 2-11-70 |
| Plasma pool: liters | 14.25 | 50.0 |
| 〃 〃 : UI/m*l* | 22[a] | 10.6[a] |
| RIGH: IU/ml. | 702[a]–406[b] | 269[a]–216[b] |
| 〃 : Assigned IU/m*l* | 550[c] | 240[c] |
| Pyrogen, sterility, identity tests | Passed | Passed |
| Safety tests—mice and guinea pigs | 〃 | 〃 |
| Protein concentration: % | 14.0 | 17.6 |
| IgG purity: % | 98.1 | 98.9 |
| Mobility: Cm²/volt/sec. | $1.21 \times 10^{-5}$ | $1.24 \times 10^{-5}$ |
| pH | 6.59 | 6.41 |
| Gelation: 4 hours at 57°C | None | None |
| Turbidity: 7 days at 37°C | 〃 | 〃 |

*a* Each number is a geometric mean of 3 determinations at Cutter Laboratories.
*b* Single determination at Center for Disease Control.
*c* Average of *a* and *b* values for RIGH.

Potency of the two lots was determined in our laboratory and also at the Center for Disease Control (CDC), through the courtesy of Dr. Keith Sikes. The values obtained for the two RIGH lots were 22- to 25-fold those of the plasma pooled, a ratio consonant with the concentration factor. The results obtained in the two laboratories were in remarkable agreement, considering the limited precision of the assay procedure. The potency assigned to each preparation was the average of the values from the two laboratories.

The potency of the two lots was well above that ordinarily found for the currently employed Antirabies Serum (Equine Origin) (Winkler *et al.*, 1969). This permitted the administration of substantially reduced volumes of RIGH to the volunteers admitted to the clinical study.

*Human dose determination*

A total of 41 volunteers participated in a study intended to determine the proper dosage of RIGH. They were divided into 5 groups, each of which received a different immunization schedule. The 5 schedules and the number of participants in each are presented in Table 2.

Table 2. Rabies Immune Globulin (Human) (RIGH)—Cutter Immunization Schedules of Five Groups of Volunteer Students

| | Group Designation | | | | |
|---|---|---|---|---|---|
| | A | B | C | D | E |
| No. of volunteers in group | 8 | 8 | 8 | 9 | 8 |
| RIGH Dose (IU/kilo)[a] | 40 | None | 40 | 20 | 10 |
| DEV Doses[b] | None | 14+2 | 14+2 | 14+2 | 14+2 |

*a* The full RIGH dose was given in a single intramuscular injection on day zero.
*b* DEV=Rabies Vaccine, Duck Embryo Origin. Administered in 14 daily injections of 1 m*l*, followed by a 1 m*l* booster dose on day 23, and another on day 33.

Regardless of the dose of RIGH to be administered, lot PR 2316 was given in all cases only once, on the day the study was initiated. A chart of weights ranging from 134 lbs. to 200 lbs. in 2- to 3-lb. increments was prepared in advance. In it the volume of RIGH equivalent to 40, 20 or 10 IU/kilo was calculated for each weight.

As each student presented himself for his first injection, a pre-immunization blood sample was withdrawn, the student was weighed, the dose he was to receive, if any, was determined from the chart, and was administered to him intramuscularly. This was followed, where applicable, by the first dose of 1.0 m*l* DEV subcutaneously.

Administration of DEV to those who were to receive it was uniform. It consisted of 14 daily injections of 1.0 m*l* each, beginning as indicated above on day zero. An additional 1 m*l* booster injection was given on day 23, and another on day 33. These booster injections were in accordance with the regimen recommended by the WHO Expert Committee on Rabies to overcome any interference by Antirabies Serum (Equine Origin) (WHO, 1966).

In addition to the zero-day bleeding, serum samples were also obtained from all participants on days 1, 3, 6, 9, 23, 30, 40, 60, 90 and 180. One last sample will be taken one year after the first injection. The sera which were frozen soon after their separation from the clot, were shipped frozen to the laboratory where they were so held until tested.

Table 3. Clinical Study with Rabies Immune Globulin (Human) (RIGH)—Cutter
Volunteer Group A: RIGH only—40 IU/kilo
Individual Serum Neutralizing Titers[a]

| Volunteer Designation | Days after RIGH | | | | | | | | | | |
|---|---|---|---|---|---|---|---|---|---|---|---|
| | 0 | 1 | 3 | 6 | 9 | 13 | 23 | 30 | 40 | 60 | 90 |
| 1. JB | <2 | 9 | 18 | 16 | 50 | 32 | 20 | 17 | 20 | 7 | 3 |
| 2. SD | <2 | 11 | 18 | 25 | 23 | 16 | 27 | 21 | 17 | 12 | 5 |
| 3. LH | <2 | 8 | 13 | 36 | 14 | 36 | 25 | 11 | 9 | 9 | <2 |
| 4. TK | <2 | 14 | 22 | 36 | 25 | 28 | 25 | 19 | 7 | 7 | <2 |
| 5. HM | <2 | 11 | 16 | 35 | 45 | 35 | 28 | 26 | 20 | 11 | 4 |
| 6. MM | <2 | 8 | 25 | 20 | 18 | 16 | 23 | 17 | 18 | 20 | 9 |
| 7. CM | <2 | 16 | 22 | 25 | 22 | 50 | 25 | 25 | 25 | 8 | 3 |
| 8. NW | <2 | 14 | 26 | 11 | 25 | 45 | 16 | 9 | 8 | 3 | <2 |
| Titer Ranges | <2 | 8–16 | 13–26 | 11–36 | 14–50 | 16–50 | 16–28 | 9–26 | 7–25 | 3–20 | <2–9 |
| Geometric Means | <2 | 11 | 20 | 24 | 26 | 30 | 23 | 17 | 14 | 9 | 3 |

*a* Reciprocal of dilutions.

The laboratory received no information about the group to which each student belonged. Thus, the study was blind in this regard. Each serum was identified simply by the student's name and the date of bleeding.

Testing for serum neutralizing antibody was begun when the 30-day sera from all participants became available. All samples from the same individual were tested at one time. The code was broken only after the 0- to 30-day specimens from all 41 participants had been tested. Then the testing of the 40-, 60- and 90-day samples began, again titrating the three sera from each student simultaneously, and repeating the 30-day sample in the same test for the sake of tying together the results from each individual.

*Group A*: As was indicated in Table 2, the 8 participants in this group received RIGH only, in a dose of 40 IU/kilo. They were to provide the rate of decline, or half-life, of the passively acquired, homologous antibody. The antibody titers of the 0- to 90-day sera are shown in Table 3 for each individual, as are the titer ranges obtained on each of the bleeding dates and the geometric mean titer calculated for these dates. The titer ranges and the geometric mean titers are also graphically plotted in Fig. 1.

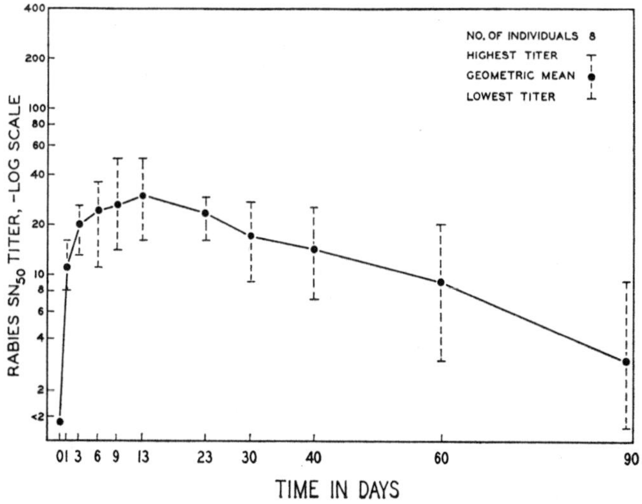


Fig. 1. Volunteer Group A: Neutralizing Antibody Response Following Administration of 40 IU/kilo Rabies Immune Globulin (Human) Only.

All participants were seronegative for rabies antibody at the initiation of the study. Twenty-four hours after RIGH injection, however, all had measurable antibody titers. Their geometric mean

Table 4. Clinical Study with Rabies Immune Globulin (Human) (RIGH)—Cutter
Volunteer Group B: DEV Only
Individual Serum Neutralizing Titers[a]

| Volunteer Designation | Days after First DEV Injection | | | | | | | | | | |
|---|---|---|---|---|---|---|---|---|---|---|---|
| | 0 | 1 | 3 | 6 | 9 | 13 | 23 | 30 | 40 | 60 | 90 |
| 1. MF | <2 | <2 | <2 | 7 | 11 | 72 | 101 | 101 | 101 | 128 | 79 |
| 2. JH | <2 | <2 | <2 | 4 | 10 | 40 | 44 | 36 | 51 | 36 | 29 |
| 3. KJ | <2 | <2 | <2 | 2 | 14 | 79 | 320 | 454 | 513 | 363 | 255 |
| 4. RN | <2 | <2 | <2 | <2 | 22 | 128 | 100 | 357 | 144 | 229 | 114 |
| 5. BP | <2 | <2 | <2 | <2 | 26 | 100 | 199 | 360 | 507 | 403 | 227 |
| 6. JR | <2 | <2 | <2 | <2 | 40 | 89 | 288 | 361 | 313 | 361 | 255 |
| 7. AS | <2 | <2 | <2 | <2 | <2 | 9 | 14 | 18 | 51 | 14 | 13 |
| 8. SV | <2 | <2 | <2 | <2 | 8 | 40 | 80 | 72 | 64 | 73 | 64 |
| Titer Ranges | <2 | <2 | <2 | <2–7 | <2–40 | 9–128 | 14–320 | 18–454 | 51–513 | 14–403 | 13–255 |
| Geometric Means | <2 | <2 | <2 | 2 | 11 | 56 | 99 | 133 | 145 | 124 | 87 |

*a* Reciprocal of dilutions.

titer was 1:11, with individual titers ranging between 1:8 and 1:16. The antibody level rose gradually to a peak geometric mean of 1:30 by the 13th day, when it began to decline. The period of antibody rise was longer than was anticipated, and no obvious reason offers itself to explain this. Be that as it may, the rate of decline of the antibody from a peak titer of 1:30 at 13 days to a titer of 1:3 seventy-seven days later conforms to the 21-day half-life estimated for homologous passive immune globulin in man.

*Group B*: The 8 students in this group received DEV only. As shown in Table 4 and in Fig. 2, no rabies antibody was detected for 3 days after the initial vaccine injection. Low levels could be measured on the 6th day in only 3 of the participants, and higher titers were obtained in 7 out of 8 on the 9th day.

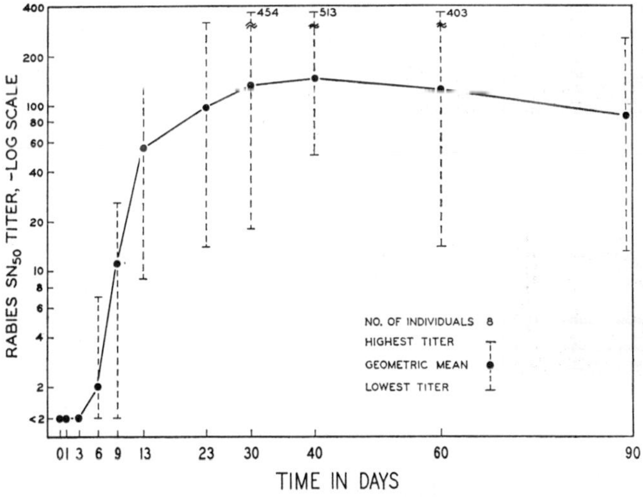


Fig. 2. Volunteer Group B: Neutralizing Antibody Response Following Administration of a Course of Rabies Vaccine, Duck Embryo Origin.

All the students were positive for rabies antibody on the 13th day, their individual titers ranging from 1:9 to 1:128. Most titers continued to rise, reaching a peak geometric mean of 1:145 on day 40. Thereafter the mean decreased to one-half by day 90, although some individual titers remained quite elevated.

*Group C*: The 8 Group C students were given 40 IU/kilo RIGH and a full course of DEV. Development of their rabies antibody titers is represented in Table 5 and Fig. 3.

Table 5. Clinical Study with Rabies Immune Globulin (Human) (RIGH)—Cutter
Volunteer Group C: RIGH—40 IU/kilo+DEV
Individual Serum Neutralizing Titers[a]

| Volunteer Designation | Days after First Injection 0 | 1 | 3 | 6 | 9 | 13 | 23 | 30 | 40 | 60 | 90 |
|---|---|---|---|---|---|---|---|---|---|---|---|
| 1. RB | <2 | 11 | 28 | 32 | 37 | 40 | 16 | 21 | 51 | 23 | 23 |
| 2. MB | <2 | 20 | 40 | 40 | 20 | 28 | 32 | 36 | 36 | 28 | 10 |
| 3. RF | <2 | 20 | 32 | 32 | 36 | 64 | 25 | 30 | 40 | 23 | 32 |
| 4. MR | <2 | 3 | 25 | 22 | 32 | 32 | 23 | 54 | 91 | 45 | 45 |
| 5. TS | <2 | 13 | 18 | 45 | 20 | 28 | 28 | 13 | 16 | 13 | 13 |
| 6. SS | <2 | 20 | 20 | 32 | 70 | 126 | 203 | 157 | 114 | 72 | — |
| 7. ST | <2 | 18 | 28 | 32 | 28 | 32 | 22 | 21 | 32 | 14 | 11 |
| 8. CT | <2 | 16 | 40 | 40 | 323 | 643 | 641 | 570 | 513 | 641 | 647 |
| Titer Ranges | <2 | 3–20 | 18–40 | 22–45 | 20–323 | 28–643 | 16–641 | 13–570 | 16–513 | 13–641 | 10–647 |
| Geometric Means | <2 | 13 | 28 | 34 | 43 | 60 | 47 | 48 | 61 | 39 | 31 |

*a* Reciprocal of dilutions.

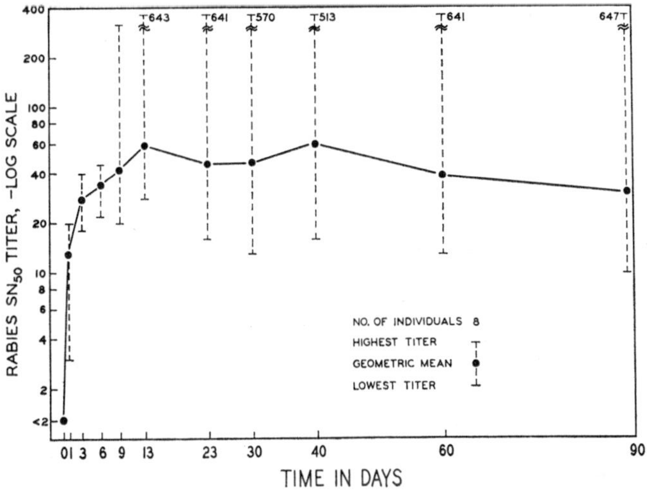


Fig. 3. Volunteer Group C: Neutralizing Antibody Response Following 40 IU/kilo Rabies Immune Globulin (Human) and a Course of Rabies Vaccine, Duck Embryo Origin.

As was the case for the two previous groups, all the students in this one also were seronegative before immunization. Twenty-four hours later, their geometric mean titer was 1:13, a level comparable to that of Group A after the same time interval. Also, as in this latter group, the geometric mean titers continued to rise until day 13. After a slight decline on days 23 and 30, the titers resumed their rise to peak on day 40, probably as a result of the booster injections on days 23 and 33. Titers became gradually lower on days 60 and 90. Although the geometric mean on day 90 was about ten times that of Group A on the same day, it was less than half the one achieved by Group B, this despite the exceedingly high antibody response of one of the 8 volunteers (CT). The consistently lower titers of 7 of the 8 participants in Group C between days 23 and 90, as compared to those of Group B subjects, suggest that a RIGH dose of 40 IU/kilo did interfere with the full expression of active immunity.

*Group D*: Students in Group D each received 20 IU/kilo RIGH and a course of DEV. Of the 9 comprising the group, one (EW) was found to have a low but definite rabies antibody titer before any immunizing injection. This individual had no history of rabies vaccination. The rapid climb of his antibody level on day 3 suggested an anamnestic response to the vaccine. The titers of this student

Table 6. Clinical Study with Rabies Immune Globulin (Human) (RIGH)—Cutter
Volunteer Group D: RIGH—20 IU/kilo+DEV
Individual Serum Neutralizing Titers[a]

| Volunteer Designation | Days after First Injection | | | | | | | | | | |
|---|---|---|---|---|---|---|---|---|---|---|---|
| | 0 | 1 | 3 | 6 | 9 | 13 | 23 | 30 | 40 | 60 | 90 |
| 1. TA | <2 | 6 | 16 | 40 | 31 | 22 | 82 | 23 | 57 | 40 | 20 |
| 2. SB | <2 | 6 | 16 | 20 | 18 | 16 | 18 | 12 | 13 | 9 | 5 |
| 3. DB | <2 | 6 | 18 | 22 | 13 | 51 | 127 | 227 | 509 | 509 | 255 |
| 4. CG | <2 | 5 | 8 | 14 | 25 | 9 | 11 | 227 | 80 | 90 | 90 |
| 5. WH | <2 | 8 | 17 | — | 32 | 18 | 24 | 72 | 90 | 90 | 40 |
| 6. GH | <2 | 9 | 11 | 10 | 18 | 28 | 100 | 162 | 456 | 361 | 516 |
| 7. LL | <2 | 4 | 9 | 16 | 8 | 18 | 20 | 23 | 90 | 72 | 32 |
| 8. BS | <2 | 6 | 22 | 20 | 30 | 71 | 76 | 229 | 203 | 161 | 93 |
| 9. EW[b] | 3.2 | 9 | 40 | 28 | 22 | 25 | 40 | 73 | 112 | 70 | 70 |
| Titer Ranges | <2 | 4–9 | 8–22 | 10–40 | 8–32 | 9–71 | 11–127 | 12–229 | 13–509 | 9–509 | 5–516 |
| Geometric Means | <2 | 6 | 14 | 19 | 20 | 23 | 41 | 74 | 111 | 94 | 59 |

*a* Reciprocal of dilutions.
*b* Omitted from titer ranges and from calculation of geometric mean titers.

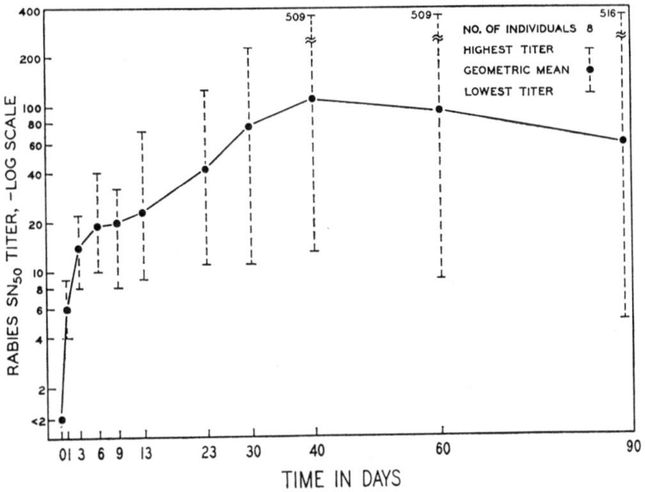


Fig. 4. Volunteer Group D: Neutralizing Antibody Response Following 20 IU/kilo Rabies Immune Globulin (Human) and a Course of Rabies Vaccine, Duck Embryo Origin.

were, therefore, omitted from the calculation of the geometric mean titers given in Table 6 and used to plot Fig. 4.

In the other 8 participants, rabies antibody was absent on the day of the first injection. It was, however, detected in all 24 hours later. Its geometric mean titer then was 1:6, about half the level noted after injection of 40 IU/kilo. The geometric mean titers rose gradully, and continued to rise through day 40 to reach a value of 1:111. This titer is almost twice that of Group C on the same day, and only slightly lower than the one achieved by Group B. The same titer relationships held through day 90, suggesting little or no interference in Group D.

*Group E*: It is evident from Table 7 and Fig. 5 that passive rabies antibody appeared late and rose slowly in this group, being barely detectable 24 hours after injection. On days 3, 6 and 9, the titers were still much lower than the corresponding values for the two preceding groups. Although rabies antibody titers continued to rise steadily through day 40, the antibody profile of this group resembled more that of Group C between days 30 and 90 than the one of Group D. The significance of this finding is uncertain, however, because of the relatively small size of the study groups.

Table 7. Clinical Study with Rabies Immune Globulin (Human) (RIGH)—Cutter
Volunteer Group E: RIGH—10 IU/kilo+DEV
Individual Serum Neutralizing Titers[a]

| Volunteer Designation | Days after First Injection | | | | | | | | | | |
|---|---|---|---|---|---|---|---|---|---|---|---|
| | 0 | 1 | 3 | 6 | 9 | 13 | 23 | 30 | 40 | 60 | 90 |
| 1. RA | <2 | 4 | 13 | 14 | 26 | 40 | 36 | 25 | 80 | 101 | 45 |
| 2. KB | <2 | 2 | 2 | 5 | 23 | 21 | 18 | 46 | 51 | 57 | 78 |
| 3. RH | <2 | <2 | 3 | 4 | 7 | 13 | 28 | 30 | 57 | 64 | 40 |
| 4. MH | <2 | <2 | 6 | 18 | 16 | 22 | 20 | 24 | 113 | 71 | 40 |
| 5. GR | <2 | <2 | 4 | 4 | 15 | 20 | 22 | 65 | 143 | 201 | 57 |
| 6. RS | <2 | 4 | 7 | 13 | 14 | 25 | 58 | 41 | 101 | 113 | 127 |
| 7. RT | <2 | 3 | 7 | 14 | 20 | 32 | 20 | 16 | 25 | 20 | 32 |
| 8. RW | <2 | 3 | 10 | 11 | 12 | 18 | 20 | 20 | 32 | 20 | 3 |
| Titer Ranges | <2 | <2–4 | 2–13 | 4–18 | 7–26 | 13–40 | 18–58 | 16–65 | 25–143 | 20–201 | 3–127 |
| Geometric Means | <2 | 2 | 6 | 9 | 16 | 23 | 26 | 30 | 65 | 63 | 37 |

*a* Reciprocal of dilutions.

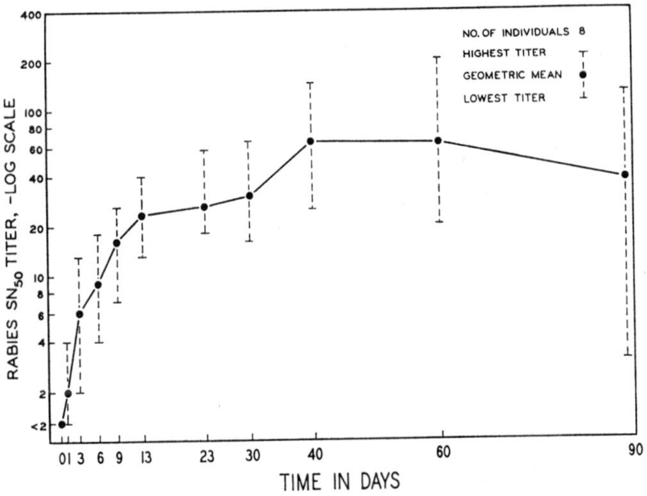


Fig. 5. Volunteer Group E: Neutralizing Antibody Response Following 10 IU/kilo Rabies Immune Globulin (Human) and a Course of Rabies Vaccine, Duck Embryo Origin.

The comparative geometric mean titers of the five study groups summarized in Table 8, and diagrammed in Fig. 6, emphasize again the apparent superiority of immunization schedule D. The seemingly lower active antibody titers achieved between days 30 and 90, in comparison with Group B, are more than compensated for by the passive immunity induced between days 0 and 9 (Fig. 6, shaded area).

Table 8. Clinical Study with Rabies Immune Globulin (Human) (RIGH)—Cutter Geometric Mean Titers[a] Achieved Following Five Different Immunization Schedules

| | | Days after First Injection | | | | | | | | | |
|---|---|---|---|---|---|---|---|---|---|---|---|
| Group | 0 | 1 | 3 | 6 | 9 | 13 | 23 | 30 | 40 | 60 | 90 |
| A | <2 | 11 | 20 | 23 | 25 | 30 | 23 | 17 | 14 | 9 | 3 |
| B | <2 | <2 | <2 | 2 | 11 | 56 | 99 | 133 | 145 | 124 | 87 |
| C | <2 | 13 | 28 | 34 | 43 | 60 | 47 | 48 | 61 | 39 | 31 |
| D | <2 | 6 | 14 | 19 | 20 | 23 | 41 | 74 | 111 | 94 | 59 |
| E | <2 | 2 | 6 | 9 | 16 | 23 | 26 | 30 | 65 | 63 | 37 |

a Reciprocal of dilutions.

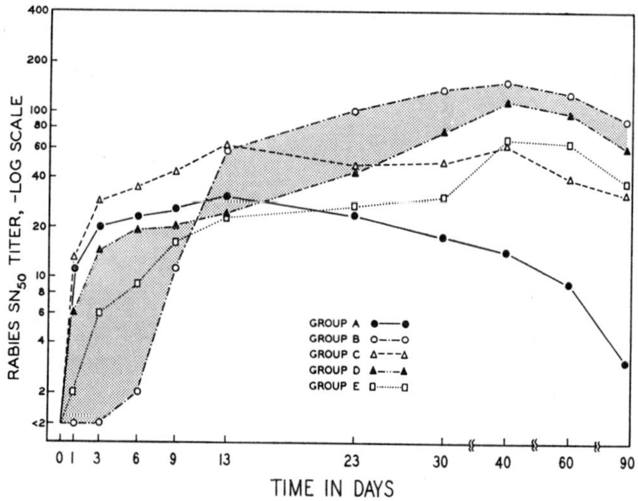


Fig. 6. Comparative Neutralizing Antibody Responses Following Five Different Schedules of Immunization against Rabies.

## SUMMARY AND CONCLUSIONS

Donors with elevated rabies antibody titers were carefully selected from among human volunteers who, because of actual past exposure to rabid animals had received one or more courses of rabies vaccine, or who, because of the nature of their occupation underwent actual preexposure immunization against rabies.

During a 7-month period, two lots of 16.5% IgG (±2.5%) Rabies Immune Globulin (Human) (RIGH) were prepared from two separate plasma pools derived from the selected donors. Concentration of the IgG was accomplished by the alcohol fractionation procedures of Cohn and associates (Cohn *et al.*, 1946; Oncley *et al.*, 1949). Besides meeting the biological and physicochemical requirements set forth for other immune serum globulin products, the two lots of RIGH had rabies antibody potencies in excess of that accepted for the currently employed antirabies serum of equine origin. The first lot contained 550 International Units of antibody per m*l* (IU/m*l*,) and the second 240 IU/m*l*.

A clinical study was carried out in five groups of volunteer students, to determine the proper dosage of RIGH when used in conjunction with Rabies Vaccine, Duck Embryo Origin (DEV). The five groups each consisted of at least 8 participants who would ordinarily have received preexposure rabies prophylaxis.

Group A received a single injection of 40 IU/kilo RIGH only. It was to serve for confirmation of the half-life of the homologous immune globulin in man. Group B received a full course of DEV only, consisting of 14 daily 1 m*l* injections, followed by 1 m*l* boosters 10 and 20 days later. All Group C, D and E participants were also given full courses of DEV but, in addition, received initially a single RIGH injection in the following dosages: Group C – 40 IU/kilo; Group D – 20 IU/kilo; and Group E – 10 IU/kilo. Serum samples for rabies antibody determination were obtained from all students on days 0, 1, 3, 6, 9, 13, 23, 30, 40, 60, 90 and 180.

Antibody testing has been completed through the 90-day samples, and the results obtained would justify the following conclusions:

1. The half-life of RIGH in Group A is in agreement with that estimated for homologous passive immune globulin in man.

2. Twenty-four hours after RIGH injection, amply detectable levels of passive rabies antibody were found in all subjects after 40 and 20 IU/kilo, but not after 10 IU/kilo. This latter dosage clearly appears to be insufficient for early protection.

3. Rabies antibody levels achieved by Groups C and D between days 30 and 90 suggest that RIGH may have interfered with optimal active antibody production when given in a dose of 40 IU/kilo and that 20 IU/kilo results in minimal, if any, interference. Under the conditions of our study, 20 IU/kilo may indeed represent an optimal dosage.

The active antibody response after a RIGH dose of 10 IU/kilo (Group E) resembled that which followed 40 IU/kilo (Group C), a rather unexpected result in view of the insufficient level of passive antibody.

## ACKNOWLEDGMENT

The authors extend their thanks to Dr. M. M. Mozen and Mr. J. Smiley for fractionation of the rabies immune plasma; to Dr. G. J. Mouratoff and Mr. W. R. Hardie for professional liaison during the clinical studies; to Mrs. Barbara Smith for able nursing assistance; to Mr. Bruce Pesis for obtaining the many blood specimens required for the study; to Mrs. Helen Hughes and Miss Mary Anderson for able record keeping and coordination of student visits; to the volunteer students of the School of Veterinary Medicine, University of California at Davis, without whose contribution these studies would not have been possible; and to Mr. A. H. Hammar, to Dr. B. I.

Wilner and to Mrs. L. I. Petter for valuable support in the preparation of this manuscript.

## REFERENCES

Anderson, G. R. and Sgouris, J. T. (1965). The preparation of rabies immune globulin and use in monkeys following virus challenge. In: International Symposium on Rabies, Talloires, Basel, Karger, p. 319 (Symposia Series in Immunobiological Standardization, Vol. I).

Archer, B. G. and Dierks, R. E. (1968). Effects of homologous or heterologous antiserum on neutralizing-antibody response to rabies vaccine. *Bull. Wld. Health Org.*, **39**, 407–417.

Atanasiu, P., Bahmanyar, M., Baltazard, M., Fox, J. P., Habel, K., Kaplan, M. M., Kissling, R. E., Komarov, A., Koprowski, H., Lépine, P., Gallardo, F. Pérez and Schaeffer, M. (1956). Rabies neutralizing antibody response to different schedules of serum and vaccine inoculations in non-exposed persons. *Bull. Wld. Health Org.*, **14**, 593–611.

Atanasiu, P., Bahmanyar, M., Baltazard, M., Fox, J. P., Habel, K., Kaplan, M. M, Kissling, R. E., Komarov, A., Koprowski, H., Lépine, P., Gallardo, F. Pérez and Schaeffer, M. (1957). Rabies neutralizing antibody response to different schedules of serum and vaccine inoculations in non-exposed persons: Part II. *Bull. Wld. Health Org.*, **17**, 911–932.

Atanasiu, P., Cannon, D. A., Dean, D. J., Fox, J. P., Habel, K., Kaplan, M. M., Kissling, R. E., Koprowski, H., Lépine, P. and Gallardo, F. Pérez. (1961). Rabies neutralizing antibody response to different schedules of serum and vaccine inoculations in non-exposed persons: Part III. *Bull. Wld. Health Org.*, **25**, 103–114.

Atanasiu, P., Dean, D. J., Habel, K., Kaplan, M. M., Koprowski, H., Lépine, P., and Serié, C. (1967). Rabies neutralizing antibody response to different schedules of serum and vaccine inoculations in non-exposed persons: Part IV. *Bull. Wld. Health Org.*, **36**, 361–365.

Babes, V. and Lepp (1889). Recherches sur la vaccination antirabique. *Ann. Inst. Pasteur*, 384–390.

Baltazard, M., Bahmanyar, M., Ghodssi, M., Sabeti, A., Gajdusek, C. and Rouzbehi, E. (1955). Essai pratique du sérum antirabique chez les mordus par loups enragés. *Bull. Wld. Health Org.*, **13**, 747–772.

Cohn, E. J., Strong, L. E., Hughes, W. L., Mulford, D. J., Ashworth, J. N., Melin, M. and Taylor, H. L. (1946). Preparation and properties of serum and plasma proteins. IV. A system for the separation into fractions of the protein and lipoprotein components of biological tissues and fluids. *J. Amer. Chem. Soc.*, **68**, 459–475.

Dean, D. J. (1966). Local wound treatment of animal bites. Proc. Nat. Rabies Symposium, Nat. Commun. Dis. Center; Atlanta, Georgia; May 5–6, pp. 85–87.

Dean, D. J., Baer, G. M. and Thompson, W. R. (1963). Studies on the local treatment of rabies-infected wounds. *Bull. Wld. Health Org.*, **28**, 477–486.

Habel,. K (1945). Seroprophylaxis in experimental rabies. *Public Health Rep.*, **60**, 545–560.

Habel, K. (1966). Post exposure vaccination and antiserum prophylaxis of rabies in man. Proc. Nat. Symposium, Nat. Commun. Dis. Center; Atlanta, Georgia; May 5–6, pp. 89–93.

Habel, K. and Koprowski, H. (1955). Laboratory data supporting the clinical trial of antirabies serum in persons bitten by a rabid wolf. *Bull. Wld. Health Org.*, **13**, 773–779.

Hosty, T. S., Kissling, R. E., Schaeffer, M., Wallace, G. A. and Dibble, E. H. (1959). Human antirabies gamma globulin. *Bull. Wld. Health Org.*, **20**, 1111–1119.

Kaplan, M. M., and Paccaud, M. F. (1963). Effectiveness of locally inoculated antirabies serum and gamma-globulin in rabies infection of mice. *Bull. Wld. Health Org.*, **28**, 495–497.

Kaplan, M. M., Cohen, D., Koprowski, H., Dean, D. and Ferrigan, L. (1962). Studies on the local treatment of wounds for the prevention of rabies. *Bull. Wld. Health Org.*, **26**, 765–775.

Koprowski, H., Van der Scheer, J. and Black, J. (1950). Use of hyperimmune antirabies serum concentrates in experimental animals. *Amer. J. Med.*, **8**, 412–420.

Koprowski, H. and Cox, H. R. (1951). Recent developments in the prophylaxis of rabies. *Amer. J. Publ. Health*, **41**, 1483–1489.

Koprowski, H. and Black, J. (1954). Studies of chick-embryo-adapted rabies virus. V. Protection of animals with antiserum and living attenuated virus after exposure to street strain of rabies virus. *J. Immunol.*, **72**, 85–93.

Kärber, G. (1931). Beitrag zur kollektiven behandlung pharmakologischer Reihenversuche. *Arch. f. exper. Pathol. u. Pharmakol.*, **162**, 480–483.

Oncley, J. L., Melin, M., Richart, D. A., Cameron, J. W. and Gross, P. W. (1949). The separation of the antibodies, iso-agglutinins, prothrombin, plasminogen and $beta_1$ lipoproteins into sub-fractions of human plasma. *J. Amer. Chem. Soc.*, **71**, 541–550.

Selimov, M., Boltucij, L., Semenova, E., Kobrinskij, G. and Zmusko, L. (1959). Results of the use of antirabies gamma globulin and vaccine in prophylaxis of rabies in the Soviet Union. *J. Hyg. Epidem., Microb. and Immunol.* (Prague), **3**, 168–180.

Spearman, C. (1908). The method of "Right and Wrong Cases" (Constant Stimuli) without Gauss' formulae. *Brit. J. of Psych.*, **2**, 227–242.

WHO Expert Committee on Rabies. (1966). WHO Technical Report Series No. 321. Fifth Report. Geneva.

Winkler, W. G., Schmidt, R. C. and Sikes, K. (1969). Evaluation of human rabies immune globulin and homologous and heterologous antibody. *J. Immunol.*, **102**, 1314–1321.

For Discussion, see page 225.

# Prophylaxis of Rabies in Rabbits by Poly I:C

BOSKO POSTIC* AND PAUL FENJE**

*University of Pittsburgh, Pittsburgh, Pennsylvania 15213
**Connaught Medical Research Laboratories, Toronto 4, Canada

The immune prophylaxis of rabies is the presently available post-exposure treatment in humans. Since this method is not effective in all cases, a search for alternate and supplementary methods is justified. The possible use of interferon in this field is yet to be defined. In Finter's hands, administered interferon failed to protect mice from infection with the CVS strain of rabies (Finter, 1967). On the other hand, Vieuchange reported that neurovaccinia virus or crude interferon partially protected rabbits against challenge with street virus (Vieuchange, 1967). Nemes and associates, from the Merck group, found moderate protection by injecting a synthetic inducer of interferon, the multistranded polyribonucleotide, polyinosinic-polycytidylic acid (poly I:C) to mice 3 hours before intraplantar injection with a low dose of the CVS virus (Nemes *et al.*, 1969; Field *et al.*, 1967). We reported recently on the protection of rabbits by poly I:C administered either before or after injection with rabies street virus (Fenje & Postic, 1970). The present report summarizes our findings using this experimental model.

The rabies street virus strain employed by us originated from an infected fox and was used in rabbits for immunization-challenge experiments in a previous study by Fenje and Pinteric (1966). The challenge consisted of an appropriate dilution of infected salivary glands of which 0.20 m*l* was injected into each of the 2 masseters of 1kg rabbits. Neutralizing antibodies and the interferon levels in rabbit sera were determined as described in previous publications (Fenje & Pinteric, 1966; Postic *et al.*, 1969).

The effect of a single intravenous injection of 1 mg of poly I:C given to rabbits challenged with 25 $LD_{50}$ of rabies virus is presented in Table 1. Significant protection could be seen at intervals before and even 6 and 24 hours after infection. The untreated rabbits died by the 16th day of infection, with the first manifestation of encephalitic symptoms appearing between the 12th and 14th days. In contrast to this effect we found that prophylaxis with poly I:C was

Table 1. Outcome of Rabies Infection in Rabbits Receiving Poly I:C[a]

| Poly I:C | Hour | Dead/Challenged | Survival (%) |
|---|---|---|---|
| None | — | 7/7 | 0 |
| 1 mg | −24 | 0/6 | 100 |
| | −3 | 0/13 | 100 |
| | 0 | 0/10 | 100 |
| | +3 | 1/10 | 100 |
| | +6 | 1/10 | 90 |
| | +24 | 5/15 | 66 |

[a] Each 1 kg rabbit received a single intravenous injection of polyI:C at the indicated hour before (−) or after (+) an intrammasseteric injection of 25 $LD_{50}$ of street rabies virus; animals were observed for 5 weeks.

less protectivc whcn a highcr challcngc dosc amounting to 125 rabbit $LD_{50}$ was used. The results of this experiment are summarized in Table 2. Protection was seen only when the treatment and the challenge with virus were administered concurrently (0 hour), as measured by the majority of rabbits surviving the challenge. In respect to the prolonged incubation we observed borderline protection when treatment was given at minus 3 days, plus 4 hours and plus 24 hours.

Table 2. Influence of Time of Prophylaxis on Rabies in Rabbits after 125 $LD_{50}$ of Virus[a]

| Poly I:C | | Dead/ Challenged | Survival % | Incuvation (Median Day) |
|---|---|---|---|---|
| Dose | Time Given | | | |
| None | — | 4/4 | 0 | 11 |
| 1 mg/kg | −7 days | 7/7 | 0 | 12 |
| | −5 days | 8/8 | 0 | 13 |
| | −3 | 5/6 | 17 | 16 |
| | 0 hour | 2/6 | 67 | 31 |
| | +4 hours | 5/7 | 29 | 15 |
| | +24 hours | 7/8 | 12 | 14 |
| | +3 days | 6/6 | 0 | 12 |

[a] Same as Table 1 (except for the virus inoculum).

To improve the protection by poly I:C, combined prophylaxis was attempted by initiating daily injections with Semple vaccine at 24 hours postinfection with 125 $LD_{50}$ of virus. No improvement over the effect of poly I:C alone was noted, although there was evidence of accentuation of neutralizing antibodies by the vaccine (Table 3).

The relationship of the dose of polyI: C given to rabbits challenged with 125, 625 and 3,125 $LD_{50}$ of rabies virus is shown in Table 4. Both treatment and challenge were administered at the same time (0

Table 3. Effect of Poly I:C and Vaccine 24 Hours after 125 $LD_{50}$ of Rabies Virus

| Postexposure[a] Treatment | Neutralizing[b] Antibody (day 7) | Dead Challenged (day 28) | Median Incubation (day) |
|---|---|---|---|
| None | — | 4/4 | 11 |
| Poly I:C Alone | 15 | 7/8 | 14 |
| Poly I:C and Semple Vaccine | 125 | 6/7 | 14 |

*a* Poly I:C (1 mg/kg) was given intravenously, Semple vaccine was injected subcutaneously in 14 daily doses.

*b* Determined in neutralization tests in mice against 100 $LD_{50}$ of CVS strain (5) and listed as reciprocals of serum dilutions.

— test not done

Table 4. Relationship of Dose of Poly I:C to the Protection of Rabbits against Rabies Infection[a]

| Poly I:C mg/kg | Dead/Challenged Rabbits, Rabies Virus $LD_{50}$: 125 | 625 | 3,125 |
|---|---|---|---|
| None | 4/4 | 4/4 | 4/4 |
| 1.0 | 2/6 | 1/6 | 5/8 |
| 0.2 | 4/8 | — | — |
| 0.04 | 3/8 | — | — |

*a* Poly I:C given I.V. to 1 kg rabbits just before (0 hour) intramasseteric injection of street virus.

— test not done

hour). It can be seen that 1 mg/kg was protective against virus challenge exceeding 625 $LD_{50}$. We found also that 0.2 and 0.04 mg/kg offered protection against 125 $LD_{50}$.

In protection experiments, rabbits received a single intravenous injection of 1 mg/kg of poly I:C before or after infection. To monitor interferon levels in sera, four rabbits were bled 2 hours following the administration of poly I:C—the time when the appearance of peak titers may be expected. Serum interferon was determined by a plaque inhibition assay using primary rabbit kidney cells and vesicular stomatitis virus.

Table 5 lists the results of interferon assays of 4 samples taken from uninfected rabbits injected with poly I:C 2 hours previously, showing the high inhibitory titers expressed as reciprocals of serum dilutions in homologous (rabbit) cells, and the absence of the inhibition in heterologous cells. The digestion of sera with trypsin and ribonuclease was done according to the procedure of Ho and Ke (1970) in order to differentiate the interferon activity from residual poly I:C. Under the conditions described in this table, interferon is destroyed by trypsin, but not by ribonuclease. The results show that the serum samples contained high levels of rabbit interferon, with detectable traces of poly I:C.

Table 5. Virus Inhibitory Activity of Rabbit Sera Following Intravenous Administration of Poly I:C[a]

| Treatment of Samples | Individual Inhibitory Titers ×100 | |
|---|---|---|
| | Cell Culture | |
| | Rabbit Kidney | Chicken Embryo |
| None | 1500, 3100, 1000, 650 | <1. <1, <1, <1 |
| Crystalline Trypsin (0.1%) | <2, <2, <2, <2 | not done |
| RNA-ase (50. μg/ml) | 1500, 3100, 1000, 650 | not done |

a Serum samples of four 1 kg rabbits bled 2 hours following the administration of 1 mg poly I:C. Sera were treated by incubation at 37° for 1 hour. Antiviral effect was assayed on monolayers; titers represent reciprocals of dilutions inhibiting 50% of VSV plaques.

The possibility that the protected rabbits became immune was examined in the following manner. Rabbits receiving poly I:C and surviving rabies infection were observed for 5 weeks and bled on 3 different occasions. Table 6 shows the titers of neutralizing antibody in their sera on day 1, 16, and 35 after first infection. At both of the latter points a significant titer was demonstrated. Following the last

Table 6. Immunity of Rabbits Surviving Rabies Infection to Repeated Challenge

| Rabbit Group[a] | Median Neutralizing Antibody Titers of Sera[b] | | | Dead/Challenged |
|---|---|---|---|---|
| | Day after 1st Infection | | | 2nd Infection |
| | 1 | 16 | 35 | |
| Poly I:C on Day 0 | <1:5 | 1:190 | 1:73 | 0/58 |
| Controls | <1:5 | (All died) | | 8/8 |

a Survivors from the treated group were rechallenged 35 days after injection with 25 $LD_{50}$ of virus, and were observed for another 5 weeks.

b Sera from groups of 5 rabbits were pooled; titers refer to the medians of 6 such pools; for method see Table 3.

bleeding on the 35th day, the rabbits were again challenged with 25 $LD_{50}$ of rabies virus. All of the rabbits surviving the first infection survived this challenge also. Controls represented by previously uninoculated rabbits showed no rabies neutralizing activity in their sera (titers<1:5) and succumbed uniformly. Thus, resistance of the survivors to the repeated challenge was associated with high levels of rabies virus neutralizing antibody.

Our data show that 1) 1 mg/kg of poly I:C given within 24 hours either before or after injection with 25 $LD_{50}$ or rabies virus protected a large proportion of rabbits, and 2) the animals become immunized and resisted a repeated challenge. We suggest that the interferon stimulated by poly I:C was protective through the suppression of virus replication possibly before the rabies infection became localized in the cells of the central nervous system. This impression is supported by the critical time of stimulation, as shown by the experiment using 125 $LD_{50}$ as challenge (Table 2), when only the concurrent injection of virus and poly I:C resulted in the survival of the majority of rabbits. Petrovic and Timm reisolated the CVS virus following intraplantar infection of hamsters from the moment of inoculation throughout the incubation lasting for 6 days (Petrovic & Timm, 1969). They recovered the highest concentration of virus from the plantar site immediately following infection, but the rather long persistence of infectivity may reflect limited extraneural viral replication. If this held true, the prospects for the postexposure prophylaxis of this disease by interferon would appear more promising. Recently, Janis and Habel communicated a somewhat improved protection of rabbits by injecting poly I:C 3 hours after street virus into the same leg muscle rather than the opposite leg. (Janis & Habel, 1970).

The infection model used by us may be pertinent to rabies in man. Street virus from a rabid animal was inoculated intramuscularly, simulating the natural transmission. Unlike the prophylaxis in humans, postexposure vaccination of rabbits is not protective, due to a shorter incubation period, reflecting the greater virulence of rabies virus for this animal host. The rabbit is more reactive to the interferon-stimulating effect of poly I:C than appears to be the case with man. Even with these reservations, our observations indicate a new approach to the incubationary treatment of rabies.

## SUMMARY

Protection of rabbits from rabies was attempted by prophylactic treatment with an inducer of interferon, the polyinosinic-polycytidylic acid complex, poly I:C. Street virus originated from a rabid fox salivary gland suspension and was injected appropriately diluted into the masseters of rabbits. The following observations were made. 1) Poly I:C at 1 mg/kg was protective when administered intravenously within 24 hours before or after 25 rabbit $LD_{50}$ of virus. It was protective partially against virus challenge consisting of 125, 625, and 3125 $LD_{50}$. However, with the high challenge consisting of 125 rabbit $LD_{50}$ of rabies virus, protection resulted only when the treatment was administered concurrently with the injection of virus and not 4 and 24 hours postinfection. 2) When 25 $LD_{50}$ of virus and poly I:C were injected simultaneously, 0.2 and 0.04 mg/kg offered partial protection. 3) Protected rabbits developed neutralizing antibodies and resisted a repeated challenge. 4) Twenty-four hours after the rabbits were infected with 125 $LD_{50}$ of virus, prophylaxis was attempted by a course of Semple vaccine initiated concurrently with the administration of poly I:C. No appreciable enhancement of the resistance of animals was noted despite higher levels of neutralizing antibodies in the serum. 5) Poly I:C quickly stimulated high levels of serum interferon, suggesting that it suppressed the replication of rabies virus before it became fixed in the cells of the nervous system, and was thus instrumental in protecting from rabies.

## ACKNOWLEDGMENTS

This work was supported in part by a grant from the U.S. National Institute of Health (AI—02953). We thank Drs. Monto Ho and William McD. Hammon of the University of Pittsburgh for their support and discussion of this work, Professor Y. Nagano of Tokyo, Japan, for his interest and Mr. V. Boggs of Connaught Laboratories for excellent technical assistance.

## REFERENCES

Fenje, P. and Pinteric, L. (1966). Potentiation of tissue culture rabies vaccine by adjurants. *Amer. J. Pub. Health*, **56**, 2106–2112.

Fenje, P. and Postic, B. (1970). Protection of rabbits against experimental rabies by poly I. poly C. *Nature*, **226**, 171–172.

Field, A. K., A. A. Tytell, G. P. Lampson and Hilleman, M. R. (1967). Inducers of interferon and host resistance. II. Multistranded synthetic polynucleotide complexes. *Proc. Nat. Acad. Sci. U.S.A.*, **58**, 1004–1010.

Finter, N. B. (1967). Of mice and men: studies with interferon. From Ciba foundation symposium on interferon, edited by G. E. W. Wolstenholme and Maeve O'Connor, pp. 204–215, J. & A. Churchill, London.

Ho, M. and Ke, Y. H. (1970). The mechanism of stimulation of interferon production by a complexed polyribonucleotide. *Virology*, **40**, 693–702.

Janis, B. and Habel, K. (1970). Polyriboinosinic and polyribocytidylic acid polymer (poly I:C) in rabies prophylaxis. *Federation Proceedings Abstracts 1970*, 29, 2:636.

Nemes, M. M., A. T. Tytell, G. P. Lampson, A. K. Field and Hilleman, M. R. (1969). Inducers of interferon and host resistance. VI. Antiviral Efficacy of poly I:C in animal models. *Proc. Soc. Exptl. Biol. and Med. U.S A.*, **132**, 776–783.

Petrovic, M. and Timm, H. (1969). Experimenteller beitrag zur pathogenese der tollwut. Zentralblatt für Bakteriologie, Parasitenkunde, *Infekionskrankheiten und Hygiene,* **211**, 149–161.

Postic, B., C. J. Schleupner, J. A. Armstrong and Ho, M. (1969). Two variants of Sindbis virus which differ in interferon induction and serum clearance. I. The phenomenon. *J. of Infect Dis.*, **120**, 339–347.

Vieuchange, J. (1967). Interférence entre le virus vaccinal et le virus rabique; rôle éventuel d'un interféron. *Archiv für die gesamte virusforschung*, **22**, 87–96.

For Discussion, see page 225.

# Discussion*

DAVENPORT: I would like to ask Dr. Koprowski a question: In your opinion, what is currently the ideal post-exposure prophylactic regimen for rabies?

KOPROWSKI: To tell you the truth, none.

DAVENPORT: What is the optimum or the best available? What would you do if you were bitten by a rabid dog?

KOPROWSKI: I would immunize myself before I was bitten. Seriously, if that were impossible, post-exposure treatment offers a good possibility of immunization. Regardless of the quality of vaccine used, a person immunized before exposure could consider himself protected. The problem lies with post-exposure immunization. It is difficult to recommend anything, because the quality of post-exposure vaccines is very poor. I have no doubt that the brain tissue vaccine used in the past causes a much higher antibody titer than does the duck embryo vaccine. I have seen too many failures of duck embryo vaccine administered post-exposure to be comfortable with its use.

Also, the combined use of immune serum and vaccine raises two problems: The serum may contain lytic antibody, which could harm the exposed person. This can be avoided by absorbing the antibody out of the serum. The second problem involves planning the serum regimen so as not to inhibit active antibody response. My recommendation is that, following a severe bite from an animal known to be rabid, one should administer the prescribed dose of serum, having first removed the lytic antibody, and follow that by an intensive course of vaccine therapy with many repeated booster injections so as to be sure of getting active immunity following passive immunization.

DAVENPORT: In the real world, those of us who are asked to handle or advise on the management of some of these problems have no

* This Discussion refers to the reports by Nomura, Koprowski, Kitamoto *et al.*, Nagano, Nomura *et al.*, Shiraki, Cabasso *et al.* and Postic *et al.*

way of knowing whether there is lytic antibody in materials furnished for the treatment of patients. As I understand it, it is not a standard procedure to test such antibody at this time.

KOPROWSKI: This procedure is not standard, though it could be rendered standard with little difficulty. Human serum may have lytic antibody; certainly horse serum does. If you absorb the antibody out of the serum using cells which have membrane rabies antigen, you would be left with all of the other antibodies minus lytic antibody. At present, this is not a recommended procedure; I only mentioned it for purposes of discussion.

Another point I would emphasize is the importance of thorough cleansing of the wound following exposure. Thorough cleansing would be followed by inoculation with serum and then with a potent rabies vaccine. In one slide from my talk, I showed the effects of treating rabbits with immune serum followed by vaccine administration 15 days later. A good antibody response was achieved by delaying vaccination for 15 days. In actual practice, however, you cannot afford a 15-day delay. All you can do is start treatment immediately, followed by booster inoculations 20, 25 and 30 days later, and hope that you will not get passive immunity interfering with active immunity.

NAGANO: In reply to Dr. Davenport's question I would like to say that the UV inactivated vaccine is the only one which has actually been shown to be more effective than the classical Pasteur vaccine in the post-exposure treatment of human subjects.

The question of the combination of vaccine and serum has been discussed in Dr. Koprowski's and Dr. Cabasso's lectures.

In an experiment carried out in our laboratory (Y. KONISHI, *Virus*, **8**, 40, 1958), groups of mice received various doses of UV inactivated vaccine and were given various doses of rabbit antiserum at different intervals. The titer of circulating neutralizing antibodies and the resistance to challenge were estimated. Vaccine and immune serum have been found to reciprocally suppress, more or less, their effects in every combination. It is natural that an antigen and corresponding antibody would interfere with each other.

Several years ago, the combined use of vaccine and serum was performed in Iran and it was said then that the combination was better than vaccine alone. But this was probably because the antigenicity of the vaccine used at the time was too poor to interfere with the effect of the immune serum. Unfortunately, injection of serum alone was not done.

KOPROWSKI: I will reply to Dr. Nagano by discussing the trials in Iran. The Fermi vaccine, used in these trials, is a powerfully antigenic vaccine, containing living virus at a titer of $10^{-2}$ or $10^{-3}$ $LD_{50}$. Following 21 injections of vaccine alone, which was the prescribed treatment in Iran, three out of five persons died. When 21 infections of the vaccine were combined with immune serum, only 1 out of 12 persons died. Since this was an actual situation and not an experiment, serum alone could not be administered. We feel that immune serum should be included with vaccine in rabies virus prophylaxis. Vaccines containing living virus have been severly condemned as a result of the unfortunate occurrence in Fortaleza, Brazil, where it was discovered that fixed virus can be lethal for man. A vaccine was produced which had a titer of $10^5$ in mice and which killed human beings who were treated with it.

I should also like to mention ultraviolet-irradiated vaccine, which you seem to favor. If UV-irradiated vaccine proves effective and safe, I think it could be used. It would be better than duck embryo vaccine, but probably not superior to Fermi or Semple vaccine. However, we should note a strange incident which occurred in South America, particularly Venezuela. Following use of UV-irradiated suckling mouse brain vaccine, 37 persons exhibited the Landry-Guillain-Barré syndrome. The cause of this paralysis is still unknown. It was proposed that demyelination occurred following injection of the vaccine, but theoretically, the suckling mouse brain vaccine should have less myelin than the adult vaccine. Any attempts to reproduce the disease in animals failed. There was not enough myelin in the incriminated vaccine lots to cause allergic encephalitis in guinea pigs, so it is not known whether there was enough to cause demyelination in man. The rabies virus was probably killed by UV-irradiation; there is the remote possibility that another agent more resistant to UV-irradiation survived, and caused the Landry-Guillain-Barré syndrome.

NAGANO: The vaccine used was so poor in potency that 3 out of 5 vaccinees died. So the vaccine did not do much to suppress the effect of immune serum. If a group had been treated with immune serum alone, the result could have been as follows:

| | |
|---|---|
| Vaccine alone | 3/5 |
| Vaccine+Serum | 1/12 |
| Serum alone | 0/12 |

Conversely, a poor serum combined with a highly potent vaccine has an effect about the same as vaccine alone.

KOPROWSKI: Mortality from rabies among non-treated people exposed to the bite of the same wolf in Iran was 47%. In other studies in Iran, 40% mortality was observed during years of observation among people who received 21 injections of Fermi vaccine. It is extremely difficult to evaluate any vaccine under such conditions. We cannot say what would happen in a comparative evaluation of duck embryo vaccine with any other vaccine; it may be that no vaccine will work. But to return to Dr. Nagano, and his data on serum alone, though we do not have any results from studies in Iran, we do have results from Dr. Sikes's post-exposure treatment of monkeys:

| | |
|---|---|
| vaccine alone | 1/8 |
| vaccine+immune serum | 1/8, 1/8 |
| immune serum alone | 5/8, 7/8 |

If I were to predict results, I would probably change Dr. Nagano's tentative results to a 11/12 ratio for the group receiving serum and vaccine.

HAMMON: I am a little bit disturbed at some of the remarks that have been made about the vaccines that are used today and their comparative evaluations. I think it would be rather a shame if this conference went on record with some of these statements that have been made without better supporting evidence. There have been statements made to the effect that this is a vaccine that has some advantages as well as disadvantages. I think to leave the impression that the duck embryo vaccine, which I believe is betapropiolactone inactivated, is no good and has been proved in human usage to be ineffective is not a scientific fact. I don't know of any comparative studies proving that there are a greater number of failures of the duck embryo vaccine than there are of the central nervous system vaccine, Semple type. We do know that by the Habel mouse test, which is the test that is used in the United States to evaluate the potency of vaccines, that the duck embryo vaccine runs on an average a little lower than the mouse embryo vaccine and that by injections in man; the neutralizing antibody response is frequently and perhaps usually a little lower than with the central nervous system vaccine. We also know that one can give more vaccine and that less danger is encountered by the person receiving this series of vaccinations with the duck embryo vaccine. Thus, the series can be made longer and the amount given can be made larger. Without any direct evidence I do not think we should go away from here with the idea that one vaccine is no good, particularly when there hasn't been any kind of a scientific trial. Before we had the duck embryo vaccine there were many indications in the literature and from reports that the central nervous system Semple type vaccine failed. The failures were usually with the short incubation period onset of disease, less than 30 days. We have indications in the literature now of a number of failures of the duck embryo vaccine and again, practically all of these are in short incubation period rabies. So I'm bothered by the fact that one vaccine is being said to be much less effective or no good at all in comparison to another when we do not have any more evidence than we do now. Excuse my long speech but to me a scientific discussion should not include these frank statements of comparison without better evidence than we have.

LENNETTE: At this point I wish to exercise the prerogative of the chair to make a couple of comments. First, I do not believe the situation which you have painted is quite as grim or as dismal as you make it, or at least as one might infer from your commentary. You may have gathered an impression which I did not, since, so far as I am aware, there have been no unequivocal statements that the duck embryo vaccine is without value. In my own case, my comment in relation to Keith Sikes's statement about the vaccine being safe, to wit "so is water" was in no sense an implication that the vaccine is valueless, but the point at issue is that of potency. The salient point with respect to any rabies vaccine is how well it meets the minimum requirements for potency and how much potency exists above that minimal level, i.e., what is the stability and the shelf life of the vaccine. This, in my estimate, was the focus of the discussion which centered around the matter of potency and its maintenance. Secondly, failures have been ascribed to all of the vaccines in current or recent use and a comparative evaluation such as you suggest, while an ideal, would probably be impossible ever to carry out.

SIKES: I would also like to clear some confusion that is coming out of the meeting about the possible misconception of what we know about duck embryo vaccine and the Semple vaccine used in the United States. The situation is that the duck embryo vaccine does have to pass the same potency test that the nervous tissue vaccine has to pass. Indeed, there is not a great deal of difference in the antigenic values of the two. On the average, the duck embryo vaccine will run between 0.3 antigenic value and 1. With the nervous tissue vaccine, Semple type which is used in the United States, it would usually run around 1, sometimes as low as 0.5. So there is not a great deal of difference as measured in the mice. As far as the antibody response in man is concerned, there is a quicker antibody response with duck embryo but not quite as high response, on the average. Further, the data of failures of the two vaccines—and one must look since 1957 when duck embryo became available—show the rates to be almost the same; if anything the rate is a little higher in failures with the nervous tissue vaccine. But according to our data, that does not mean there is any significant difference in the two. The neuroparalysis associated with Semple vaccine is something not to overlook. Indeed, the rate of about one in 8,000 is exhibited in the United States and this often or sometimes involves death caused by the vaccine. We have had no deaths associated with the reaction of the duck embryo vaccine. Adding all of this up, we have made the statement to the Public Health Service Advisory Committee on Immunization Practices that the local wound treatment plus the serum plus the vaccine, at least 14 to 21 daily doses plus at least 2 booster doses are recommended. The 2 booster doses given at 10 and 20 days following the last dose of vaccine. One can argue with these potency values and we wish we had better vaccines but we must live with what we have for at least several years; maybe one more year, as Dr. Koprowski suggests but perhaps longer than that.

TIERKEL: I think we are shedding a little more light on what Dr. Davenport has called "real life". There is no question that we want and need more antigenic vaccines. These are still on the work bench and everyone hopes of course, that they will come through one day. I would like to interpose one thought with regard to the practice of specific immunization against rabies. There are more and more people, particularly in the United States, who are undergoing the pre-exposure series of immunization for one reason or another. These, to begin with, were in the domestic "high risk" groups such as animal handlers, veterinarians and so on, and it began to expand into other population groups such as people who go overseas. Immunization has become a routine practice for our Peace Corps volunteers who go into areas where there is an extremely high incidence of rabies and now the State Department has beung this as routine practice for all of its embassy and A.I.D. personnel who work overseas. There is thus a growing number of people who are undergoing the pre-exposure series. The great majority of there are responding as shown by the SN antibody tests which are being carried out. Dr. Sikes mentioned yesterday that it is very close to 100% as far as detectable antibody is concerned. There is, of course, degradation of the antibody over the years, but as Dr. Sikes also pointed out, a booster at any point in time creates an immediate and robust response in antibody. I think this is a very important point considering that when any one of this population group is indeed exposed, one should be extremely careful not to interpose the use of immune serum and spoil the chances for an active booster response. I firmly believe that if there is a history of previous successful immunization, whether it is pre-exposure series or whether it was a post-exposure series sometime in the history of the person, a potent vaccine should be used immediately for boosting the antibody level of this person without the interposition of immune serum, no matter how serious the exposure.

LENNETTE: You made one important statement, Dr. Tierkel. You said that the antibody response was 100% following the use.

TIERKEL: I said nearly. In 4 separate study groups, using 1 m*l* of vaccine subcutaneously in a pre-exposure series of 3 or 4 inoculations, we had positive responses in 86%, 94%, 95% and 90% of each respective group.

LENNETTE: Very well, I stand corrected. However, the important point is whether the antibody response you mentioned occurs after one course of inoculations or after two. If we are talking about pre-exposure prophylaxis, the number of courses is not a critical factor. Thus, after one course of vaccine administration, an antibody titration can be done. If the individual has demonstrable humoral antibody, nothing further need be done; however, if antibody is not demonstrable, then a second course of vaccine injections is indicated. However, in the case of post-exposure situations, one is dealing with an entirely different matter. Dr. Sikes, would you care to clarify these points?

SIKES: Yes, the data that we have been putting together and the point that I was trying to make yesterday concerned these data. You can count on seroconversion in roughly 80% of those who get the 2 doses a month apart followed by a booster 3 months later; 80% of those people would get a detectable titer. It may not be high but we can detect it and we have done many thousands of these. So if the person needs to get the immunization sooner he can get the alternate schedule and have three injections a week apart and a booster 3 months later; this also will get about 80% seroconversion. This occurs if you bleed the person roughly one month after the last injection. If the person's titer results show no detectable antibody, he will take an additional booster. That means that 50% of the remaining 20%, or 10% more, will give up to 90% of the total people vaccinated to get rabies antibody. Ultimately we recommend at least two more of these boosters then making sure that as many as possible can get the titer. We think about 95% will ultimately get a titer like this. If those people are then exposed, they get the 1–5 daily injections plus a booster 20 days later. If the person in that 5% group still does not respond, the only choice is to give serum plus vaccine to that person, following exposure. Those points were made clearly in committee by the United States Public Health Service Advisory Committee on Immunization Practices and those are the recommendations.

HUMPHREY: I want to add that in treatment of an exposed individual, there is one procedure that can be carried out which is not often remembered or emphasized enough, and that is good local treatment. Soap and water or detergent with thorough swabbing or flushing have been shown to help considerably and the earlier done, the better. Sometimes we rush to emphasize specific systemic treatment, but I still believe that thorough swabbing and flushing of the bite wound is the first thing that should be done and can be very beneficial. Early and efficient local treatment may mean the difference between success and failure even when combined with adequate systematic treatment.

KITAOKA: On the basis of results on serum therapy in rabbits infected by the sciatic nerve route (Matsui, *Niigata Med. J.*, **64**, 522, 1950) I have always recommended the cleaning of the local lesion and injection of immune serum in man, except if prepositive, immediately after being bitten by a rabid animals. I have no experience of a marked interference in the combined use of serum and vaccine in rabies vaccination as observed in the cases of measles and Japanese encephalitis vaccines (Mitamura *et al.*, Nihonigaku Kenkohoken, No. 3208, 737, 1940).

DAVENPORT: I wish to ask Dr. Cabasso what the relationship is between the doses of human serum which he used in the experiments he showed and the amounts used in prophylaxis after exposure. In other words, how do these two compare? You showed a regimen which you felt was quite acceptable. How does that amount compare to the amount used in post-exposure?

CABASSO: The dosage of horse serum recommended today is 40 International units (I.U.) of horse serum antibody per kilo, plus the series of vaccine injection. However, we have to take into consideration that horse serum has a half-life of only 9 days, whereas homologous human antibody would have a half-life of 21 days. We feel, therefore, that 40 I.U. of human antibody may perhaps act as a much higher dose of horse antibody, and may perhaps also interfere. Our data showed that there may be some interference with 40 I.U. and less interference with 20.

KOPROWSKI: In our discussions of duck embryo, Semple or other vaccines, no one has condemned one vaccine as compared to any other. All that was said was that probably the present treatment is inadequate because of low antigenicity of existing vaccines. Neutralizing antibody responses following duck embryo vaccination, range from 50% to 90%. The antibody levels are low—in the range of 1–10, to 1–30 dilutions of serum. I do not know whether the neutralizing antibody is the protective antibody, but if any conclusion can be drawn from the post-exposure trials in monkeys, it is that it is necessary to achieve a high antibody response. Those animals which died, had antibody levels within the lower range on the third day after exposure.

We sorely need a much better vaccine. We must, however, deal also with the problem of stability. A lot of duck embryo vaccine which passes the NIH potency test when first produced may not pass the test at a later time. Our aim is to improve the quality of the vaccine and the method of treatment as well.

NAGANO: I have two comments on Dr. Postic's paper. First, this work gives us much hope that interferon may be effective in the post-exposure prophylaxis of rabies. I hope Dr. Postic will soon develop a procedure available for humans. One other point concerns the pathogenesis of rabies. Production of interferon begins several hours after poly I:C is injected, in other words, in the earlier stage of the incubation period of the rabies virus. According to Dr. Postic's data, interferon exerts its effect in this early stage. It is well known that interferon does not inactivate a free virion but only interferes with its intracellular replication. Considering this fact on the one hand, and the paper presented by Dr. Richard Johnson, which suggests that the rabies virus may be passing through peripheral nerves, on the other, Dr. Postic's paper seems to support the possibility that the rabies virus particle is not simply travelling through peripheral nerves but is replicating before it arrives at the central nervous system.

JOHNSON, R. T.: Dr. Postic and I have been in correspondence about this very subject.

Poly I : C was used on the assumption that there was extraneural replication, since interferon is largely excluded from the central nervous system. Yet we have no definitive evidence of replication in the muscle or in the peripheral nerve. An interesting point, however, in the studies of Yamamoto and Shiraki, Otani, and of my own, is that the initial antigen development was not in the central nervous system per se but in the afferent dorsal root ganglia. The dorsal root ganglia in rabbits and guinea pigs, the only two animals on which we have data, is permeable to large molecular weight dyes and proteins. They are external to the blood-brain barrier. Therefore, circulating interferon which would be excluded from the nervous system would have ready access to these ganglia. It is therefore not necessary to postulate extraneural replication, for the effect of Poly I : C. It could occur at a ganglia level. As I mentioned yesterday, replication in the ganglia seemed, in all of our initial studies, a very inconsequential point. Explaining the efficacy of Poly I:C, this may be an important point. This might also be relevant to the use of immune serum, since, I believe the use of systemic immune serum is as effective, if not more so, than the local use of immune sera. If one finds that systemic immune sera are as effective, they must be acting at some site other than at the site of inoculation.

HAMMON: To add a little bit, we know of course that Poly I:C is not quite ready for use in man by a parenteral rot. If and when Poly I:C or something that is equally effective becomes available, I think this will offer a rather exciting prospect of a very effective new tool in the control of post-exposure rabies. The work that Dr. Postic and Dr. Fenje did with the rabbits obviously cannot be translated directly into what is going to happen in man. There has been some work to indicate that it is not nearly as effective in the mouse. Is the mouse or the rabbit closer to man? We do not know. And until this has been tried in primates and man, we cannot do very much in the way of guessing how effective it will be, but there are several suggestions of its advantages in man. For one thing the incubation period is considerably longer in man and therefore a small dose of Poly-I:C could be given anywhere up to 12 or 24 hours in man. It is quite possible that the delay in time could be much greater, and it would still be effective. And if the virus has to get to the dorsal ganglia before the critical effect takes place, there may be lots of time to give Poly I:C. The work, of course, has to be done in other animals and Dr. Postic and Dr. Fenje are planning and going ahead with this in other animals, dogs and monkeys, and I am sure that others will as well. But it is a good lead and I am quite hopeful that Poly I:C can be used in this way; I can see no reason personally why it can not be combined with vaccine or even combined with serum to provide one other tool—perhaps one of great advantage in treating post-exposure rabies.

# General Epizootiology of Rabies

HARALD NORLIN JOHNSON

*Viral and Rickettsial Disease Laboratory, California State Department of Public Health, Berkeley, California 94704*

There are two epidemiological types of rabies, the natural infection as it occurs in wild animals and the aberrant type which is maintained in domestic dogs. Dogs revert easily to a semiwild or scavenger existence and the number of stray dogs increases rapidly in any community unless an organized effort is made to collect and destroy them. The propagation of rabies in dogs is dependent on the presence of a large population of owned and ownerless dogs running at large in urban communities. It has been difficult to enforce dog control regulations such as leashing and muzzling because dogs kept about human habitation for protection are not effective watch dogs unless they are allowed to run at large. In view of the present high population of dogs and the extensive epizootic of rabies in wildlife, dog rabies would be a serious public health problem if we did not have an effective rabies vaccine for dogs.

The early history of rabies in Europe and Asia tells us that the disease appeared from time to time among foxes and wolves in certain regions. Such foci served as starting points for recurrent migrating epizootics of fox rabies. The disease was limited by certain geographical barriers, such as mountain ranges and water, as well as by the abundance and distribution of suitable hosts capable of spreading the infection. Once established in domestic dogs, these limiting factors were much less effective as dogs could travel with their masters over great distances and so introduce the disease into areas far removed from the original source of the infection. Rabies in wolves, foxes and jackals, has been known since ancient times but epizootics of rabies in domestic dogs were not recorded until the middle of the 18th century. Dog rabies reached its greatest intensity in the Old World during the first half of the 19th century.

The current prevalence of rabies in wildlife in many parts of the world is an example of the cyclical character of diseases derived from wildlife. About 100 years ago there was a similar epizootic of rabies. During such epizootics a great variety of wild animals are infected and the source of the disease in nature becomes obscured. We can learn much about the ecology of the virus by reviewing reports of sporadic cases of rabies in man and domestic animals resulting from the bite of wild animals. In this type of situation we can ascertain the various species and relative numbers of each species of animal living in the same area and we can assume that one of these is the reservoir host of the infection.

In reviewing the literature we find that the middle of the 19th century marks the beginning of a period of widespread rabies in wildlife in different parts of the world. For example, in 1858, a 10-year-old girl died of rabies in Greenville, Texas, after she had been bitten by a spotted skunk, *Spilogale putorius*, at night while sleeping (DeJernett, 1859). It was noted that over a period of 6 years there had been a total of 4 cases of human rabies from the bite of this animal. Only one dog was known to have developed rabies during the same period and there were no cases of rabies in man from dog bite exposure. During the same year a man died of rabies in Tanjore, India, after he was attacked and bitten in daytime by a mongoose (Moodelly, 1859). In 1859 there was an epizootic of rabies in foxes and eskimo dogs in Greenland (Colan, 1881). In each of these regions there followed a period of enzootic rabies in wildlife. There were 17 human cases of rabies from skunk bite in western Kansas during the period 1866–1876 (Roberts, 1884). Ten persons died of rabies from skunk bite in Arizona during the period 1907–1910 (Yount, 1910). The occurrence of sporadic cases of rabies in man from skunk bite in regions where there was no evidence of enzootic rabies in dogs or wild canines gives us information about the presence of a reservoir host system in southwestern United States and that the infection can be maintained in skunks or some animal that is associated with them. There is a tradition in western United States that the spotted skunk is a carrier of rabies and this animal is known as the "phobey cat," because many persons were known to have died of hydrophobia following the bite of this animal during the period 1850–1910. The earliest reference to skunk rabies in North America is that of Duhaut-Cilly who, when he visited Lower California in 1826, noted that the people there told him that skunks sometimes entered houses and bit people and gave them hydrophobia (Nelson, 1918).

The current epizootic of rabies in wildlife in North America began in 1940 when rabies appeared in epizootic proportions in foxes in Georgia (Johnson, 1945). During the next ten years other epizootics of fox rabies developed in southern and eastern United States where foxes were abundant. There was evidence of rapid dieoffs of foxes in any one local area but the disease progressed as a migrating epizootic for several years. There had been sporadic cases of fox rabies in previous years but these were thought to be related to the enzootic disease in dogs and there was no evidence of transmission of the disease in dogs and there was no evidence of transmission of the disease among foxes prior to the epizootic. There was a history of sporadic cases of rabies in skunks and these continued to occur. For example, in New York State single cases of skunk rabies were identified in 1929, 1934 and 1937. There were single cases of fox rabies in 1941 and 1943. An epizootic of fox rabies developed in Chautauqua County in 1944. This outbreak lasted only one year. In 1945 another epizootic developed in Broome County and from here the disease spread into nearby counties. Subsequently the epizootic spread further westward and northward and has continued to the present time. Sporadic cases of skunk rabies have been identified each year from 1948 to 1965, with the exception of 1952 (Friend, 1968). Since 1960 there has been a gradual decrease in the incidence of fox rabies in southern United States but new foci of epizootic fox rabies have appeared in east central and northeast United States. The abandonment of millions of acres of farmland in southern and eastern United States during the past 50 years and gradual reforestation in these regions resulted in a marked increase in the population of wildlife. Foxes became unusually abundant and this seems to have been a precipitating factor in the development of epizootics of rabies.

In 1942, an eskimo died of rabies in Noorvik, Alaska, following wolf bite. Subsequent studies confirmed the presence of rabies in foxes and wolves in Alaska. The diagnosis of the disease was difficult because it was not possible to demonstrate characteristic Negri bodies in the brains of the affected animals. The occurrence of rabies in foxes on St. Lawrence Island off the coast of Alaska during the period 1949–1957 is of particular interest because of its isolated location (Williams, 1949; Rausch, 1958). Fox rabies appeared in epizootic proportions in the Northwest Territories of Canada during the period 1947–1952 (Plummer, 1954). An outbreak of rabies in foxes in northern Alberta in 1952 coincided with the peak of the 8-year cycle of the fox population (Ballantyne & O'Donoghue, 1954). Fox rabies appeared in Ontario in 1954 and has continued to the present time, spreading to the provinces of Quebec and New Brunswick (Johnston & Beauregard, 1969). In 1957–1960 there was an epizootic of rabies in Greenland affecting dogs and foxes. There was one human case of rabies from dog bite (Lassen, 1962).

There has been a large scale epizootic of rabies in wildilfe in Europe following the same pattern as that described in North America. The major focus of fox rabies has been in East and West Germany but there have been epizootics of fox rabies in Poland, Czechoslovakia, Switzerland, Austria, Belgium, France, and the U.S.S.R. More than 18,000 cases of fox rabies were identified in East and West Germany during the period 1955–1962. Among mustelids there were 301 cases in martens, 72 in ferrets and 18 in weasels (Pitzsehke, 1963). From 1953–1956, rabies was prevalent among arctic foxes and wolves in the northern U.S.S.R. (Kantorovich, 1957). There was an outbreak of rabies in wolves and foxes in Kazakstan in 1950 (Pavlovsky, 1960).

Skunk rabies has been known in North America for 144 years. Sporadic cases of rabies in skunks have been reported in the United States every year since modern diagnostic facilities have become available. Beginning in 1952 there was a general increase in the incidence of rabies in skunks and there were many local epizootics of rabies in striped skunks, *Mephitis mephitis*. Rabies in the spotted skunk has continued at a sporadic level with no evidence of epizootics in this species. In 1969 there were 1,156 cases of skunk rabies in the United States. Rabies was identified in skunks in 32 states. Wyoming can be cited as an example of the presence of skunk rabies with little involvement of other species. There were 54 cases of rabies in skunks, one in a cow and one in a cat (NCDC Annual Summary, Rabies, 1969). In California there were 321 cases of rabies in animals in 1969. Of these, 241 were in skunks. There were only 3 cases of dog rabies, all single cases in different counties. There were 8 cases in foxes but there was no evidence of fox to fox transmission of the disease. In 12 counties, only skunks were found to be infected with rabies (State of California, Department of Public Health, Reported Cases of Animal Rabies, 1969).

There have been 7 cases of rabies from skunk bite in the United States and 2 in Canada since 1952. Three of these occurred in South Dakota, 2 in California, 1 in Ohio, 1 in Minnesota and 2 in Ontario, Canada. One of the deaths following skunk bite in South Dakota is presumed to have been due to rabies. This is the case of an 11-year-old girl who was bitten by a skunk while asleep in a tent in July 1960. The first symptoms were pain and paraesthesia in the arm where the bite occurred and the clinical course was compatible with rabies. The child became comatose and did not die until 3 months after the onset of the disease. She did have a course of rabies vaccine. Specimens taken during the acute illness and at autopsy were negative for rabies. Many persons have been bitten by rabid skunks during the past 15 years and the number of cases of rabies from skunk bite would have been much greater if the combined serum and vaccine treatment had not been available. For example, early on the morning of April 19, 1959, a rabid skunk invaded a Boy Scout camp in Sacramento County, California. The skunk attacked the boys, all asleep in sleeping bags. One boy was bitten on the scalp at the base of the skull, one was bitten under the right eye, one was bitten on the temple and finger, one was bitten on the knuckle and one had contusions and scratches on the back of one hand. The skunk was killed and proved to be positive for rabies. The five boys were treated with antirabies serum and vaccine and all remained well (California Surveillance Report, May, 1959).

The occurrence of sporadic cases of rabies in man in southwestern United States from the bite of the spotted skunk is perhaps the most spectacular illustration of rabies derived from wildlife. A woman died of rabies in California in 1954 after she had been bitten by a spotted skunk when sleeping in a tent when on a hunting trip with her husband (Johnson, 1959). There had been no known cases of rabies in the area where the exposure occurred. The skunk brain was negative for Negri bodies and the woman decided not to take the rabies vaccine treatment, although she was advised to do so. The skunk brain was tested for virus by the mouse inoculation test but a month elapsed before it was found that the skunk was positive for rabies. The vaccine treatment was started but the woman developed symptoms of rabies after having had only a few injections of vaccine. The rabies virus obtained from the skunk and the woman infected by it was unusual in that the disease produced by it in mice was characterized by a long incubation period, and the absence of Negri bodies. There were some atypical intra-cytoplasmic inclusion bodies but a definite diagnosis could not be made by the microscopic examination. Only a few spotted skunks have been submitted to the California State Health Department for virus isolation studies. The rabies virus strains isolated from this animal are similar to that obtained from the case noted above. One of these strains, M400, has been isolated and maintained in hamster kidney cell culture. This non-neuroadapted virus is used as a type strain of the natural skunk virus. This virus is characterized by a tropism for certain organs such as the brain, submaxillary salivary glands, lungs, pancreas, mammary glands, kidneys and muscle tissue.

Some strains of rabies virus isolated from skunks are relatively nonpathogenic for adult mice. The salivary gland of M1942, a striped skunk obtained from El Dorado County in 1957, had a titer of $> 10^{-6}/0.015$ m*l* when tested in infant mice. The titer in adult mice was $< 10^{-1}/0.015$ m*l*. This strain of virus does not produce characteristic Negri bodies (Johnson, 1966). It is obvious that such virus strains would have been missed in previous years when the laboratory examination was limited to the search for Negri bodies or animal inoculation using adult mice.

The history of mongoose rabies is much like that of skunk rabies. There is a history of persons being bitten by mad mongooses in India. Often it has been necessary to kill the animal in order to get it to let go. There were 32 cases of mongoose bite treated at Kasuili from 1922 to 1931. One girl living in Jullundur District was attacked by a mongoose in May 1932 and the animal had to be killed before it would let go. This animal was found positive for rabies. The child was given the rabies vaccine and survived. A woman, aged 35, was bitten on the left great toe by a mongoose on September 21, 1929. The patient became ill on October 31 and died November 4. The disease began with symptoms of pain in the left leg and subsequently she developed hydrophobia and convulsions. She was not given the vaccine treatment (Greval, 1932).

In South Africa there are sporadic cases of rabies in man from the bite of the yellow mongoose, *Cynictus penicillata*. Of 33 cases of human rabies which occurred from 1916 to 1936, 19 were from the bite of the yellow mongoose (Thomas & Neitz, 1936).

Mongoose rabies has been known in Puerto Rico for over ten years and there is no evidence that the disease is maintained in dogs or other animals. In 1969 there were 21 cases of rabies in mongooses in Puerto Rico. There was only 1 case of rabies in a dog, 1 in a cat, 5 in cattle and 3 in horses (NCDC, Annual Summary, Rabies, 1969).

During the 1870s, 7 pairs of mongooses were introduced into Grenada from Jamaica for rat control. By 1955 the mongoose population had become excessive and it was noted that domestic animals bitten by mongooses sometimes developed a fatal disease resembling rabies. Beginning in 1965 the Trinidad Regional Virus Laboratory began testing animal brain specimens from Grenada by the FRA test and by animal inoculation using infant mice. During the period

1965 through 1968, 16 of 20 mongooses killed when acting in an abnormal manner were proved to have been infected with rabies virus. Among routinely trapped mongooses, 29 of 600 were found positive for rabies. Only 12 cattle, 5 dogs and 8 other domestic animals were found positive for rabies (Jonkers *et al.*, 1969). A girl and an adult woman died of rabies in Trinidad in 1919 after bites by a "strange mad cat." These cases occurred during a time when rabies was otherwise unknown on the island (Pawan, 1959). It is presumed that the biting animal was a mongoose. Dr. F. Kasse has informed me that a person died of rabies in the Dominican Republic in 1961 following a bite on the mouth by a mongoose. The Indian mongoose, *Herpestes javanicus auropunctatus* (Hodgson) was introduced into the West Indies to reduce the number of rats. The natural range of this animal is northern India. The information cited above indicates that the Indian mongoose found in the West Indies is able to maintain rabies virus over long periods of time with only rare sporadic cases of disease attributable to the infection.

There have been sporadic cases of rabies in weasels in North America. The long tailed weasel, *Mustela frenata*, the short tailed weasel, *Mustela rixosa*, and the ermine, *Mustela erminea*, are all commonly called weasels. There are occasional reports of weasels acting abnormally and attacking man or domestic animals in daytime. Only two weasels have been found positive for rabies in California. A weasel was found infected with rabies in Minnesota in 1969 (NCDC Annual Summary, Rabies, 1969). There is a history of cases of unusual behavior of weasels in Minnesota. For example, in June, 1952, a weasel entered a farmyard in Mower County in daytime and bit a dog. The weasel did not appear vicious but could not be chased away. It was killed but was not tested for rabies. In June, 1955, a weasel entered a farmyard in Freeborn County during the early afternoon and began chasing a dog. The weasel was killed and it was found to be positive for rabies. In July, 1958, a weasel was killed on a farm in Yellow Medicine County when fighting with cats in the farmyard in daytime. It was not tested for rabies. Mink, *Mustela vison*, have also been found infected with rabies (Johnson, 1959). I cite these reports because I wish to encourage virus isolation studies of weasels which are observed acting in an abnormal manner, hoping to obtain more information about their role in the maintenance of rabies in nature. There is no evidence of epizootics of rabies in weasels and this would seem to be in accord with what one would expect of a reservoir host. It has been noted that weasels are sometimes found infected with rabies in Canada (Ballantyne & O'Donoghue, 1954; Plummer, 1954; Rausch, 1958). In the tundra regions of the Far North, in Greenland and on St. Lawrence Island, the ermine seems to be the most likely reservoir host of rabies. Knowing the nature of the rabies virus strains isolated from foxes and wolves in the Far North, it is likely that the identification of rabies in ermine requires modern laboratory diagnostic methods such as the FRA test and the use of infant mice as test animals.

When we look for sporadic cases of rabies in carnivores in Europe to see whether there is anything like skunk, weasel or mongoose rabies there, we find that polecats, martens and weasels have been found infected with rabies. During 1968, rabies was identified in polecats in Belgium, Czechoslovakia, Germany and Switzerland, in martens in Austria, Belgium, Czechoslovakia, Germany and Switzerland and in a weasel in Germany (WHO World Survey of Rabies for 1968). In Europe the wild ferret, *Mustela putorius*, is known as a polecat. During a survey of wildlife for rabies in the U.S.S.R. in 1967–1968, rabies virus was isolated from an ermine, *Mustela eversmanni* (Rudakov *et al.*, 1969). The mottled polecat, *Vormela peregusna*, fills the ecologic niche in southern U.S.S.R., occupied by the spotted skunk in North America. It is also very similar to the African polecat, *Ictonyx striatus*.

There is also information about sporadic cases of rabies in the polecat, *Ictonyx striatus*, and the civet cat, *Civettictis civetta*, in Africa (Thomas & Neitz, 1936; Adamson, 1954). The 1969 WHO report on rabies listed cases of rabies in the civet cat in Kenya and Cameroon. In Malaya there are weasels (*Mustelidae*) and civets (*Viverridae*) which should be considered as possible vectors of rabies. The civets are native to rain forest. The viverrids may be divided into two groups, the ground dwellers, *Viverra* and *Viverricula* which are called "civets," and the tree dwelling forms called "palm civets" or "musangs." These animals fit the same ecological niche in the rain forest as that occupied by the mongoose in drier parts of Asia.

I will review briefly the history of bat rabies because this will be covered extensively in another paper at this meeting. I do not believe that bats are a part of the natural reservoir host system for rabies virus. The large scale epizootics of rabies in vampire bats in South America and in *Tadarida brasiliensis* colonial bats in North America can be cited as examples of successful parasitism in an aberrant host. There is no evidence that bats play a role in the maintenance of rabies virus in wildlife in Europe, Africa, Asia or Australia. In the tropical evergreen forest of South America, Africa and Asia there are enormous numbers of bats, including insectivorous, fruit eating and carnivorous species. There is no worldwide pattern of parasitism of bats by rabies virus. It is also difficult to relate bats to the reservoir host system in the Far North, especially in the tundra regions.

The early studies of vampire bat rabies in Trinidad and Brazil have been cited as proving that the vampire bat can act as a symptomless carrier of rabies virus. I have had considerable experience with vampire bat rabies, having isolated rabies virus from vampire bats in Mexico in 1944, and in 1967 I conducted a field investigation of vampire bat rabies in northern Argentina (Johnson, 1948). These studies make me believe that the epizootics of rabies in vampire bats follow the same pattern as those in wild canines, that is, the disease appears to arise abruptly, revealing itself by the occurrence of epizootic paralytic rabies in cattle on which the bats normally feed. The epizootic is short-lived in any one local area, and then the disease moves as a migrating epizootic, killing both vampire bats and cattle. There is no definite information of transmission of the disease among cattle but this should be considered. The epizootic in cattle at any one ranch is usually over in 3 to 6 months. The epizootic of vampire bat rabies which began in northern Argentina in 1960 has progressed slowly southward and is still continuing on a reduced scale. On the basis of past experience, by the time the disease is identified in cattle on a ranch, the great majority of exposures have occurred and the infected vampire bat population has died of the disease. Killing of the bats will have little effect on the course of the epizootic on that ranch, that is, the animals that die will have been bitten before the control work was started. With a mean incubation period of about 3 months, the dieoff will continue for about that length of time. If the animals are vaccinated with a live virus rabies vaccine, one can expect that a good level of immunity will develop within 4 to 6 weeks, and then the dieoff will stop. No effect can be expected during the first month after vaccination because some of the animals exposed prior to vaccination will die before a high grade of immunity develops from the vaccination. It is this situation which has led to suspicion that vaccination of cattle with some live virus rabies vaccines has produced vaccine-induced rabies. For comparison one can cite vaccination of thousands of cattle with the same vaccine in other areas with no evidence of disease caused by the vaccine.

The introduction of cattle into Central and South America resulted in a gradual increase in the vampire bat population because cattle furnish a ready source of blood. In a way, the vampire bat is a domesticated animal, living in hollow trees, caves, wells or mines near cattle ranches and feeding almost entirely on cattle. In many regions of Central and South America there are high populations of vampire bats with no evidence of the presence of rabies in the bats or the cattle. This was true for northern Argentina for a long time prior to the epizootic of 1960–1970. In some regions there are vampire bats and isolated cases of rabies in domestic animals. If one investigates such outbreaks one usually finds that there is rabies in dogs and foxes and the affected animals do not exhibit the characteristic paralytic disease which is caused by rabies virus transmitted by vampire bats. Farmers are apt to call all bats "vampiros." It is important to look for evidence of bite wounds on the cattle. These are usually obvious if there are vampire bats nearby because they feed each night.

The research studies on vampire bat rabies done prior to the age of antibiotics and the use of the mouse inoculation test are subject to criticism and the reputed rabies carrier state is open to question. We are well aware of the many reported isolations of rabies virus from animals and which now are regarded as due to experimental error. The major criticism of the early studies of vampire bat rabies was that virus isolation studies could not be carried out on saliva specimens because if the saliva was inoculated intracerebrally into experimental animals they died of bacterial infection. The use of cattle for feeding experiments in Trinidad made it possible for the animals to be exposed before or after the experimental test feeding because they were from an area where vampire bats were abundant and some were infected with rabies virus. There is no recent experimental evidence that rabies virus is present in the saliva or salivary glands of naturally infected vampire bats which do not die of rabies. I have studied over 150 vampire bats collected in foci of paralytic rabies of cattle and we did not isolate rabies virus from salivary gland specimens where the brain specimens were negative for the virus.

The current epizootic of rabies in insectivorous bats in North America dates to 1953, when the disease was identified in a bat in Florida (Johnson, 1958). There has been a major epizootic of rabies in the colonial bat, *Tadarida brasiliensis* in southwestern United States. There have been instances of small epizootics of rabies in other bat species such as free-living *Lasiurus* bats, and the colonial big brown bat, *Eptesicus fuscus*. A large percentage of the rabies positive bats are isolated in location and occur in a sporadic fashion. There have been 485 cases of bat rabies in California. The peak incidence was reached in 1965 when there were 72 positive bats. Most of the cases of bat rabies have occurred in the fall when the bats are migrating southward. This is especially marked in the cases of rabies in hoary bats, *Lasiurus cinereus*, and silver-haired-bats, *Lasionycteris noctivagans*. I suspect that most of the bats of these species found to have rabies in California, were infected in northern United States or Canada. Sporadic cases of bat rabies observed in the spring and summer tend to occur in counties where rabies is enzootic in wildlife. The known habit of some bats to feed on insects collected on the ground, such as crickets and beetles, makes them accessible to exposure by rabid skunks. Weasels and spotted skunks are good climbers and can expose bats by bite when trying to capture them in trees, in rock crevices or caves.

Rabies virus obtained from insectivorous bats is of two distinct types. The virus from *Tadarida* bats is characterized by a short incubation period of the disease in mice and the presence of abundant Negri bodies. This virus produces an acute excitement stage in infected mice. The virus from other species of bats, especially the free-living bats, is characterized by a long incubation period in infected mice and a lack of Negri bodies in the brains of the mice. These strains of rabies virus are like those obtained from skunks, while those from *Tadarida* bats are like those obtained from dogs.

We have found no evidence of a carrier state of rabies in California bats. We do find other viruses in bats such as Rio Bravo virus and Kern Canyon virus. I have routinely tested the salivary glands, lungs and kidneys of bats submitted to the California State Health Department for rabies diagnosis and which are negative for rabies virus in the brain. These were all negative for rabies virus by the mouse inoculation test. We have also studied the tissues of a large number of bats collected in surveys looking for arboviruses. I have studied various tissues of 45 rabid insectivorous bats where the brain was positive for rabies. Twenty-seven of 41 tested, or 66%, had rabies virus in the submaxillary salivary glands. Eighteen of 36, or 50%, had rabies virus in the lungs. Four of 38, or 10%, had rabies virus in the kidneys. Twelve of 34, or 35%, had rabies virus in the pectoral muscle. Only 2 of 22 tested had rabies virus in the brown fat specimen. These two isolations were obtained during the early part of this study and it is possible that there was some contamination of the specimen from the brain case, salivary glands or mammary glands. Only one of 8 and two of 6 infant mice died after inoculation with the positive brown fat specimens. Subsequently, great care was taken in dissecting away other tissues from the brown fat specimen and thorough rinsing in saline solution, and the other brown fat specimens taken from rabid bats have all been negative by the mouse inoculation test (Johnson, 1967).

The natural capacity of rabies virus to produce encephalitis becomes the means by which it can adapt to the canine host, which normally attacks and kills by biting. The selection of this highly neurotropic variant of the virus eventually kills off the host until the chain of infection is broken. The virus must invade the submaxillary salivary glands in order to be successful in maintaining this aberrant cycle. On the other hand, the invasion of the lung is not necessary, so the tropism of the virus for this organ is lost by passage in the canine host. In bats, especially in cave bats such as *Tadarida brasiliensis*, the tropism of the virus for the lung is maintained and possibly increased. In this instance aerosol exposure seems to be the means of transmission. This has led to the development of a highly dangerous variant of rabies virus which can be transmitted from animal to animal by inhalation (Constantine, 1962). If this variant should become established in man it could cause a devastating epidemic of rabies.

The main purpose of this presentation is to point out some possible lines of investigation which could lead to our obtaining more knowledge about the natural reservoir host system of rabies, particularly in Asia. Rabies virus may be present in small carnivores such as skunks, mongooses, civets and weasels without any evidence of disease in man or domestic animals. Therefore, the lack of recognized cases of rabies in a country does not prove that rabies virus is not present in wildlife. On the basis of our general knowledge of parasitology we do not expect to see epizootics of disease in a natural reservoir host of a parasite. We can expect to find occasional instances of disease and death in the reservoir host. If we pursue the investigation of obscure cases of disease in small carnivores, especially instances where these animals act in an unusual manner, appearing in farmyards and about houses and acting tame, we may be able to locate foci of rabies infection and thus be able to study the wildlife population to learn which animal is the source of the virus. There is need for investigation of the mode of transmission of rabies in the immediate post natal period. Concurrent with the outbreak of skunk rabies in California we began receiving reports of bites by rabid pet skunks. Upon investigating these cases, it was learned that these animals had been collected in the wild as infants and had been taken to a veterinarian for removal of the scent glands. Some had been vaccinated with the live virus rabies vaccine. Others had not been vaccinated. For example, 3 infant skunks were found at Vallejo, Solano County, April 16, 1957. These were raised as pets and had not been vaccinated. All 3 died of rabies between July 10 and July 29. The incubation period in all three was over 3 months. When infant skunks are found wandering about in daytime, we can expcct that the mother animal is dead. During the course of the epizootic of skunk rabies in California there have been many instances where infant skunks have been found in this way and where persons have subsequently been exposed to rabies by skunk bite. Because of this, the sale of wild caught skunks for pets has been prohibited in California.

The use of primary cell culture for isolation of latent viruses in small mammals has been useful in my studies of arboviruses (Johnson, 1970). I have done some preliminary cell culture studies of small carnivores such as spotted skunks and weasels in California. I have not isolated any strains of rabies virus, but I have isolated a variant of Powassan virus from the cell culture of the kidney of a spotted skunk. Knowing the natural tropism of rabies virus, I recommend doing cell cultures of the submaxillary salivary glands, a pool of trachea and lung tissue and the kidneys of animals suspected as reservoir hosts of rabies. The cell cultures can be examined for rabies virus by the FRA test.

I do not know where rabies virus persists in nature between outbreaks of rabies. I do believe that the study of sporadic cases of rabies in wildlife offers a key to the location of the reservoir host (Johnson, 1966). The dog and related wild canines can be regarded as sentinel animals which reveal the presence of rabies from time to time by the occurrence of spectacular epizootics of rabies. In the investigation of the epizootiology of rabies especial attention should be given to the foci where the epizootics began. The tendency has been to study the migrating epizootic and by the time the investigation gets under way the disease problem may be far from the natural source of the virus.

We are apt to pride ourselves on our knowledge of the epizootiology of wildlife diseases transmissible to man and domestic animals but reviewing the literature on this subject one finds that we know very little about the natural history of the parasites that cause these diseases. With the newer techniques now available, such as the FA test and a variety of virus isolation systems, there is a wide-open field for the young adventurous biologist in the study of the life history of wildlife viruses.

## REFERENCES


Adamson, J. S. (1954). Ecology of rabies in southern Rhodesia, *Bull. WHO*, **10**, 753–759.

Ballantyne, E. E., and O'Donoghue, J. G. (1954). Rabies control in Alberta, *J. A. V. M. A.*, **125**, 316–326.

Colan, T. (1881). The dog disease, or canine madness of the Arctic regions, viewed in connection with hydrophobia; together with the measures used and suggested for its extinction, from information collected, and observations made in the country, *Vet. J. Ann. Comp. Path., London*, **13**, 324–325.

Constantine, D. G. (1962). Rabies transmission by nonbite route, *Pub. Health Rep.*, **77**, 287–289.

DeJernett, R. (1859). A case of hydrophobia from the bite of a pole-cat-tracheotomy, *South. Med. Surg. J.*, **15**, 3–6.

Friend, M. (1968). History and epidemiology of rabies in wildlife in New York, *New York Fish & Game J.*, **15**, 71–97.

Greval, S. D. S. (1932). Rabies in the mongoose (reports from records, including a report on the first positive brain of mongoose examined at Kasauli. Comments including speculation and bearing on treatment). *Indian Med. Gaz.*, **67**, 451–453.

Johnson, H. N. (1945). Fox rabies, *J. M. A. Alabama*, **14**, 268–271.

Johnson, H. N. (1948). Derriengue; vampire bat rabies in Mexico, *Am. J. Hyg.*, **47**, 189–204.

Johnson, H. N. (1958). Rabies in insectivorous bats of North America, Proc. 6th Int. *Congr. Trop. Med. Malaria*, **5**, 559–567.

Johnson, H. N. (1959). The role of the spotted skunk in rabies, Proc. 63rd Annual Meeting U.S. Livestock San. Assn., pp. 267–274.

Johnson, H. N. (1966). Sporadic cases of rabies in wildlife: Relation to rabies in domestic animals and character of virus, Proc. National Rabies Symposium, NCDC, Atlanta, pp. 25–30.

Johnson, H. N. (1967). Patogenesis de la Rabia, Primer Seminario Internacional sobre rabies para las Americas, OPS, OMS, pp. 68–72.

Johnson, H. N. (1970). Long-term persistence of Modoc virus in hamster-kidney cells, *Am. J. Trop. Med. & Hyg.*, **19**, 537–539.

Johnston, D. H. and Beauregard, M. (1969). Rabies epidemiology in Ontario, *Bull. Wildlife Disease Assoc.*, **5**, 357–370.

Jonkers, A. H., Alexis, F. and Loregnard, R. (1969). Mongoose rabies in Grenada, *W. I. Med. J.*, **18**, 167–170.

Kantorovich, R. A. (1957). The etiology of "madness" in Polar animals, *Acta Virol. (Eng.)*, **1**, 220–228.

Lassen, H. C. A. (1962). Paralytic human rabies in Greenland, *Lancet*, **1**, 247–249.

Moodelly, P. S. M. S. (1859). Hydrophobia from mongoose bite, *Indian Ann. Med. Sc.*, **6**, 201–202.

Nelson, E. W. (1918). Wild Animals of North America, p. 579, Nat. Geograph. Soc., Washington D.C., Judd & Detweiler.

Pavlovsky, Y. N. (1960). Natural foci of disease and ecology of the zoonoses, European Seminar on Veterinary Public Health, Warsaw, pp. 183–216, Copenhagen, WHO.

Pawan, J. L. (1959). Paralysis as a clinical manifestation in human rabies, *Caribbean Med. J.*, **21**, 157–165.

Pitzschke, H. (1963). Verlauf der Tollwut in Mitteleuropa 1959–1962 mit besonderer Berucksichtigung Deutschlands, Arch. Exp. Vet. Med. Leipzig, **17**,1031–1048.

Plummer, P. J. G. (1954). Rabies in Canada, with special reference to wildlife reservoirs, *Bull. WHO*, **10**, 767–774.

Rausch, R. (1958). Some observations on rabies in Alaska, with special reference to wild canidae, *J. Wildlife Management*, **22**, 246–260.

Roberts, H. S. (1884). Hydrophobia, Tr. Med. Soc. Kansas 1860–1877, *Lawrence*, **1**, 378–387.

Rudakov, V. A., Malkov, G. B. and Kantorovich, R. A. (1969). Experience of epidemiological reconnaissance of natural foci of rabies in Western Siberia, Symposium on Rabies, Academy of Med. Sc., U.S.S.R., Moscow, pp. 93–94 (In Russian).

Thomas, A. D. and Neitz, W. O. (1936). Wild carnivora as carrier of rabies, *J. Royal Sanitary Instit. Transactions*, **56**, 754–760.

Williams, R. B. (1949). Epizootic of rabies in Interior Alaska 1945–47, *Canad. J. Comp. Med.*, **13**, 136–143.

Yount, C. E. (1910). Rabies: with reports of cases from skunk bites, *South. California Pract.*, **25**, 105–116.

For Discussion, see page 263.

# Bat Rabies: Current Knowledge and Future Research

DENNY G. CONSTANTINE

*Cell Culture Laboratory, Naval Biomedical Research Laboratory, Oakland, California 94625*

Any general discussion of bat rabies should be preceded by a few remarks about the host, the bat. There are about 2,000 kinds of these mammals. They vary in size from those with a wingspread of several inches to species with a wingspan in excess of 5 feet. The various species are specialized in food habits. They may be categorized as insect-eating, fruit-eating, fish-eating, nectar- or pollen-eating, meat-eating, or blood-drinking. Some are omnivorous. Bats are found throughout the world to the limits of tree growth. They increase in kinds and numbers as the tropics are approached. They are active throughout the year in the tropics. They hibernate during winter in temperate zones or migrate to warm areas instead. Many species of bat are essentially cold-blooded when at rest, assuming the temperature of their environment. The majority of species are gregarious, living in colonies of hundreds or millions in dark, confined areas such as caves. Other species live as solitary individuals, usually in open places, such as tree foliage.

The bat rabies problem may be divided into (1) the problem involving the vampire bat, and (2) the problem in insect-eating bats and several other species. Vampire bat rabies constitutes a direct public health menace and a formidable economic problem because these bats deliberately seek out and bite sleeping persons and livestock in order to obtain their sole dietary item: blood. The vampire inhabits tropical America. Rabies in insectivorous bats is a lesser public health problem, because the infected bats rarely attack man without provocation. Rabies is known from numerous species of nonvampire bats in the Americas. It has been reported from several bats in Europe and Asia but reports from those areas are few and, in some cases, questionable. Studies of bat rabies have partially clarified the direct hazard to man. More importantly, they have produced evidence that the virus may be maintained in certain populations of gregarious bats as an inapparent infection transmitted by respiratory route. These findings appear to relate to a reservoiring pattern of the virus, a system that may prove to be duplicated in cretain terrestrial carnivorous mammals.

## RABIES IN VAMPIRE BATS

Evidently, vampire bats were infected with rabies virus prior to the discovery of America, since many of the conquering troops and their livestock perished with rabies-like symptoms following bites by vampires. Natives were accustomed to avoiding the disease by washing the wound and cauterizing it with wood embers. (De Oviedo y Valdes, 1526).

The problem in cattle was not diagnosed as rabies until 1908 (Carini, 1911). However, as early as the mid-17th century, the problem in man was attributed to bat-transmitted rabies (Piso, 1658), but that opinion was forgotten, and it was not until the present century after the human disease had been routinely misdiagnosed as polio, botulism, and others illnesses that Hurst and Pawan (1931) made the laboratory diagnosis of rabies.

The most striking aspect of the infection reported in vampires was that of survival of many infected bats, i.e., evidence of a nonlethal infection (Pawan, 1936; Torres & Queiroz Lima, 1936). Though some data were obtained from laboratory infections, others were compiled from observations of naturally-acquired infections. The bats could infect each other by bite. The virus appeared in saliva 2 weeks after exposure, and it could be detected there for periods that sometimes exceeded 3 months, after which it disappeared. Bats might be asymptomatic throughout the infection, or they might show signs of paralysis and later recover. Some bats died. These early studies lacked the precision now possible with modern techniques, and they should be repeated for verification. The vampire-transmitted disease in men and livestock is characterized by paralysis; it lacks the excitative or aggressive phase.

Vampires naturally bite each other frequently, precluding the necessity for furious rabies signs to effect viral transmission between the bats, probably explaining the reported absence of disease signs in some infected vampires and the absence of furiousness in victims of vampire-borne rabies. One may expect that the absence of encephalitis would increase the host's potential for survival. Airborne or other nonbite viral transmission routes between the bats would similarly bypass dependence on encephalitis to effect transmission by bite. In other words, encephalitis and consequent death of the host could be profitably cancelled out of the equation, and indeed that may be what happens.

The infection in vampires appears to be a closed cycle (with the posssible exception of viral exchange with other bat species), though man and livestock are infected tangentially. Surveys for the virus in brain and salivary gland tissues of clinically-normal vampires usually disclose infection rates of about 1% (Sugay & Nilsson, 1966; Williams, 1960).

Vampires are said to prefer to feed on man and livestock in the following decreasing order of preference: cattle, horses, goats, swine, poultry, sheep, dogs, and man (Goodwin & Greenhall, 1961). Vampire populations have grown with the increasing livestock populations; they are particularly concentrated in cattle-producing areas. The annual blood loss caused by each vampire is about 5.75 gallons, a figure that includes the bleeding that occurs after the bat has finished feeding.

Species known to be infected by vampire-borne rabies include man, cattle, horses, swine, goats, and sheep. Most noticeable have been outbreaks in cattle that may claim lives of 80% of the local population. Endemic zones are characterized by 1 to 10 week outbreaks every 2 or 3 years, with or without intervening sporadic cases (Ruiz Martínez, 1963).

Some 151 human rabies deaths caused by bites of vampire bats have been reported (Constantine, in press). The record can hardly be considered complete. This problem could not compete for the attention of officials overburdened with more significant causes of human mortality.

The WHO Expert Committee on Rabies (1966) declared vampire-borne rabies to be the primary livestock disease problem of Latin America and a major obstacle to the expansion of its agricultural economy. A survey of the problem by the Food and Agricultural Organization of the United Nations indicated that more than one million animals are lost annually, causing a direct loss exceeding 100 million dollars (Steele, 1966).

Control of vampire-borne rabies has been attempted through repelling bats, bat-proofing sleeping quarters of man and livestock, destroying bat roosts, destroying bats, vaccination of cattle, and postexposure treatment of man, but the problem persists, and improved methods of combating it are being sought (Constantine, in press).

## RABIES IN OTHER BATS

The first diagnosis of rabies viral infection in a bat was made in 1916 in reference to infection in a Brazilian fruit-eating bat (Haupt & Rehaag, 1921). Since then, rabies infection in nonvampire bats has been reported throughout South America, Middle America, North America, and Europe and Asia. Though first discovered in the United States in 1953, the problem may not have been new; numbers of infected bats that were detected increased from 8 in 1953 to 484 in 1966, but the percentage of rabies-suspect bats proved to be infected did not change (Constantine, 1967b). In other words, the denominator increased in proportion with the numerator. Thus, the numbers of rabies-positive bats reflected the degree of human interest in the problem.

Evidently these bats experience intraspecific rabies cycles because flightless, suckling bats, associated with no other known source, have been found infected in bat shelters (Constantine, 1967a, 1967b; Constantine *et al.*, 1968; Schneider *et al.*, 1957). It appears then that rabies virus is maintained in isolation within certain species of bats. Moreover, at least two kinds of bat species-specific cycles are recognizable, one that usually does not kill the bat and another that does (Constantine, 1967b).

The nonlethal infection is typified by the cycle in the highly gregarious free-tailed bat; the bats usually survive without symptoms, developing serum antibodies. If disease signs develop, they are those of paralysis, not furiousness. Viral transmission evidently occurs in the course of normal behavior, probably by aerosol, possibly by casual biting (Constantine, 1962, 1966a, 1967a).

The lethal infection is typified by the disease manifested in certain small, solitary species of bat such as the California myotis. It resembles the disease observed in dogs. The bats become furious, attack without provocation, and die with encephalitis. Evidently this cyle can be perpetuated only if the virus incites these solitary bats to deliberately seek out and attack others of their kind.

The virus has been found in every species of North American bat that has been adequately sampled. Of the 41 different species of bat known from the United States, rabies has been found in 25. Infection rates in brain and salivary gland tissues of clinically-normal bats usually are about 1%.

We have scant knowledge of the characteristics of rabies cycles in many species of bat. It is probable that cyles typified by nonlethal infections will be seen in the highly gregarious species.

Rabies viruses from different species of bat have been partially characterized by the responses of laboratory animals and captive wild animals to the viruses (Constantine, 1966a; Constantine and Woodall, 1966; Constantine *et al.*, 1968a). The data indicate that the virus differs according to the species of host from which it originates, further supporting the view that it cycles independently within each species.

Rabies virus can survive for prolonged periods in bats, even when the bats seem destined to die from the infection (Constantine, 1967b). Bats, captured as they were about to awaken naturally from winter hibernation in caves, died of the disease 2 months later. Other bats, captured just before they migrated southward, died of the disease as long as 3 months later, time enough to have migrated southward and returned. This demonstrates two methods by which the virus can winter in bats.

The susceptibility of mammals like foxes, skunks, dogs, and cats to the rabies viruses of bats is irrelevant to the closed cycles in bats, and as such the responses of these carnivorous species vary according to the bat species origin of virus. The susceptibility of these terrestrial carnivores to the bat viruses is of importance to man, however, and experimental transmission of virus has been attempted from several species of bat. Relatively few experiments have been done. Foxes, coyotes, ringtails, and opossums were infected when exposed to the air of densely-populated bat caves (Constantine, 1962, 1967a). Foxes and coyotes were infected through bites inflicted by one species of bat (Constantine, 1966b). We do not know whether or not any species of bat succeeds in infecting terrestrial carnivores naturally. Evidently, two persons were infected by aerosolized virus in a bat cave, and four persons were infected by bites of insectivorous bats. If man can be infected through bat bites, it is likely that some wild animals can be similarly infected.

Potential rabies exposures have been experienced by a surprisingly great proportion of persons and pets that encountered infected bats (Constantine, 1967b). Human beings investigating live, infected bats were bitten at a rate of 14 bites/100 bats. Since the recognized bat-transmitted rabies deaths in man, bitten persons have been treated.

Infected bats observed by man contacted pets at a rate of 30 pet contacts/100 bats. Generally the exposed pets had been vaccinated or were destroyed after contact. Wild animals must be exposed to a similar or greater extent. However, we lack knowledge of the frequencies or the result.

Control procedures have been to warn the public to avoid bat bites and the atmospheres in densely-populated bat caves. It has been recommended that bats be eliminated from dwellings and school buildings, where sick bats are likely to be handled by children.

## THE NEED FOR FUTURE RESEARCH

It has been observed that rabies virus is opportunistic, like other forms of life. It survives by any route of transmission that will support it. It can readily survive in a nonlethal cycle, since the host is not destroyed. In a lethal cycle, it can survive periods of host population depletion through the occasional prolonged incubation period reported by various authors (Parker & Wilsnack, 1966; Sikes, 1962; Steele, 1969; Tierkel, 1963).

It seems reasonable to expect a nonlethal rabies cycle to be of paramount importance in viral maintenance and ultimate viral survival. "Leaks" from that cycle to animal populations whose behavior does not support airborne transmission, for example, would limit subsequent transmission to infected individuals that develop encephalitis and transmit by bite, quickly selecting for the lethal viral variants that thus survive. Outbreaks of lethal rabies would follow, but they would subside as infected populations or susceptibles are depleted, similar to rabies outbreaks seen in many species of carnivorous mammals.

Of the facts we have learned from the study of bat rabies, the most important may be the recognition of host species-specific rabies cycles, one kind of cycle characterized by death of the host, and another kind of cycle characterized by survival of the host. The latter kind of cycle would not deplete the host population and, consequently, it resembles the kind of pattern one might expect to see in a natural reservoir.

Parker (1969) pointed out that host species-specific rabies cycles are evident in terrestrial carnivorous mammals, and Tierkel (1963) gave evidence that survival from rabies infection sometimes occurs naturally in these animals. Moreover, Johnson (1965) theorized that rabies exists as an inapparent respiratory infection of certain wild carnivorous mammalian species.

On the basis of geographic distribution, Johnson suspected that the natural hosts for rabies were members of the families Mustelidae and Viverridae. The coughing or "spitting" behavior that certain of these animals display when they meet and threaten each other would readily support respiratory transmission. Behavioral aberrations such as encephalitis and consequent biting would have a destructive effect on maintanance of such a cycle, so one would expect that viral strains maintained in a respiratory cycle would not often stimulate encephalitis in the host. One would expect the virus to be nonlethal for this kind of host and perhaps but not necessarily nonlethal for other species. Viral lethality for other species would be largely irrelevant to the basic cycle and probably variable until selected for in epizootics sustained by bite-transmission.

Carnivores can be infected with the virus by respiratory route, as previously noted. Recent events indicate that airborne rabies viral transmission evidently can occur between carnivores. An epizootic of airborne rabies was accidentally started in captive foxes and other animals in 1967 (U.S.P.H.S., 1968). Foxes had been experimentally exposed to a laboratory-generated aerosol of bat rabies virus. After exposure, the foxes were housed in a building that contained numerous unchallenged animals, each caged separately. Subsequent to deaths of the experimentally-infected animals, 37 unchallenged animals (primarily foxes) died of rabies viral infection over a period of six months. Evidently, the epizootic in unchallenged animals was initiated by aerosolized virus emitted by the experimentally-infected animals, and it was subsequently transmitted similarly between the unchallenged animals.

The foregoing reports indicate that all that is needed to complete the equation for a silent reservoir among Carnivora is a virus that regularly produces a nonlethal infection in the reservoir carnivore host. It appears entirely feasible to expect such a rabies virus and nonlethal cycle to exist, as theorized by Johnson.

One should not overlook implications for direct accidental involvement of man in airborne rabies viral infection. We have seen that two persons were evidently infected by this route in a bat cave. Should infected persons transmit the virus by airbone route to other persons, paralleling the epizootic in caged foxes, epidemics in man might result. Such outbreaks might be difficult to control.

Past experience indicates that effective control of wildlife rabies will have to await the results of studies in the pathogenesis and epizootiology of the different kinds of rabies cycles that exist in the various kinds of wildlife hosts. We need to know the characteristics of these cycles and how they interact to cause outbreaks that affect man. We may anticipate that effective rabies control will follow only when the reservoiring cycles have been identified and disrupted.

I am conducting a preliminary study of the pathogenesis of air-borne rabies viral infection in colonial bats. It is apparent that the respiratory system plays a leading role in this cycle. I would expand this investigation to thoroughly study the pathogenesis and epizootiology of the infection, not only to clarify the status of that cycle as a reservoir but to apply the knowledge thus gained to identify reservoir systems in other mammalian populations, such as terrestrial carnivores.

The investigation in bats requires field and laboratory studies of the host, the virus, and the environment. Special attention must be paid to determining the sites of viral invasion, replication, and release to the environment. We must determine if environmental factors such as noxious cave gases predispose the bat populations to infection.

Concurrent, parallel studies of aerosolized viral stability must be done, with special attention given to the influences of heat, humidity, and atmospheric gases on viral survival. A sensitive method must be developed to detect and quantitate the aerosolized virus (Constantine, 1967a; Winkler, 1968). In addition, it is necessary to investigate methods that may be used efficaciously for control of atmospheres that contain the aerosolized virus.

The asymptomatic rabies cycle in colonial bats appears to be one of many viral cycles similarly maintained in these gregarious mammals. Rio Bravo virus, serologically classified as an arbovirus, was the second of many viruses to be discovered in bats (Johnson, 1962). Evidently, it is transmitted in bat saliva, either by bite or aerosol. It is not known to cause disease in the bats, and they can liberate the virus in saliva for years (Constantine & Woodall, 1964). To date, 28 kinds of viruses have been found in bats, and antibodies for 32 additional viruses have been reported in bats (Constantine, in press). The viruses were isolated from colonial bats. Nineteen of the viruses that were isolated have been serologically characterized as arboviruses. Fifteen of the viruses were sought in salivary gland tissues, where all but one of the viruses were found. These data indicate that many arboviruses may exist in basic asymptomatic cycles in colonial bats without being transmitted by arthropods. However, some infections in bats were probably accidental and of little consequence. Several of the arboviruses isolated from bats are prominent: chikungunya, western equine encephalomyelitis, Venezuelan equine encephalomyelitis, Japanese B encephalitis, Saint Louis encephalitis, and yellow fever.

It appears then that the ecological model or niche typified by the airborne rabies viral cycle may be an unsuspected hiding place for a great many other viruses and relevant studies are indicated if reservoirs are to be identified.

## REFERENCES


Carini, A. (1911). Sur une grande épizootie de rage. *Ann. Inst. Pasteur*, (Paris) **25**, 843–846.

Constantine, D. G. (1962). Rabies transmission by nonbite route. *Public Health Rep.*, (U.S.) **77**, 287–289.

Constantine, D. G. (1966a). Transmission experiments with bat rabies isolates: Reaction of certain Carnivora, opossum, and bats to intramuscular inoculations of rabies virus isolated from free-tailed bats. *Amer. J. Vet. Res.*, **27**, 16–19.

Constantine, D. G. (1966b). Transmission experiments with bat rabies isolates: Bite transmission of rabies to foxes and coyote by free-tailed bats. *Amer. J. Vet. Res.*, **27**, 20–23.

Constantine, D. G. (1967a). Rabies transmission by air in bat caves. U.S. Public Health Serv. Public. No. 1671. p. 51.

Constantine, D. G. (1967b). Bat rabies in the southwestern United States. *Public Health Rep.*, (U.S.) **82**, 867–888.

Constantine, D. G. (In press). Bats in relation to the health, welfare, and economy of man. In "Biology of Bats." (W. A. Wimsatt, ed.), Vol. II, pp. 319–449, Academic Press, New York.

Constantine, D. G., Solomon, G. C. and Woodall, D. F. (1968a). Transmission experiments with bat rabies isolates: Responses of certain carnivores and rodents to rabies viruses from four species of bats. *Amer. J. Vet. Res.*, **29**, 181–190.

Constantine, D. G., Tierkel, E. S., Kleckner, M. D. and Hawkins, D. M. (1968b). Rabies in New Mexico cavern bats. *Public Health Rep.*, (U.S.) **83**, 303–316.

Constantine, D. G. and Woodall, D. F. (1964). Latent infection of Rio Bravo virus in salivary glands of bats. *Public Health Rep.*, (U.S.) **79**, 1033–1039.

Constantine, D. G. and Woodall, D. F. (1966). Transmission experiments with bat rabies isolates. Reactions of certain Carnivora, opossum, rodents, and bats to rabies virus of red bat origin when exposed by bat bite or by intramuscular inoculation. *Amer. J. Vet. Res.*, **27**, 24–32.

De Oviedo y Valdes, F. (1526). "Sumario de la Natural Historia de las Indias." Reprinted by Fondo de Cultura Economica, Mexico, 1950.

Goodwin, G. G. and Greenhall, A. M. (1961). A review of the bats of Trinidad and Tobago. *Bull. Amer. Mus. Natur. Hist.*, **122**, 187–301.

Haupt, H., and Rehaag, H. (1921). Durch Fledermäuse verbreitete seuchenhafte Tollwut unter Viehbeständen in Santa Catharina (Süd-Brasilien). *Z. Infektionskrankh. Haustiere*, **22**, 76–88 and 104–127.

Hurst, E. W. and Pawan, J. L. (1931). An outbreak of rabies in Trinidad. *Lancet II*, 622–628.

Johnson, H. N. (1962). The Rio Bravo virus: Virus identified with group B arthropod-borne viruses by hemagglutination inhibition and complement fixation tests. *Proc. 9th Pacific Science Congress*, Bangkok, 1957, **17**, 39.

Johnson, H. N. (1965). Rabies virus. In "Viral and Rickettsial Infections of Man." (F. L. Horsfall, Jr., and I. Tamm, eds.), pp. 814–840, Lippincott, Philadelphia and Montreal.

Parker, R. L. (1969). Epidemiology of rabies. *Arch. Environ. Health*, **19**, 857–861.

Parker, R. L. and Wilsnack, R. E. (1966). Pathogenesis of skunk rabies virus: Quantitation in skunks and foxes. *Am. J. Vet. Res.*, **27**, 33–38.

Pawan, J. L. (1936). Rabies in the vampire bat of Trinidad, with special reference to the clinical course and the latency of infection. *Ann. Trop. Med. Parasitol.*, **30**, 401–422.

Piso, G. (1658). "Historía Natural e Médico da India Ocidental." (Portuguese version). Inst. Nac. Livro. Rio de Janeiro, 1957.

Ruiz Martínez, C. (1963). "Epizootología y Profilaxis Regional de la Rabia Paralítica en las Américas." Mongrafías, Ediciónes Protinal, Caracas.

Schneider, N. J., Scatterday, J. E., Lewis, A. L., Jennings, W. L., Venters, H. D. and Hardy, A. V. (1957). Rabies in bats in Florida. *Amer. J. Public Health*, **47**, 983–989.

Sikes, R. K. (1962). Pathogenesis of rabies in wildlife. I. Comparative effect of varying doses of rabies virus inoculated into foxes and skunks. *Am. J. Vet. Res.*, **23**, 1041–1047.

Steele, J. H. (1966). International aspects of veterinary medicine and its relation to health, nutrition and human welfare. *Mil. Med.*, **131**, 765–778.

Steele, J. H. (1969). Understanding the disease is vital to rabies control. *J. Environ. Health*, **31**, 471–483.

Sugay, W. and Nilsson, M. R. (1966). Isolamento de vírus da raiva de morcegos hematófogos do estado de São Paulo, Brasil. *Bol. Of. Sanit. Panamer.*, **60**, 310–315.

Tierkel, E. S. (1963). Rabies. In "Diseases Transmitted from Animals to Man." (T. G. Hull, ed.), pp. 293–349. Thomas, Springfield, Illinois.

Torres, S. and de Queiroz Lima, E. (1936). A raiva e os morcegos hematophagos. *Rev. Dep. Nac. Prod. Anim., Brazil*, **3**, 165–174.

United States Public Health Service. (1968). Rabies outbreak—Southwest Rabies Investigations Station. *CDC Veterinary Public Health Notes* (*Atlanta, Ga.*) June, 1968. pp. 2–3.

Williams, H. E. (1960). Bat-transmitted paralytic rabies in Trinidad. *Can. Vet. J.*, **1**, 20–24 and 45–50.

Winkler, W. G. (1968). Airborne rabies virus isolation. *Bull. Wildlife Disease Assoc.*, **4**, 37–40.

World Health Organization Expert Committee on Rabies. (1966). Fifth report. World Health Organ., Tech. Rep. Ser. **321**.

For Discussion, see page 263.

## Discussion*

Koprowski: I should like to ask Dr. Constantine two questions: Do you consider the isolation of rabies virus from bats in Europe to be *bona fide*, and if so, how do you think the virus reached Europe? Second, has any progress been made in the eradication of rabid bats, either vampire or insectivorous?

Constantine: In reference to the infection of European bats, I think there is at least one reliable report, possibly two. As far as the source of virus for bats is concerned, what is the source in America? We do not know. Evidently it is now maintained in America bats, however. In reference to the eradication of bats, I feel that there has been some progress in development of techniques, but in application, that is something else again. Actually, I make my statement on the basis of a trap that I devised and designed so that it could be built by anybody for relatively little money. I placed it in the hands of a rancher who subsequently accounted for destroying over 500 vampire bats in several evenings. As I understand it, this compares with a vampire bat destruction rate on Trinidad of something like 2,000 bats per year by the entire bat-collecting crew, so I feel that on that basis, some progress has been made. I recently published this, but I do not know that it has been applied, at least on a large scale.

Davenport: I gather there is a difference of opinion between yourself and Dr. Johnson on the importance of the bat in the natural history of rabies. How do you expect to resolve this question? What kinds of evidence would either person accept as definitive to ascertain whether rabies in bats is an interesting phenomena in its own right or whether it has anything to do with a reservoir which spills over to ground mammals and finally to man?

Johnson, H. N.: Dr. Constantine and I are not in any basic disagreement. We are experiencing in North America a large epizootic of rabies in bats, but as he brought out, there is no evidence

* This Discussion refers to the reports by H. N. Johnson and Constantine.

of a similar epizootic in Europe. There is a single definite isolation of virus there, and as in the Middle East and Asia, there is no evidence of a similar outbreak of rabies in bats. In Africa or Australia, heavily populated with bats there is also no outbreak. I think he also will agree with me that in all the work that I have done and he has done, and his is a great deal more, I do not know of any instance in which rabies virus was isolated from the saliva or any other organ where the virus was also not present in the brain. Is that correct?

CONSTANTINE: With the exception of one sample, it is correct, and we were encouraged to discard that result because we could not rcpcat it.

JOHNSON, H. N.: I say this because in California, in Dr. Lennette's laboratory we have had for some years 484 rabid bats. I have tested all bats that came into the surveys and those found negative for rabies by the brain tests for arboviruses, which would also pick up rabies virus in salivary gland, lung, or kidney. We have been unable to isolate rabies virus from these organs unless the virus is also present in the brain.

DOWNS: In the whole discussion of rabies in wildlife, I am curious about the omission of one group of animals: the shrews. From some of the mammalogical works which I have read, it appears that in various parts of the world, the shrews, which are very rarely seen, difficult to collect, and usually almost impossible to maintain in the laboratory, nonetheless constitute in sheer weight the most significant fraction of the mammalian bio-mass. They are intense carnivores. What is the position of shrews vis-a-vis rabies?

JOHNSON, H. N.: There is certainly a large number of shrews in the world but the fact is that we do not know of a single human case of rabies stemming from shrew bite. There is also no evidence that animals which have been bitten by shrews, such as dogs and cats, become infected with rabies. I have tested salivary gland, lung, and kidney of as many shrews as we could obtain in California, and some in India, where there is a large shrew, *Suncus Murinus*. We have not isolated rabies virus from shrews. There is no record of human rabies from the bite of rats. There have been reports of isolation of many strains of rabies virus from Rattus, in certain places in the world. If there is an outbreak of rabies in rats, we would expect some to daytime acting in an abnormal manner, others to be found dead from rabies, and rat bites that produced rabies in man or some other animal. It is not uncommon for people to be bitten by shrews, both the small ones we have in North America, and the ones in India.

# The Quarantine of Dogs Imported to Japan

KENZO NOBUTO

*Animal Health Division, Bureau of Animal Industry, Ministry of Agriculture and Forestry, Tokyo*

Rabies has been legally designated as a notifiable disease of domestic animals since 1896, but we do not know what the incidence of rabies was up to that time. After 1897 the incidence of rabies in dogs and other animals was recorded almost every year, and in 1912 there were 83 human cases of rabies. In 1914 when World War I broke out, the incidence of rabies in human and dogs reached a peak. In 1918 prophylactic vaccination of dogs with inactivated vaccine was started and as a result, there was a temporary decline in the incidence of rabies. In 1923, however, the great Kanto earthquake brought about major social and economic unrest and the number of stray dogs increased. The situation became disastrous by 1924, with 3,205 dogs, 235 humans and 84 other animals infected: a total of 3,524 cases of rabies. After that time the use of prophylactic vaccination began to be effective and in 1935 the incidence of rabies in dogs decreased considerably while no human cases of rabies were reported. The incidence of rabies in 1950 was 875 dog, 54 human and 55 animal cases, arising in part from conditions after World War II, and stimulating the establishment of the rabies prevention law in the same year.

The rabies prevention law stipulates that owners of dogs of 91 days or older as of April 1st must apply every year for registration of their dogs to the governor of the prefecture through the mayor of the city, town or village in which they reside. The mayor then notifies dog owners of the specified date for vaccination of their dogs. The vaccination is carried out in a place designated for assembling and vaccinating all the dogs in the area by practising veterinarians. It is given twice a year, in the spring and autumn. Dog owners are given a certificate of vaccination and a mark showing that the dog has been vaccinated. Dog owners bear the vaccination fee.

The Ministry of Health and Welfare has jurisdiction over rabies prophylactic vaccination, and the actual work is done by the rabies control officers of the prefectural or metropolitan health centers. All dogs that have not been registered or vaccinated are caught by dog catchers under the direction of the rabies control officers.

The Ministry of Agriculture and Forestry has jurisdiction over licenses and permits of vaccine manufacturing plants, and administers the approval, assay and test of vaccines. In Japan three types of vaccines are presently authorized: ultraviolet ray irradiated inactivated vaccine, phenolized inactivated vaccine and thymerosol inactivated vaccine. Seven private companies are manufacturing approximately 15,000 *l* of these vaccines yearly. Each time a vaccine is manufactured, a sample must be sent to the National Veterinary Assay Laboratory for official assay, and only those vaccines which have passed the national assay are sold. The potency test used is the Habel index, and those having a protective value of over 1,000 are given authorization.

Japan has been a rabies-free country since 1957. Surrounded by the sea on all sides, it is limited in area and has a very small number of wild animals which could constitute a rabies reservoir. We have been able to prevent rabies by carrying out regular vaccination twice a year.

Table 1 shows the total number of registered dogs, the estimated rate of vaccination, and also the number of stray dogs caught since 1950. Recently the number of families that own pets has increased sharply. As compared with the total of dogs for 1950, 1,066,739, the number for 1969 was 2,836,285 an increase of 2.8 times. The number of vaccinated dogs was 4,569,821, including both spring and autumn vaccinations. This means that the vaccination rate is 80.6%, which may be considered sufficient to maintain the necessary immunity against a major outbreak. But we can not neglect the fact that there are many unregistered and stray dogs. In 1969 the number of dogs that were detained was 687,821 and assuming that the total number of dogs in Japan is over 4,000,000, the vaccination rate would then be less than 60%. If the virus entered the country from abroad there would be danger of an outbreak spreading through the stray dog population.

Table 1. Number of Registered Dogs and Vaccination Rate

| Year | Registered ($A$) | Vaccinated ($B$) | $B/2A \times 100$ | Detained |
|---|---|---|---|---|
| 1950 | 1,066,789 | 1,831,303 | 85.8% | 179,828 |
| 1957 | 1,736,736 | 2,811,564 | 80.9 | 452,823 |
| 1960 | 1,905,080 | 3,075,417 | 80.7 | 396,790 |
| 1963 | 2,087,483 | 3,550,379 | 85.9 | 444,602 |
| 1966 | 2,699,474 | 4,295,503 | 79.6 | 597,793 |
| 1969 | 2,836,285 | 4,569,821 | 80.6 | 687,821 |

The general situation of rabies control in Japan in 1968 appears in Table 2. More than 20,000 cases of persons being bitten by dogs and 279,227 cases of complaints against dogs occurred. Therefore, extreme care must be taken to prevent the introduction of the virus from abroad.

Table 2. General Situation of Rabies Control in Japan (1968)

| | |
|---|---|
| Number of Dogs Registered | 2,775,677 |
| Number of Dogs Vaccinated against Rabies | 4,461,492 |
| Number of Rabies Prevention Officers | 2,750[a] |
| Number of Rabies Prevention Assistants | 893 |
| Number of Dogs Detained | 697,748 |
| Number of Dogs Biting Persons | 20,428 |
| Number of Persons Bitten by Dogs | 21,075 |
| Reported Protests and Complaints Against Dogs | 279,227 |

*a* As of Sept. 1967. These figures also include food hygiene inspectors and meat inspectors who serve concurrently as rabies control officers.

Table 3 shows the figures of dog imports from 1965 to 1969. The Import-Export Quarantine of dogs as stipulated by the Rabies Prevention Law comes under the jurisdiction of the Minister of Agriculture and Forestry. The Animal Quarantine Service has its headquarters in Yokohama and 18 stations in the major sea and air ports throughout the country. There are 59 full-time veterinary inspectors engaged in quarantine service at these stations. There were more than 10,000 dogs imported in 1968 but the figure for 1969 was slightly lower. The bulk of these imports come in through Tokyo's Haneda Airport, and the port of Yokohama is second.

Table 3. Importation of Dogs by Ports

| Name of Port | No. of Vet. Inspectors | 1965 | 1966 | 1967 | 1968 | 1969 |
|---|---|---|---|---|---|---|
| Tokyo | 15 | 763 | 986 | 2,834 | 9,648 | 7,020 |
| Itami | 3 | 1 | 7 | 6 | 16 | 45 |
| Itazuke | 1 | 1 | – | – | – | 3 |
| Yokohama | 11 | 37 | 63 | 114 | 703 | 203 |
| Shibaura | 2 | 2 | 3 | 3 | 2 | 5 |
| Nagoya | 5 | 2 | 4 | 4 | – | 4 |
| Kobe | 8 | 8 | 8 | 17 | 25 | 13 |
| Osaka | 4 | 2 | 2 | 2 | – | 6 |
| Moji | 3 | 1 | 1 | 2 | – | – |
| Kagoshima | 3 | – | 4 | 1 | – | – |
| Nase | 2 | – | – | 1 | 1 | – |
| Yokkaichi | 2 | – | – | – | – | 1 |
| Total | | 817 | 1,078 | 2,984 | 10,395 | 7,300 |

The means of transportation of imported dogs is shown on Table 4. Most of them (97%) come in as air cargo and only 3% enter as passenger hand baggage.

Table 4. Means of Dog Importation

| Year | Sea Cargo | | Air Cargo | | Hand Baggage | | Total |
|---|---|---|---|---|---|---|---|
| | No. dogs | % | No. dogs | % | No. dogs | % | |
| 1965 | 39 | 5 | 712 | 87 | 66 | 8 | 817 |
| 1966 | 74 | 7 | 906 | 84 | 98 | 9 | 1,078 |
| 1967 | 44 | 2 | 2,784 | 93 | 156 | 5 | 2,984 |
| 1968 | 9 | – | 10,206 | 98 | 180 | 2 | 10,395 |
| 1969 | 29 | – | 7,081 | 97 | 190 | 3 | 7,300 |

In principle, import quarantine means the detention of the dog in the quarantine kennels of the Animal Quarantine Service, in accordance with Item 2 of Article 3 of the regulations. However, dogs that have no possibility of being infected with rabies may be confined in a place designated by the veterinary inspector; for example, the home of the owner. This home quarantine is subject to the following conditions: 1) the quarantined dog must be kept in doors, 2) no other dogs may be kept with the quarantined dog, 3) the instructions given by the veterinary inspector must be observed while the dog is under quarantine, and 4) a transportation vehicle for dogs must be used solely for this purpose. The dog must also be taken to the nearest Quarantine Service for inspection by a veterinary inspector once a week during the period of quarantine.

The period of detention is determined as follows: 1) A dog must be detained for thirty days if it received the prophylactic vaccination against rabies, as certified by the competent authority of the exporting country, during a period not less than thirty days and not more than one hundred and fifty days prior to arrival at the port of entry; and in case a dog was accompanied by a certificate issued by competent authorities of the exporting country, stating that it is not infected with rabies, the period of detention may be reduced to fourteen days. Furthermore, vaccination with the chick-embryo live virus vaccine is considered valid up to 3 years. 2) If thirty days have not lapsed since the date of the rabies vaccination, as certified by competent authorities of the exporting country, the number of days left until the 30th day is added to the 30-day detention period and the dog must be detained for 31 to 61 days. However, the detention period may be reduced to 16 to 45 days if a certificate issued by competent authorities of the exporting country, certifying that it is not infected with rabies accompanies the dog. 3) The period of detention may be reduced to 12 hours for a dog or dogs imported directly from the following countries designated by the Minister of Agriculture and Forestry:

| | |
|---|---|
| Okinawa | Finland |
| Cyprus | Portugal |
| Iceland | Northern Ireland |
| Ireland | Australia |
| Sweden | New Zealand |
| Norway | The Fiji Islands |

4) Dogs other than those in the above categories must be detained and quarantined for 120 days.

In the past five years dogs were imported from 64 countries. In recent cases where many dogs are imported for commercial purpose, the persons importing the dogs do not want to have lengthy detention and the majority of these dogs are imported from the countries designated as rabies-free by the Minister of Agriculture and Forestry.

In 1969, as seen in Table 5, 7,300 dogs were imported. Of these, 5,500 were released after 12 hours and 1,800 (24.7%) were detained. Of the detained dogs, 792 were detained in the quarantine kennels of the Animal Quarantine Services and the rest, 1,008 (56%), were kept under home quarantine.

Table 5. Number of Dogs by Type of Quarantine

| Year | Dogs Imported (*A*) | Released by Prompt Insp. (*B*) | Subjected to Quarantine (*C*) | *C/A* | Type of quarantine: at station (*D*) | Type of quarantine: home-quarantine (*F*) | *F/C* |
|---|---|---|---|---|---|---|---|
| 1965 | 817 | 319 | 498 | 61.0% | 197 | 301 | 60.4% |
| 1966 | 1,078 | 499 | 579 | 53.7 | 238 | 341 | 58.9 |
| 1967 | 2,984 | 2,160 | 824 | 27.6 | 393 | 431 | 52.3 |
| 1968 | 10,395 | 7,927 | 2,468 | 23.7 | 980 | 1,488 | 60.3 |
| 1969 | 7,300 | 5,500 | 1,800 | 24.7 | 792 | 1,008 | 56.0 |

In November of 1969 England was taken off the list of rabies-free countries designated by the Minister of Agriculture and Forestry due to the recent outbreak of rabies there.

Despite the fact that England has been a rabies-free country and has undertaken strict import quarantine for a long time, there was a case of an imported dog being infected with rabies. This served as a warning for Japan. If necessary, the existing system of import quarantine procedures might be reconsidered in light of the experience in England.

Table 6. Number of Dogs Imported by Countries (1965–1969)

| No. | Country | No. of Dogs | No. | Country | No. of Dogs |
|---|---|---|---|---|---|
| 1 | U.K. | 15,873 | 11 | Canada | 58 |
| 2 | U.S.A. | 4,997 | 12 | Netherlands | 54 |
| 3 | Ireland | 319 | 13 | France | 48 |
| 4 | West Germany | 292 | 14 | U.S.S.R. | 41 |
| 5 | Australia | 228 | 15 | Thailand | 38 |
| 6 | Okinawa | 87 | 16 | Philippines | 26 |
| 7 | Switzerland | 79 | 17 | Korea | 25 |
| 8 | Hong Kong | 67 | 18 | New Zealand | 17 |
| 9 | China (Taiwan) | 60 | 18 | Indonesia | 17 |
| 10 | India | 59 | 20 | Italy | 15 |

For Discussion, see page 273.

## Discussion*

TIERKEL: My question, Dr. Nobuto, does not have anything to do with rabies. Your tables showed something like a tenfold increase in the number of dogs that came into Japan in a period of about three years. To what do you attribute this?

NOBUTO: This is because social conditions and the way of life in Japan have changed and more families want to own pets. The increase in income has also brought about a desire to own purebred dogs, and this is why there is an increase in the number during this three-year period.

JOHNSON, H. N.: Have you had any dogs which die in quarantine and what are the procedures if they die? Are the brains tested for rabies?

NOBUTO: The person in charge of quarantine is present here and I would like to refer the question to him.

YAMANO: When a dog dies at the airport, we carry out an autopsy and if there are no lesions, we burn it in our furnace. We do not carry out any virus isolations because we trust the health certificates that come with the dogs.

JOHNSON, H. N.: We can be quite certain that some dogs will die in quarantine, and the question is whether each dog that dies is tested for rabies virus by inoculation of mice and by the fluorescent antibody test.

LENNETTE: It might be interesting to know what they died of, Dr. Beran.

BERAN: Doctor, do you have any regulations here in Japan on internal shipment of dogs, for example, from one island to another? Are there any health or vaccination certificates or anything of this kind required?

---

* This Discussion refers to the report by Nobuto.

NOBUTO: No certificates are required for domestic shipment in Japan.

HAMMON: You mentioned, and I didn't understand all of it, the types of vaccines that are permitted for use in dogs today. I remember the Semple type and the irradiated type and what else?

NOBUTO: Phenol inactivated, and ultraviolet inactivated, and thimerosal inactivated vaccines.

HAMMON: I'd like to ask about the potency tests. What potency tests are the licensed vaccines for dogs required to pass and who is responsible for them?

SAZAWA: The National Veterinary Assay Laboratory is responsible for National tests on biological products. Each lot of vaccine is subjected to required tests at the laboratory. We get about 100 lots of vaccine per year, 60 lots of phenolized vaccine, 20 lots of thimerosal vaccine, and 20 lots of UV inactivated vaccine. These are all tested by the Habel test and 1,000 is the minimum requirement. However, the majority of these vaccines are of the order of 10,000 to 100,000.

The Habel test is carried out by immunizing 50 mice, using 30 for control. The immunization is carried out 6 times using 0.5% tissue concentration. On the 14th day, we challenge the mice with a virus dilution. And those on the order of 1,000 and above are considered acceptable. Dogs are vaccinated twice a year, with a dose of 3–5 m*l*.

HADDOCK: In the discussion of rabies in Japan, so far only dogs have been mentioned. I understand that there is at least one wild carnivore in Japan, the Japanese weasel. I would like to ask if there is any routine surveillance of wild animals in Japan, and if so, what the results have been.

NOBUTO: We in the veterinary field do not carry out surveillance of weasels.

JOHNSON, H. N.: In the WHO Chronicle (1968, June, 22, No. 6, pp. 254-256) there is an article on the use of weasels in rat control and it says, "The idea of using Japanese weasels for rat control is not new to the Ryukyus, for they were first introduced into Kikaijima in 1942 with encouraging results. On Zamami-shima about 40 of these animals were introduced in 1957 and crop damage by rats, formerly heavy,—is now negligible." I bring this up because I have mentioned the introduction of mongooses into the Caribbean area in my paper. It took almost 100 years before it was discovered that they were harboring rabies virus and I believe this introduction of weasels onto some of these islands will be an excellent opportunity to study the ecology of this introduced animal. I also believe that warning should be given to proper authorities on these islands to be on the lookout for animals acting in an abnormal manner and have these tested for rabies by the tests I mentioned, the fluorescent antibody test and the inoculation into infant mice.

LENNETTE: Dr. Haddock and Dr. Johnson have brought up an extremely interesting point. I would like to add to that by suggesting, as Dr. Johnson already has, the use of very young animals for test animals, not adult mice but suckling or weanling mice:

DAVENPORT: Dr. Johnson—may I ask if it is known what the non-canine vectors of rabies might be in places like Thailand, Cambodia, or Southeast Asia in general?

JOHNSON, H. N.: I just had a discussion here with one of my colleagues about the paper published on rabies in rats and shrews in Thailand. I think this will come up in the panel discussions. But at the present time there is really nothing known or any work going on in trying to elucidate the information on natural hosts other than canines in Asia, that I know of. The reason probably is because in places like Thailand and India or say, the Philippine Islands where rabies exists in canines, the problem is so acute in the canine host that there is really no time or money to look into the background of where this virus may be maintained.

# Field Control of Animal Rabies

A Sixty-One-Year (1909–1969) Review of
the Disease and Measures Applied for
Its Control in the State of California

George L. Humphrey

*Veterinary Section, California Department of Public Health, Berkeley, California 94704*

The basic principles of operational programs for the control of animal rabies are well known and have been widely disseminated throughout the world in reports of the World Health Organization Expert Committee on Rabies (1950, 1954, 1957, 1960): 1) elimination of stray dogs, 2) canine vaccination and 3) control of wildlife vector populations. In addition, the WHO Expert Committee on Rabies (1950, 1954, 1957) has recommended application of the following specific measures in areas affected with rabies: 1) registration, licensing, and taxation of dogs, 2) elimination of stray animals, 3) restraint of dogs while the control campaign is underway, 4) mass vaccination of dogs free of charge, 5) provision of adequate facilities for diagnosis, 6) reduction in number of wildlife species where these are a reservoir of the disease, and 7) a continual and energetic publicity campaign.

While the foregoing basic principles and specific measures are simply set forth, their implementation to form effective operational control programs are frequently difficult to achieve. The details of essential promotional work which must precede the successful implementation of a control program are seldom the subject of published papers and constitute undocumented stories underlying various publications describing the successful results of program application.

There are reasons for the absence of published descriptions of how most control programs are brought into existence. Disease control programs such as those for rabies are seldom the product of the effort of a single person. Usually the support and work of many persons, both in and out of government, as well as various organizational groups, are necessary for successful implementation of a control program. Regulatory officials concerned with the development and implementation of a rabies control program must deal with a variety of factors, many of which will be unique to the particular area and

Table 1. Annual Report of Local Rabies Control Activities (California, 1956–1968)

| Year | Vaccination Program | | | | |
|---|---|---|---|---|---|
| | Dogs Vaccinated | | | | Registration |
| | Total | Private Vaccinations | Low-Cost Public Clinics | Low-Cost Clinics Held | Dogs Licensed for Which Valid Vaccination Certificates Were Submitted |
| 1956 | 131,030 | 50,362 | 18,221 | NA | 406,095 |
| 1957 | 115,765 | 56,481 | 35,354 | NA | 534,517 |
| 1958 | 303,223 | 149,850 | 139,602 | 599 | 488,353 |
| 1959 | 198,507 | 116,117 | 73,473 | 758 | 538,759 |
| 1960 | 277,645 | 153,451 | 107,307 | 1,456 | 628,120 |
| 1961 | 311,188 | 151,846 | 151,908 | 905 | 692,029 |
| 1962 | 335,142 | 196,713 | 135,727 | 958 | 745,461 |
| 1963 | 422,174 | 259,519 | 162,655 | 1,183 | 863,524 |
| 1964 | 480,616 | 290,298 | 188,990 | 1,240 | 960,066 |
| 1965 | 518,441 | 303,511 | 210,052 | 1,281 | 958,561 |
| 1966 | 511,242 | 308,234 | 203,008 | 1,348 | 1,079,615 |
| 1967 | 494,041 | 326,423 | 226,686 | 1,417[a] | 1,229,064 |
| 1968 | NA | NA | 229,820 | 1,407 | 1,260,414 |

NA: Not Available.

*a* Estimated.

Source: State of California, Department of Public Health, Annual Reports of Local Rabies Control Activities. Figures for 1956–1957 were collected under a voluntary program. Those since 1958 were collected under provisions of regula-

political jurisdictions involved. Such factors may include, but are not limited to, political, legislative, judicial, social, cultural, religious, racial, ecological, environmental, economic, educational, public relations, and public opinion considerations.

Rabies control is a proper task of government, since it is beyond the capability of individual action to control the disease. Rabies in animals often affects wide geographic areas and does not recognize political boundaries and its control is most properly a responsibility of central government—countries and states—in partnership with local government—counties, cities, boroughs, districts. The role of central government is to provide needed authority (legislation) and leadership to extend uniform rabies control measures over the large geographic area necessary to insure disease control success. The role of local government is to enforce control measures within their respective jurisdictions.

A factor lacking in the control of rabies in dogs in the United

| Canine Rabies Control | | | | | | | Animal Bites Reported | | |
|---|---|---|---|---|---|---|---|---|---|
| Stray Dog Control | | | | Enforcement | | | | | |
| Impounded | Redeemed | Sold or Given Away | Destroyed | Warning Issued for Violations | Number Brought to Court | Convictions Obtained | Dog | Other Domestic Animal | Wild Animal |
| 126,472 | 20,540 | 20,567 | 82,054 | 11,463 | 1,919 | 314 | 31,721 | 5,237 | 263 |
| 172,151 | 26,104 | 28,867 | 113,592 | 18,687 | 1,505 | 620 | 44,708 | 4,263 | 576 |
| 238,375 | 31,501 | 36,187 | 169,407 | 30,246 | 2,717 | 1,253 | 45,785 | 5,386 | 1,237 |
| 235,001 | 33,601 | 42,557 | 172,328 | 53,389 | 4,076 | 1,823 | 36,835 | 5,952 | 1,557 |
| 311,211 | 45,198 | 47,469 | 222,701 | 62,393 | 7,018 | 1,553 | 43,340 | 8,368 | 1,884 |
| 320,700 | 46,978 | 55,078 | 214,169 | 130,624 | 4,680 | 1,625 | 43,272 | 7,663 | 1,910 |
| 328,677 | 51,125 | 57,819 | 226,880 | 180,088 | 4,288 | 1,739 | 42,640 | 7,643 | 1,906 |
| 381,920 | 50,760 | 63,586 | 270,026 | 189,041 | 4,842 | 2,849 | 55,758 | 9,067 | 2,433 |
| 412,711 | 64,490 | 79,558 | 298,633 | 202,017 | 7,351 | 6,374 | 56,990 | 7,712 | 2,408 |
| 370,418 | 65,368 | 84,487 | 268,067 | 258,221 | 9,363 | 5,673 | 45,056 | 7,573 | 2,675 |
| 458,739 | 66,457 | 86,492 | 315,166 | 500,662 | 9,730 | 6,547 | 53,117 | 9,267 | 3,486 |
| 452,065 | 72,451 | 78,453 | 304,070 | 551,344 | 11,441 | 7,093 | 58,856 | 9,724 | 3,562 |
| 552,836 | 80,641 | 89,548 | 367,202 | 294,430 | 13,451 | 6,676 | 61,032 | 10,049 | 3,761 |

tions adopted pursuant to new rabies control legislation implemented on December 2, 1957. Figures are not statewide but represent those received from counties under declaration as *rabies endemic areas* from October 10, 1955, to December 1, 1957, or under declaration as *rabies areas*, December 2, 1957 to December 31, 1968.

States is the absence of essential federal legislation to require the various rabies affected states to implement adequate control programs (Sikes, 1968). Currently, only 14 of the 48 continental states have adopted legislation requiring rabies vaccination of dogs. The state of California adopted legislation requiring rabies vaccination of dogs and establishing minimum standards for local (city and county) control programs in counties declared *rabies areas* in 1957. The legislation adopted in 1957 required eight years of work to achieve passage. Results of the program have been outstanding (Tables 1 and 2) (Humphrey, 1966).

## DESCRIPTION OF STATE

The borders of California enclose 158,693 square miles; its length from extreme north to south is 800 miles and its extreme width, east to west, 375 miles. The 1970 population of the state is approximately

Table 2. Animal Rabies, California, 1909–1969[a]

| Year | Total Cases Reported | Cases Reported in Domestic Animals: Case of Rabies in Dogs: Total Dogs | In Mexico Border Area[1] | In Balance of State[2] | Other Domestic Species |
|---|---|---|---|---|---|
| 1909–1969 | 26,544 | 20,879 | – | – | 1,799 |
| 1909–1921 | 1,587 | 922 | – | – | 163 |
| 1922–1937 | 12,943 | 12,069 | – | – | 770 |
| 1938–1953 | 7,858 | 7,104 | – | – | 613 |
| 1954–1969 | 4,156 | 784 | – | – | 253 |
| 1954 | 85 | 34 | 1 | 33 | 7 |
| 1955 | 425 | 246 | – | 246 | 13 |
| 1956 | 303 | 141 | – | 141 | 36 |
| 1957 | 197 | 49 | – | 49 | 8 |
| 1954–1957 | 1,010 | 470 | 1 | 469 | 65 |
| 1958 | 173 | 4 | – | 4 | 8 |
| 1959 | 167 | 34 | 29 | 5 | 20 |
| 1960 | 123 | 14 | 10 | 4 | 11 |
| 1961 | 253 | 20 | 15 | 5 | 16 |
| 1958–1961 | 716 | 72 | 54 | 18 | 55 |
| 1962 | 293 | 46 | 45 | 1[b] | 22 |
| 1963 | 309 | 86 | 84 | 2 | 12 |
| 1964 | 328 | 36 | 34 | 2 | 12 |
| 1965 | 229 | 18 | 16 | 2 | 21 |
| 1962–1965 | 1,159 | 186 | 179 | 7 | 67 |
| 1966 | 311 | 24 | 20 | 4 | 21 |
| 1967 | 264 | 21 | 16 | 5 | 16 |
| 1968 | 375 | 8 | 8 | – | 14 |
| 1969 | 321 | 3 | 1 | 2 | 16 |
| 1966–1969 | 1,271 | 56 | 45 | 11 | 67 |

*a* Figures for 1909 cover the period November 2-December 31 only.

*b* Dog in Butte County developed clinical symptoms five days after return from a 7-week stay in Mexico.

1 Cases in California-Mexico Border area, Imperial and San Diego Counties.

2 California excluding Imperial and San Diego Counties.

3 Rabies in animals imported from out-of-state: 1956, skunk shipped into Riverside County from Texas; 1959, dog shipped into Sonoma County from Georgia; 1961, monkey shipped into Los Angeles County from Peru; 1963, dog shipped into Los

20 million, an increase of over 9 million above the 1950 population of 10,586,000, and some 5,000,000 above that for 1960 (Rand McNally, 1962, 1967).

The backbone of the state is the Sierra Nevada Range. This range of mountains extends 400 miles along the eastern border, south from the Cascade Range in the north to the Tehachapi Mountains in the south. The foregoing mountains together with the Klamath Moun-

| Cases Reported in Wild Animals | | | | | | | | | |
|---|---|---|---|---|---|---|---|---|---|
| Total Wild-life Cases | Skunk | Bat | Fox | Coy-ote | Bobcat | Other Wild-life | Species not Spec-ified | Animals Imported from Out-of-state[3] | Rodents[4] |
| 3,366 | 2,459 | 484 | 188 | 160 | 49 | 26 | 462 | 12 | 26 |
| 105 | – | – | 2 | 100 | 3 | – | 392 | 4 | 1 |
| 32 | 4 | – | 2 | 24 | – | 2 | 68 | – | 4 |
| 118 | 50 | – | 33 | 17 | 8 | 10 | 2 | – | 21 |
| 3,111 | 2,405 | 484 | 151 | 19 | 38 | 14 | – | 8 | – |
| 44 | 32 | 1 | 8 | – | 2 | 1 | – | – | – |
| 166 | 141 | 2 | 19 | – | 3 | 1 | – | – | – |
| 125 | 119 | 4 | 2 | – | – | – | – | 1 | – |
| 140 | 130 | 2 | 7 | – | – | 1 | – | – | – |
| 475 | 422 | 9 | 36 | – | 5 | 3 | – | 1 | – |
| 161 | 145 | 8 | 7 | – | 1 | – | – | – | – |
| 112 | 82 | 18 | 8 | 1 | 1 | 2 | – | 1 | – |
| 98 | 83 | 12 | 2 | 1 | – | – | – | – | – |
| 216 | 174 | 34 | 3 | 3 | – | 2 | – | 1 | – |
| 587 | 484 | 72 | 20 | 5 | 2 | 4 | – | 2 | – |
| 225 | 189 | 29 | 4 | 1 | – | 2 | – | – | – |
| 209 | 145 | 53 | 5 | 1 | 4 | – | – | 3 | – |
| 280 | 208 | 53 | 14 | 2 | 1 | 2 | – | – | – |
| 190 | 113 | 72 | 2 | – | 2 | 1 | – | – | – |
| 903 | 655 | 207 | 25 | 4 | 7 | 5 | – | 3 | – |
| 266 | 154 | 55 | 43 | 4 | 10 | – | – | – | – |
| 227 | 158 | 43 | 14 | 4 | 8 | – | – | – | – |
| 351 | 291 | 52 | 5 | – | 3 | – | – | 2 | – |
| 302 | 241 | 46 | 8 | 2 | 3 | 2 | – | – | – |
| 1,146 | 844 | 196 | 70 | 10 | 24 | 2 | – | 2 | – |

Angeles County from Wisconsin, cat shipped into Los Angeles County from Pennsylvania, and a monkey shipped into San Joaquin County from Peru; 1968, a fox shipped into Los Angeles County from Texas, an ocelet shipped into Alameda County from Peru.

4 Reported cases in rodents (squirrels-9, gophers-6, rats-6, rabbits-4 and hamster-1) not laboratory confirmed; diagnosis questionable, probably not rabies.

Source: State of California, Department of Public Health, Morbidity Records.

tains in the north and the Coast Ranges on the west form the Central Valley, a 450 mile long alluvial trough.

A narrow coastal strip fronts the Coastal Ranges along the Pacific Ocean. East of the Cascades and the Sierra Nevada Range, in the northeastern portion of the state, lies a high arid lava plateau; to the south, barren mountain ranges separate a populous coastal plain from a large desert basin containing Death Valley, the Mojave and Colorado deserts, the Imperial Valley and the Salton Sea.

The southeastern deserts receive only 2–5 inches of rainfall annually, the Sierra Nevada Range over 500 inches of snowfall and the north coastal areas more than 100 inches of rainfall.

The Sacramento and San Joaquin Rivers drain the Central Valley, from the north and the south, respectively, along with flow from the western slope of the Sierra Nevada Range, to the ocean via the San Francisco Bay.

Prevailing westerly winds bring fog and rainfall to the coast ranges and heavy snow to the Sierra Nevada. The Central Valley is cooled by the ocean winds and protected from the continental cold by the Sierra Nevada Range. Rainfall in the Central Valley is about 20 inches in the north and 10 inches in the south. Some 20 national forests include about 25,000,000 acres of fir, pine and redwood timber in the Sierra Nevada, the Cascades, and the northern coastal ranges.

The state includes ten principal metropolitan areas: 1) Los Angeles-Santa Ana-Pomona-Ontario-San Bernardino-Riverside, 2) San Diego, 3) Ventura-Oxnard, 4) Santa Barbara, 5) Bakersfield, 6) Fresno, 7) Stockton, 8) Sacramento, 9) San Francisco-Oakland-San Jose, and 10) Modesto. Over 80% of the state's population resides in the above 10 metropolitan areas.

The state is bounded on the west by the Pacific Ocean, the state of Oregon on the north, to the east by the state of Nevada, on the southeast by the state of Arizona, and on the south by the state of Baja California del Norte, Mexico.

California includes 58 counties and over 400 incorporated city governments. Dog control, other than rabies control, has historically been a prerogative of local government.

## RABIES IN CALIFORNIA

### *Early history*

It is not known how long rabies has been present in California. The first laboratory confirmation of the disease was made in 1898 in a dog, one of several involved in a small outbreak in Los Angeles (Black & Powers, 1910). There is little doubt, however, that rabies existed in California prior to 1898.

Nelson (1918), in his book *Wild Animals of North America*, relates instances of rabies transmission from spotted skunks to man in Arizona in 1910 and on Cape San Lucas at the tip of Lower Baja California, Mexico, in 1905. Nelson further noted that when the voyager Duhun-Cilly visited Cape San Lucas in 1826, the natives feared the spotted skunk because they entered houses at night, biting people and infecting them with hydrophobia.

Lyman (1930), in his book *John Marsh, Pioneer*, refers to the occurrence of rabies in dogs, and to cases of hydrophobia in man being cared for by Marsh, the first American to practice medicine in California, in Los Angeles in 1836. So great was the menace of rabid dogs, at that time in Los Angeles, a decree was issued by Mexican officials ". . . that no man should keep more than two dogs and that both should be securely tied. The others were poisoned."

The book *Fur Bearing Animals* (1877) contains an article reprinted from the *American Journal of Science and Art* for May 1874 entitled "Rabies Mephitica" in which the author, Reverend Horace C. Hovey (1874), makes reference in a footnote to the occurrence, ostensibly in California, of a disease in man like hydrophobia following a bite by the spotted skunk *Spirogale putorius.*

The above references strongly suggest that rabies existed in wildlife on the Pacific slope of North America more than 144 years ago (Nelson, 1918) and in dogs in California at least 134 years ago (Lyman, 1930).

The 1898 outbreak in dogs in Los Angeles was apparently limited in extent. The city council adopted a dog muzzling ordinance on February 23 1898. The ordinance was enforced for about three months and then repealed, as there was no longer any evidence of the disease. The first laboratory confirmation of rabies in California was made in a dog in the 1898 outbreak (Black & Powers, 1910). In April 1899, a man previously bitten by his own dog died of rabies in Pasadena (Table 3) (Black & Powers, 1910). Rabies was confirmed by rabbit inoculation. No additional cases of rabies were observed in dogs in the Los Angeles area until 1906 (Black & Powers, 1910).

In March 1906, a pet dog bit a man, five horses, several dogs, and hogs 12 miles southwest of Los Angeles (Black & Powers, 1910). Rabies in the dog was confirmed by the finding of Negri bodies and rabbit inoculation done at the Pasteur Institute in Chicago. Two of the five horses and a hog bitten by the rabid dog subsequently died of rabies. No further cases, however, were observed until 1909 (Black & Powers, 1910).

*Initial spread of canine rabies throughout California (1909–1913)*

In June 1909, a suspect rabid dog was shot by a policeman near the center of the city of Los Angeles (Black & Powers, 1910). In less

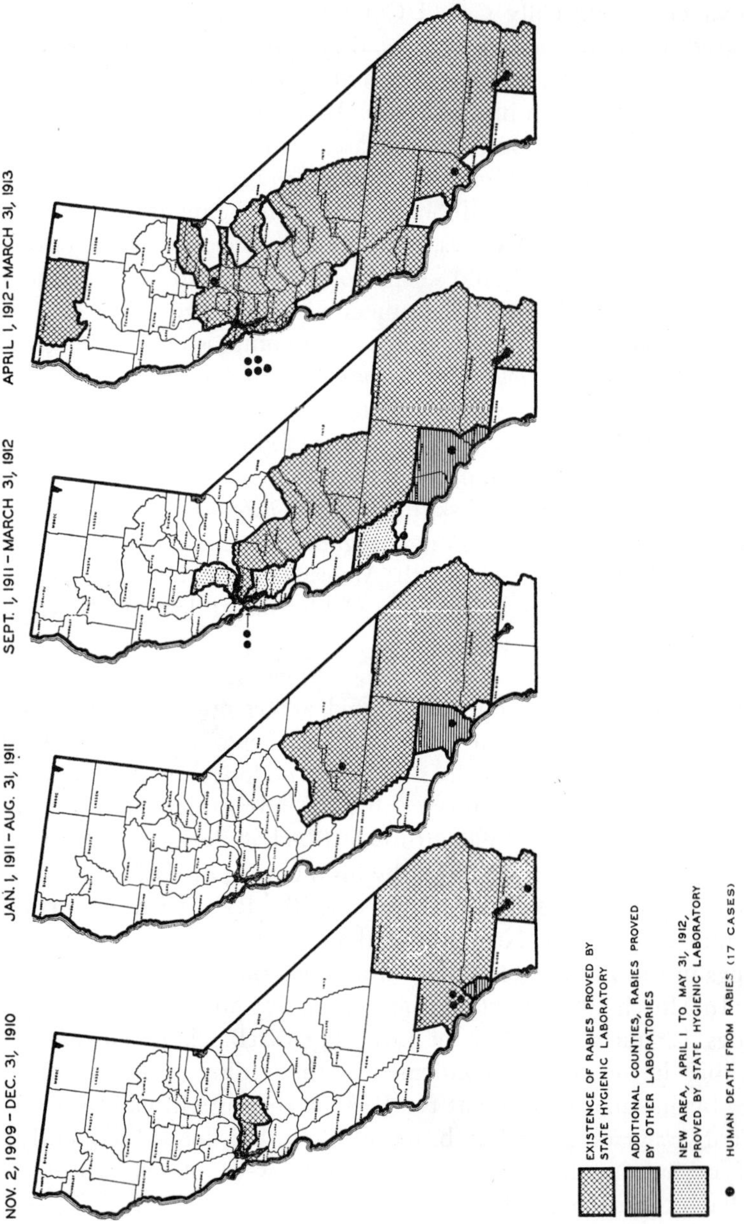


Fig. 1. Initial Spread of Canine Rabies in California by Counties, November 2, 1909–March 31, 1913

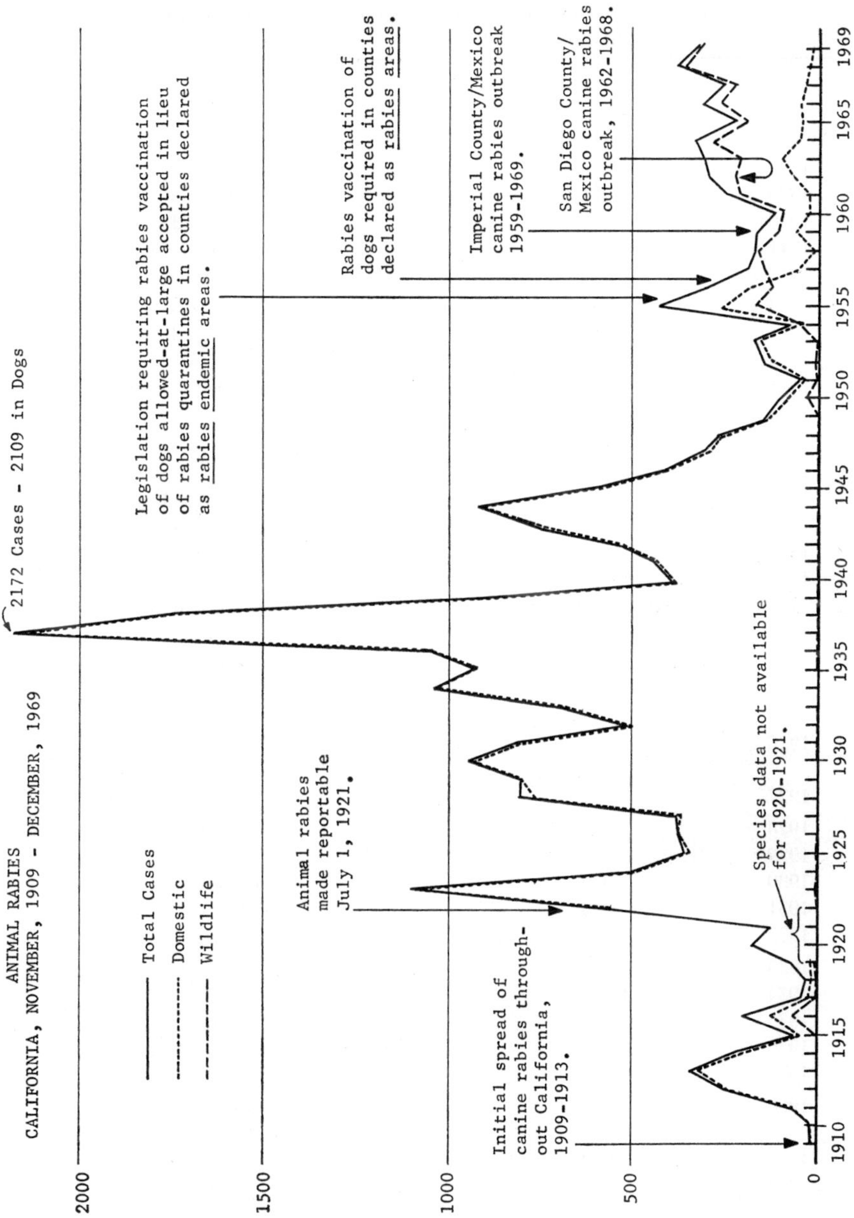
ANIMAL RABIES
CALIFORNIA, NOVEMBER, 1909 - DECEMBER, 1969
2172 Cases - 2109 in Dogs
Total Cases
Domestic
Wildlife
Legislation requiring rabies vaccination of dogs allowed-at-large accepted in lieu of rabies quarantines in counties declared as rabies endemic areas.
Rabies vaccination of dogs required in counties declared as rabies areas.
Imperial County/Mexico canine rabies outbreak 1959-1969.
San Diego County/ Mexico canine rabies outbreak, 1962-1968.
Animal rabies made reportable July 1, 1921.
Species data not available for 1920-1921.
Initial spread of canine rabies throughout California, 1909-1913.
2000
1500
1000
500
0
1910
1915
1920
1925
1930
1935
1940
1945
1950
1955
1960
1965
1969

Fig. 2.

Table 3. Animal and Human Rabies with Source of Human Infection (California, 1898–1969)

| Year | Animal | Human | Human Source |
|---|---|---|---|
| Totals | 26,544 | 111 | — |
| 1899 | NA | 1 | Dog |
| 1909 | 14[a] | 1 | Cat |
| 1910 | 18 | 3 | Dogs-3 |
| 1911 | 66 | 3 | Unknown |
| 1912 | 244 | 9 | Dogs-9 |
| 1913 | 330[b] | 8 | Dogs-8 |
| 1914 | 212 | 3 | Dogs-3 |
| 1915 | 63 | 5 | Dogs-5 |
| 1916 | 197[c] | 1 | Dog |
| 1917 | 41 | – | — |
| 1918 | 29 | – | — |
| 1919 | 73 | – | — |
| 1920 | 176 | 4 | (Dogs-3) (Unknown-1) |
| 1921 | 124 | 5 | Dogs-5 |
| 1922 | 566 | 4 | (Dogs-3) (Unknown-1) |
| 1923 | 1,092 | 11 | (Dogs-9) (Unknown-2) |
| 1924 | 500 | 5 | Dogs-5 |
| 1925 | 353 | 1 | Dog |
| 1926 | 375 | 5 | (Dogs-4) (Unknown-1) |
| 1927 | 376 | 1 | Dog |
| 1928 | 791 | 3 | Dogs-3 |
| 1929 | 787 | 2 | Dogs-2 |
| 1930 | 929 | 1 | Dog |
| 1931 | 800 | 2 | Dogs-2 |
| 1932 | 508 | 2 | Dogs-2 |
| 1933 | 681 | – | — |
| 1934 | 1,035 | 1 | Dog |
| 1935 | 926 | 1 | Dog |
| 1936 | 1,052 | 1 | Dog |
| 1937 | 2,172 | 3 | Dogs |
| 1938 | 1,730 | 4 | { (Dogs-3) (Cow-1) |
| 1939 | 899 | 1 | Dog |
| 1940 | 396 | 2 | { (Dog-1) (Cat-1) |
| 1941 | 442 | 1 | Dog |

| Year | Animal | Human | Human Source |
|---|---|---|---|
| 1942 | 531 | 1 | Dog |
| 1943 | 740 | 2 | (Dog-1) (Skunk-1) |
| 1944 | 911 | 3 | Dogs-3 |
| 1945 | 581 | 1 | Dog |
| 1946 | 413 | – | — |
| 1947 | 303 | 1[i] | Dog |
| 1948 | 279 | – | — |
| 1949 | 152 | 1 | Dog |
| 1950 | 111 | – | — |
| 1951 | 54 | – | — |
| 1952 | 142 | 1[j] | Skunk |
| 1953 | 174 | – | — |
| 1954 | 85 | 1 | Skunk |
| 1955 | 425 | – | — |
| 1956 | 303[d] | – | — |
| 1957 | 197 | 1 | Dog[k] |
| 1958 | 173 | 1 | Bat |
| 1959 | 167[e] | 1[l] | Bats |
| 1960 | 123 | – | — |
| 1961 | 253[f] | 1 | Dog |
| 1962 | 293 | – | — |
| 1963 | 309[g] | – | — |
| 1964 | 328 | – | — |
| 1965 | 229 | 1[m] | Dog |
| 1966 | 311 | – | — |
| 1967 | 264 | – | — |
| 1968 | 375[h] | – | — |
| 1969 | 321 | 1 | Bobcat |

NA Not available.
*a* Figures for 1909 cover the period November 2-December 31 only.
*b* Includes 3 cases from out-of-state.
*c* Includes bovine from out-of-state.
*d* Includes one skunk from Texas.
*e* Includes one dog from Georgia.
*f* Includes one monkey from Peru.
*g* Includes one dog from Wisconsin, one cat from Pennsylvania and one monkey from Peru.
*h* Includes one fox from Texas and one ocelot from Peru.
*i* Case occurred in a seaman bitten by a dog in Shanghai, China.
*j* Bitten by a skunk in Fresno, California; died in Oklahoma.
*k* Source unknown but occurred in an area affected by dog rabies.
*l* Probably aerosol transmission incurred in Frio Cave, Texas.
*m* Bitten by dog in Ensenada, Mexico; died in San Diego, California.
Source: State of California, Department of Public Health, Morbidity Records.

than a month, three other suspect rabid dogs were shot within 4–5 blocks of the first dog. In September 1909, a horse and a dog were confirmed rabid by the finding of Negri bodies and animal inoculation (Black & Powers, 1910).

A muzzling ordinance was passed by the Los Angeles city council on September 15, 1909, but was soon repealed, due to strong public opposition (Black & Powers, 1910). No effective control measures were thereafter adopted; and many cases of rabies in animals subsequently occurred throughout the Los Angeles area. The 1909 outbreak was the beginning of an epizootic of rabies in dogs which, by March 31, 1913, had spread throughout the state to the Mexico and Oregon borders, affecting 31 of the 58 counties in the state (Fig. 1) (Sawyer, 1912; Gieger, 1913). Seventeen human deaths due to rabies were recorded during the period November 2, 1909, to March 31, 1913 (Fig. 1).

California has been continuously afflicted by rabies in animals since June 1909, over 61 years (Fig. 2). A total of 110 cases of human rabies have been recorded in California during the 61-year period 1909–1969, and one case in 1899. Of the 111 cases, three incurred infections outside California, one in China in 1947, one in Texas in 1959 and one in Mexico in 1966. One case, incurred in California, died in the state of Oklahoma in 1952 (Table 3).

*Epizootic rabies in coyotes (1915–1917)*

While the presence of rabies in wild animals had been hypothesized as the source of the outbreak of dog rabies in Los Angeles in 1898 (Black & Powers, 1910; Calif. State Board of Health, 1910), the first available reference to laboratory confirmation of the disease in wildlife in California is that by Sawyer (Sawyer, 1912). Sawyer reported Negri bodies in the brain of a large grey fox, killed in April 1912 in the mountains of Ventura County. The second identification of rabies in wildlife was made by the State Hygienic Laboratory (California Department of Public Health) in a coyote from Tulare County in April 1913 (Sawyer, 1912).

In March 1915 the above laboratory reported rabies in two coyotes submitted from Lake County, Oregon. Lake County adjoins Modoc County, California, on the eastern portion of the Oregon-California border (Calif. State Board of Health, 1915). The report proved to be the forerunner of an extensive outbreak of rabies in coyotes which extended over southeastern Oregon, northeastern California, Nevada, and western Utah during the period 1915–1917 (Calif. State Board of Health, 1915).

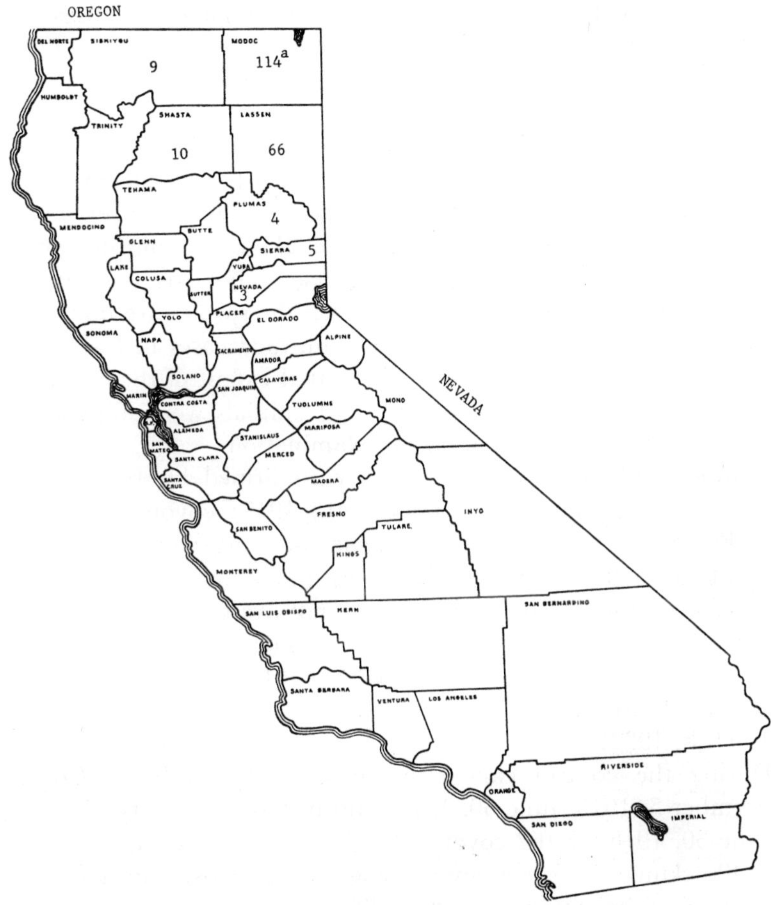


| Species | cases | Species | cases | Species | cases |
|---|---|---|---|---|---|
| Coyote | 94 | Horses | 6 | Human | 1 |
| Cattle | 64 | Bobcats | 3 | Unknown | 2 |
| Dogs | 31 | Cat | 1 | Total | 211 |
| Sheep | 8 | Goat | 1 | | |

Total cases 211
Counties affected 7
Areas affected by the 1915–1917 outbreak in coyotes included southeastern Oregon, Nevada, and western Utah as well as northeastern California

Fig. 3. Confirmed Rabies Cases, Outbreak among Coyotes, Northeastern California, October, 1915–December, 1917
*a* Includes one human case
Source: State of California, Department of Public Health, Laboratory Records

In October 1915 seven months after confirmation of the disease in Oregon, rabies was identified in four coyotes, three from Modoc County and one from Lassen County in northeastern California (Calif. State Board of Health, 1915). During the ensuing period from October 1915 through December 1917 a total of 211 cases of rabies were laboratory confirmed from seven northeastern California counties: Lassen-66 cases, Modoc-114, Nevada-3, Plumas-4, Shasta-10, Sierra-5, and Siskiyou-9 (Fig. 3). These 211 cases consisted of 94 coyotes, 64 cattle, 31 dogs, 8 sheep, 6 horses, 3 bobcats, one cat, one goat, one human, and two cases in which the species are unknown. The foregoing figures for laboratory confirmed cases in California, while large, are not indicative of the actual extent of the outbreak. Only a small proportion of the affected animals were shipped the 200–350 miles to the laboratory for examination.

Another 313 cases were laboratory confirmed by the state of Nevada during the 3-year period 1915–1917: coyotes-192 cases, dogs-43, cattle-43, cats-21, horses-6, sheep-6, and swine-2 (Records, 1932). Figures on incidence of the disease in animals in the other two affected states of Oregon and Utah are not available.

It is reported that livestock owners in Lassen and Modoc Counties alone lost an estimated $150,000 worth of cattle and horses as a direct result of the 1915–1917 outbreak in California (Calif. State Dept. of Pub. Hlth, 1932).

During the control campaign carried out in Modoc County (December 3, 1915–June 30, 1916) and in Lassen County (January 1–June 30, 1916), 7,162 coyotes, 1,091 dogs, 790 cats, 430 bobcats, and 496 skunks were destroyed using spring traps; and a total of 66,910 poison baits were placed (Calif. State Board of Health, 1916; Mallory, 1915). The control campaign in California was directed by the State Board of Health and carried out in cooperation with the United States Biological Survey and the United States Forest Service (Mallory, 1915). A total of 21 trappers were employed at the peak of the campaign in the two counties which together total 8,639 square miles (Calif. State Board of Health, 1916). The work was aided by a United States Congress appropriation of $75,000 which was applied toward control, done in the adjoining states affected by the outbreak, as well as in California (Calif. State Board of Health, 1916).

By 1918 the outbreak in dogs which had spread throughout California during the period 1909–1913, and that in wildlife during the period 1915–1917 in northeastern California, had largely subsided, and only 29 cases of rabies were recorded during the year, the lowest number since 1910.

To what degree dogs may have been responsible for the occurrence of the above rabies outbreak in coyotes is unknown. Records (1932) stated that "the disease (in dogs) gradually spread, traveling northward through California and being introduced into Oregon in 1912 by a sheep dog taken across the mountains from Redding, California, to Wallowa County in that state, where this infected dog in a fight with a coyote, first introduced the disease in wild animals." On the other hand, Mallory (1915) stated that there is reason to believe rabies may have been present in southern and eastern Oregon, with coyote involvement, as early as 1910 (Mallory, 1915). Documentation of the spread of rabies from dogs to wildlife is nearly impossible to obtain. Transmission of the disease from wildlife to dogs is more easily documented than the reverse. Transmission from wildlife to dogs can have long-term serious consequences such as the 12-year epizootic-enzootic occurrence of dog rabies along the California-Mexico border from 1959 to date (Humphrey & Hebert, 1960; Hebert & Humphrey, 1961). This extensive outbreak in dogs had origin in an epizootic of coyote rabies in Northern Baja California, Mexico, in 1958. The long-term consequences of the outbreak will be touched upon later in this paper.

*Second cycle of rabies in dogs (1919–1957)*

The year 1919 marks the beginning of a second cycle of canine rabies in California, one which persisted with varying annual incidence for over 40 years. Wildlife were little involved during this extended second cycle in dogs (Fig. 2). Complete figures on species of animals found rabid during the three years 1919–1921 are not available. However, regulations adopted in 1921, requiring the reporting of cases of rabies in animals, have provided relatively complete data since 1922. Reported figures for the 32-year period 1922–1953 show a total of 20,801 cases of animal rabies, 19,173 or 92% of which were in dogs. During the same 32-year period, only 150 cases or 0.7% were reported in wild animals (Table 2). Only in seven instances during the 32-year period 1922–1953 did the number of rabies cases reported in wildlife exceed six cases annually: 1923 (11 cases), 1947 (7), 1949 (8), 1950 (28), 1951 (10), 1952 (13), and 1953 (13).

Canine rabies reached epizootic peaks in California in 1923-977 cases, 1930-859, 1937-2,109, and 1944-854 (Fig. 2). The 7-year period 1945–1951 was one of decreasing annual incidence of rabies in dogs and a total of only 54 cases were reported during 1951, 33 of which were in dogs and 10 in wildlife. A remaining outbreak focus of canine rabies in Los Angeles and Orange Counties persisted until the end of 1957. However, the disease in dogs since 1958 has not been a problem in California with the exception of the areas immediately adjacent to the Mexican border.

## PRESENT PROBLEM OF RABIES IN WILDLIFE

In retrospect, the increased incidence of rabies reported in wild animals in 1947 (7 cases) and during the 5-years 1949–1953 (8, 28, 10, 13, and 13 cases, respectively) gave warning of a potential problem in wild animals. No one could have foretold, however, the extent and long duration of the disease in wildlife which has ensued since 1954. Rabies in wild animals broke with great rapidity in 1954–1955 with 44 and 166 cases, respectively, reported in wildlife during the 2-year period. The annual incidence of rabies in wild animals has remained high since 1955 (Fig. 2 and Table 2). Cases of the disease in wildlife during the 16-year period 1954–1969 number 3,111 or 75% of the total of 4,156 cases of animal rabies reported (Table 2).

The current occurrence of rabies in wildlife in California is not a singular phenomenon. Epizootics of the disease in wildlife have emerged in many other areas of the United States, Canada, Alaska, Greenland, the U.S.S.R., Europe, and other parts of the world since 1940 (See Johnson, General Epizootiology of Rabies, this meeting).

Wild species affected in California during the 16-year period 1954–1969 have been skunks-2,406 cases (Fig. 5), bats-484 (Fig. 6), foxes-152 (Fig. 7), bobcats-38 (Fig. 8), coyotes-19 (Fig. 9), racoons-9, badgers-3, and opossums-2 (Fig. 10). Two additional cases in wildlife were shipped into California—a skunk, and a fox from the state of Texas.

The distribution of reported cases of rabies in wildlife in California is similar for most affected species with only several exceptions (Figs. 4-13). The disease in skunks is one affecting primarily the Central Valley with extension into the western foothills of the Sierra Nevada to below snowline and the Coastal Ranges and valleys (Fig. 5). The occurrence of rabies in skunks in the Imperial Valley was first recognized in May 1969. By the end of 1969, 14 cases were reported in skunks in the valley. The outbreak continued into 1970 with an even greater number of cases recognized (46 cases through June 30, 1970).

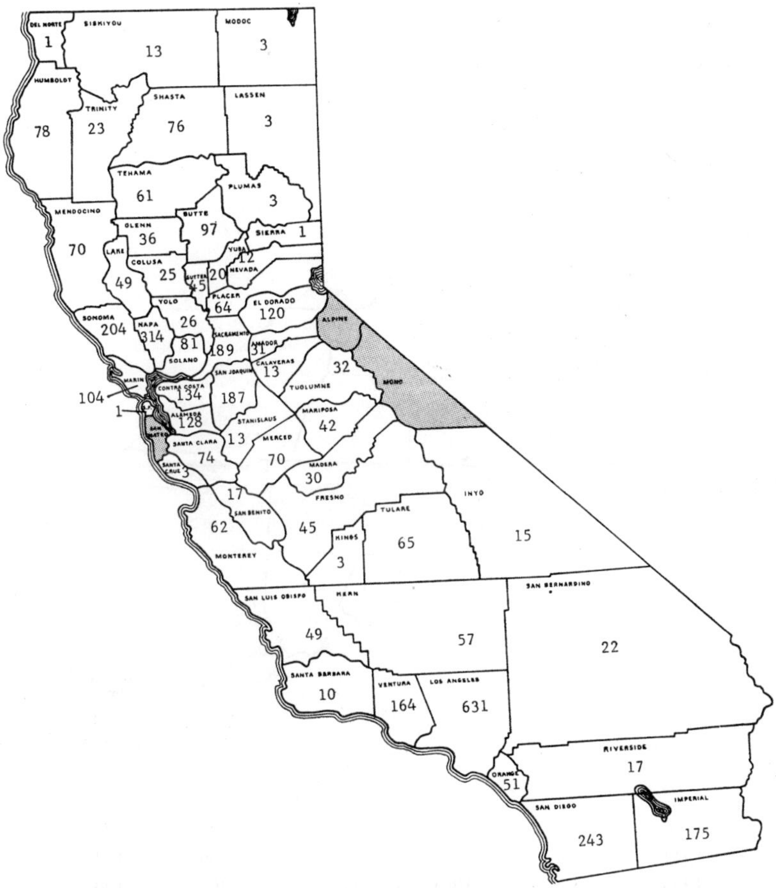


| year | cases | year | cases | year | cases |
|---|---|---|---|---|---|
| 1954 | 85 | 1960 | 123 | 1966 | 311 |
| 1955 | 425 | 1961 | 253 | 1967 | 264 |
| 1956 | 303 | 1962 | 293 | 1968 | 375 |
| 1957 | 197 | 1963 | 309 | 1969 | 321 |
| 1958 | 173 | 1964 | 328 | Total | 4156 |
| 1959 | 167 | 1965 | 229 | | |

Total cases 4156 ▩ Counties not reporting cases 3
Counties reporting cases 55

Source: State of California, Department of Public Health, Morbity Records

Fig. 4. Animal Rabies, California, 1954–1969

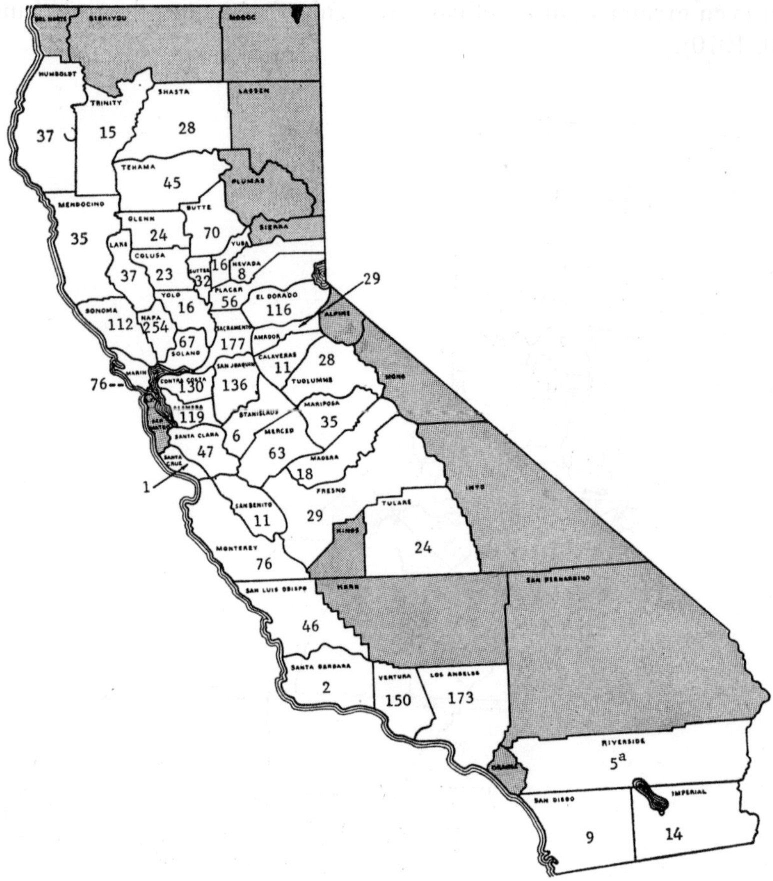


| year | cases | year | cases | year | cases |
|---|---|---|---|---|---|
| 1954 | 32 | 1960 | 83 | 1966 | 154 |
| 1955 | 141 | 1961 | 174 | 1967 | 158 |
| 1956 | 120[a] | 1962 | 189 | 1968 | 291 |
| 1957 | 130 | 1963 | 145 | 1969 | 241 |
| 1958 | 145 | 1964 | 208 | Total | 2406 |
| 1959 | 82 | 1965 | 113 | | |

Total cases 2406 ■ Counties not reporting cases 15
Counties reporting cases 43

*a* Texas source of one case in 1956
Source: State of California, Department of Public Health, Morbidity Records

Fig. 5. Rabies in Skunks, California, 1954–1969

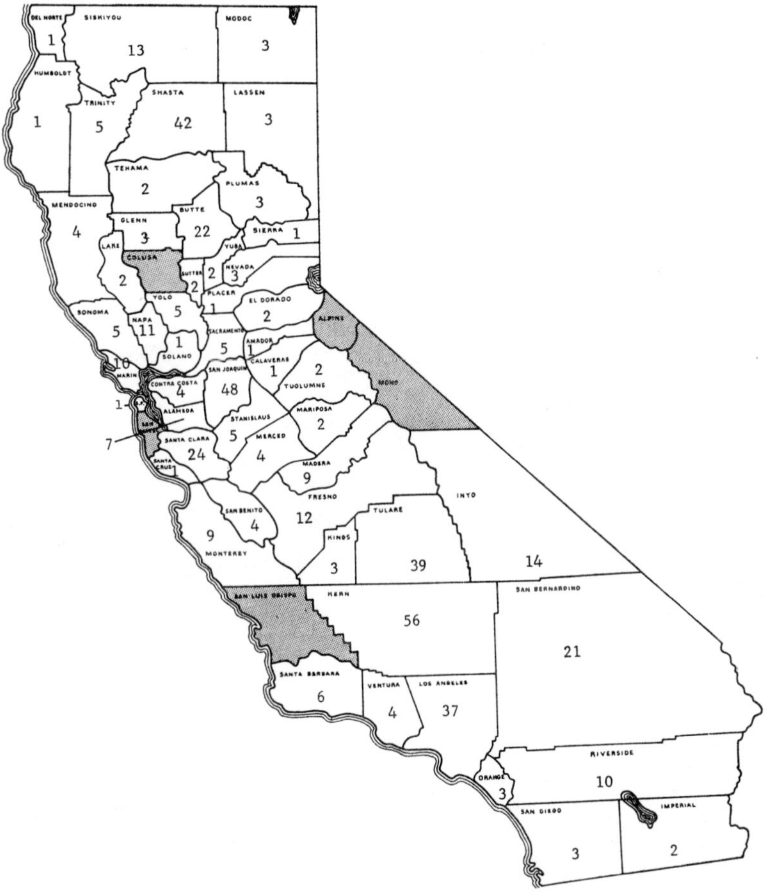


| year | cases | year | cases | year | cases |
|---|---|---|---|---|---|
| 1954 | 1[a] | 1960 | 12 | 1966 | 55 |
| 1955 | 2 | 1961 | 34 | 1967 | 43 |
| 1956 | 4 | 1962 | 29 | 1968 | 52 |
| 1957 | 2 | 1963 | 53 | 1969 | 46 |
| 1958 | 8 | 1964 | 53 | Total | 484 |
| 1959 | 18 | 1965 | 72 | | |

Total cases 484 ▩ Counties not reporting cases 5

Counties reporting cases 53

*a* First case of bat rabies recognized in California

Source: State of California, Department of Public Health, Morbidity Records

Fig. 6. Rabies in Bats, California, 1954–1969

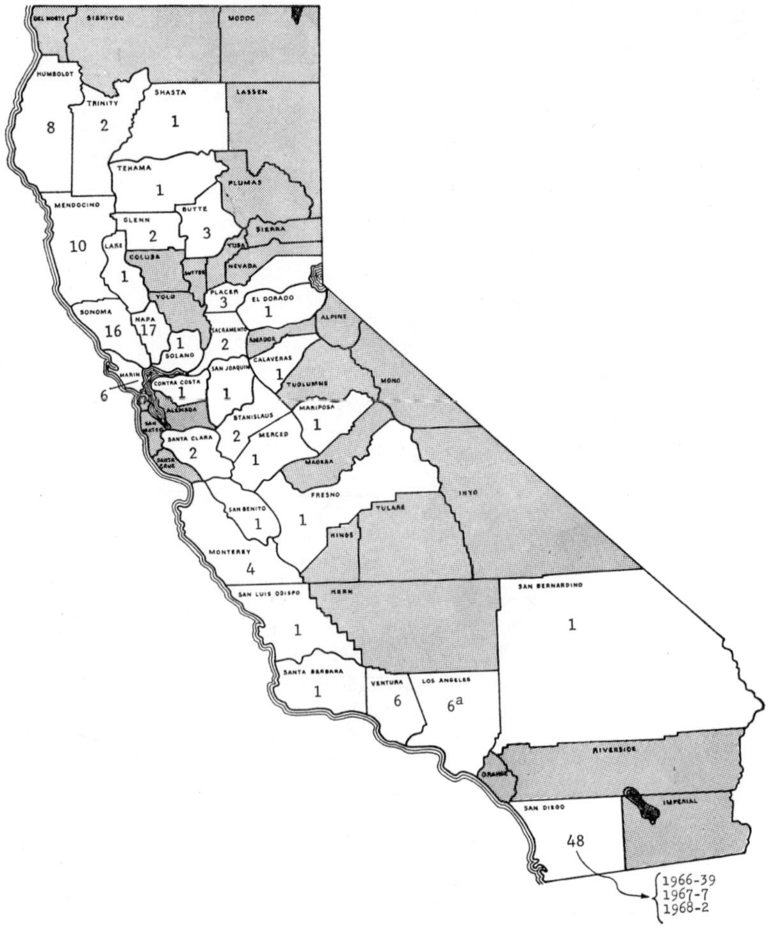


| year | cases | year | cases | year | cases |
|---|---|---|---|---|---|
| 1954 | 8 | 1960 | 2 | 1966 | 43 |
| 1955 | 19 | 1961 | 3 | 1967 | 14 |
| 1956 | 2 | 1962 | 4 | 1968 | 6[a] |
| 1957 | 7 | 1963 | 5 | 1969 | 8 |
| 1958 | 7 | 1964 | 14 | Total | 152 |
| 1959 | 8 | 1965 | 2 | | |

Total cases 152 ▨ Counties not reporting cases 27

Counties reporting cases 31

*a* Texas source of one case in 1968

Note: (1) The five counties of Humboldt, Mendocino, Sonoma, Napa and Marin account for 57–37.5% of cases.

(2) The San Diego County outbreak accounts for 48–31.6% of cases.

Source: State of California, Department of Public Health, Morbidity Records.

Fig. 7. Rabies in Foxes, California, 1954–1969

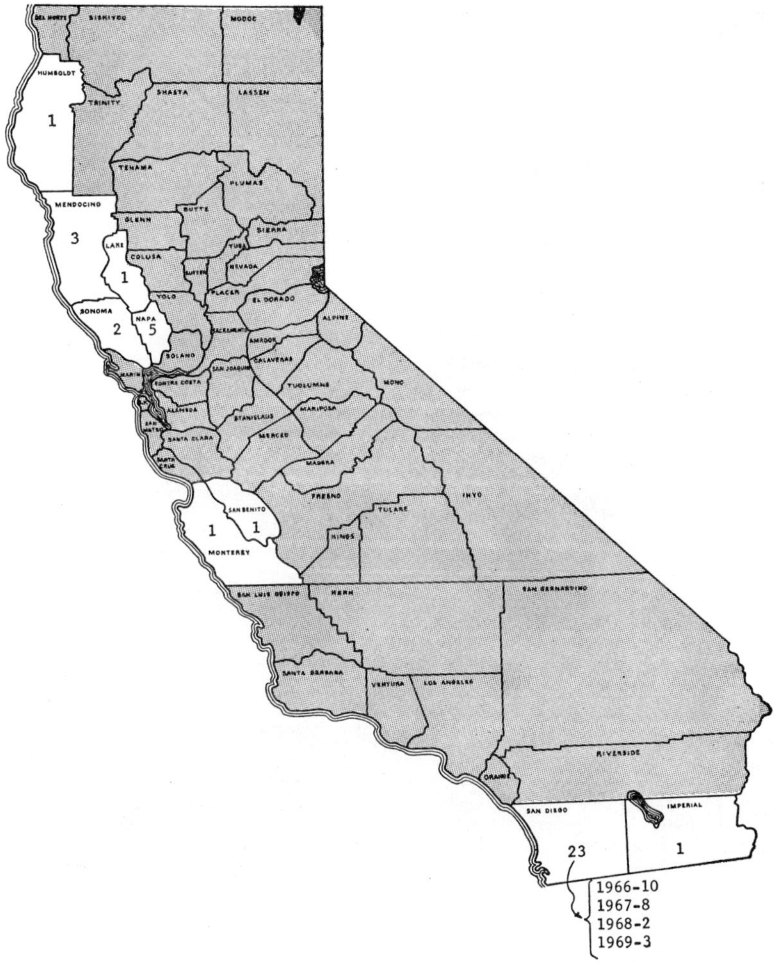


| year | cases | year | cases | year | cases |
|---|---|---|---|---|---|
| 1954 | 2 | 1960 | — | 1966 | 10 |
| 1955 | 3 | 1961 | — | 1967 | 8 |
| 1956 | — | 1962 | — | 1968 | 3 |
| 1957 | — | 1963 | 4 | 1969 | 3[a] |
| 1958 | 1 | 1964 | 1 | Total | 38 |
| 1959 | 1 | 1965 | 2 | | |

Total cases 38 ▩ Counties not reporting cases 49

Counties reporting cases 9

*a* One of the three cases reported in San Diego in 1969 was source of infection for a human case. San Diego County accounts for 23–61% of the cases.

Source: State of California, Department of Public Health, Morbidity Records.

Fig. 8. Rabies in Bobcats, California, 1954–1969

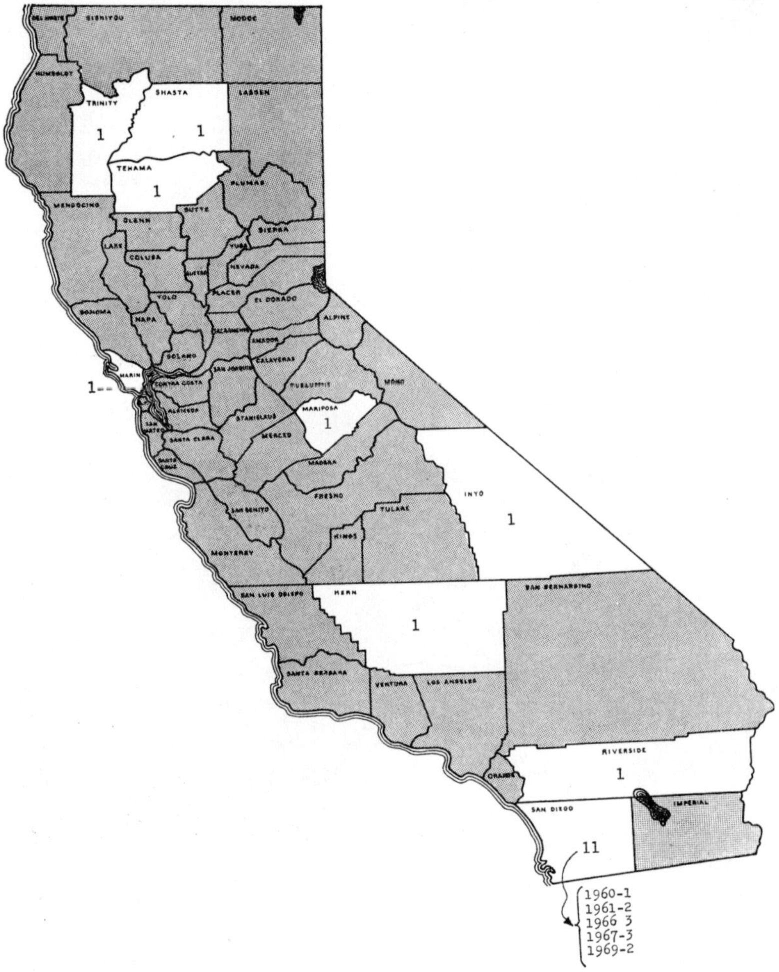


| year | cases | year | cases | year | cases |
|---|---|---|---|---|---|
| 1954 | — | 1960 | 1 | 1966 | 4 |
| 1955 | — | 1961 | 3 | 1967 | 4 |
| 1956 | — | 1962 | 1 | 1968 | — |
| 1957 | — | 1963 | 1 | 1969 | 2 |
| 1958 | — | 1964 | 2 | Total | 19 |
| 1959 | 1 | 1965 | — | | |

Total cases 19 ▩ Counties not reporting cases 49

Counties reporting cases 9

Source: State California, Department of Public Health, Morbidity Records.

Fig. 9. Rabies in Coyotes, California, 1954–1969

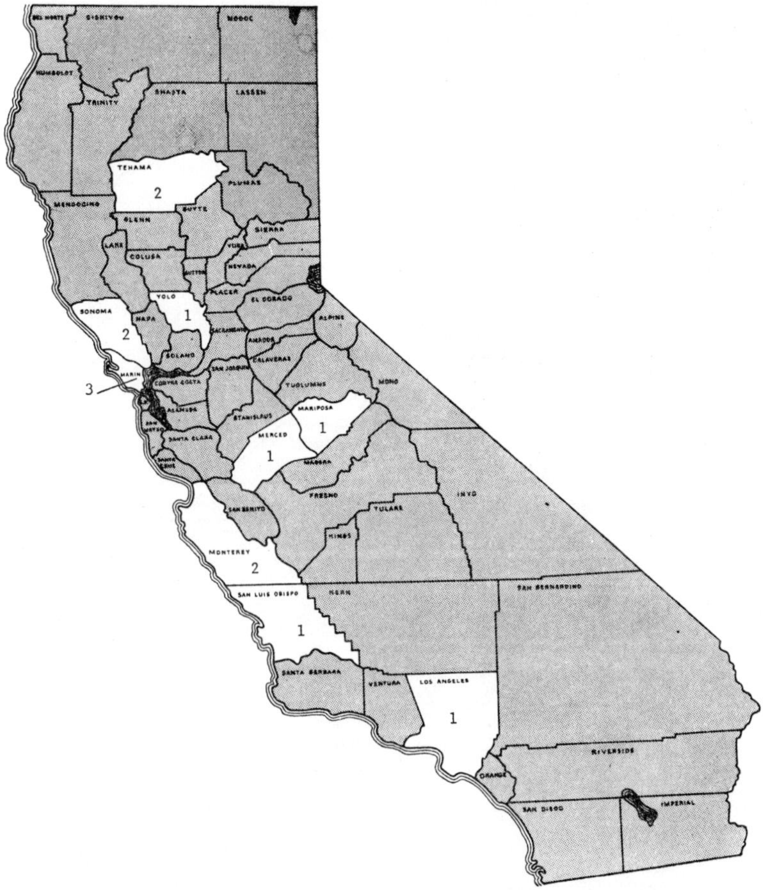


| year | cases | species | year | cases | species |
|---|---|---|---|---|---|
| 1954 | 1 | Racoon | 1963 | — | |
| 1955 | 1 | Racoon | 1964 | 2 | Racoon |
| 1956 | — | | | | Badger |
| 1957 | 1 | Racoon | 1965 | 1 | Opossum |
| 1958 | — | | 1966 | — | |
| 1959 | 2 | Racoon | 1967 | — | |
| | | Badger | 1968 | — | |
| 1960 | — | | 1969 | 2 | Racoon |
| 1961 | 2 | Racoon | | | Opossum |
| 1962 | 2 | Racoon | Total | 14 | |
| | | Badger | | | |

Total cases 14

Counties reporting cases 9

▨ Counties not reporting cases 49

* Excludes skunk, bat, fox, coyote and bobcat.

Source: State of California, Department of Public Health, Morbidity Records.

Fig. 10. Rabies in Other Wildlife* Species, California, 1954–1969

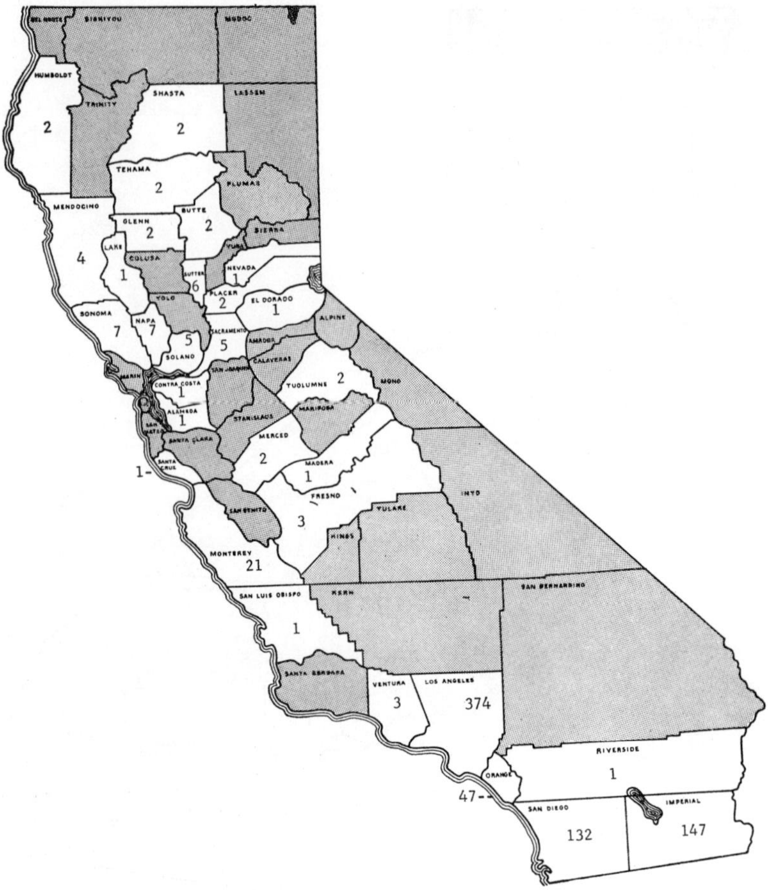


| year | cases | year | cases | year | cases |
|---|---|---|---|---|---|
| 1954 | 34 | 1960 | 14 | 1966 | 24 |
| 1955 | 246 | 1961 | 20 | 1967 | 21 |
| 1956 | 141 | 1962 | 46 | 1968 | 8 |
| 1957 | 49 | 1963 | 87[b] | 1969 | 3 |
| 1958 | 4 | 1964 | 36 | Total | 786 |
| 1959 | 35[a] | 1965 | 18 | | |

Total cases 786 ▨ Counties not reporting cases 28

Counties reporting cases 30

*a* Georgia source of one case in 1959

*b* Wisconsin source of one case in 1963.

Note: 1) 414 or 92% of the total of 421 cases of dog rabies reported from Los Angeles and Orange Counties occurred during the 4-year period 1954–1957.

2) 278 or nearly 90% of the total of 310 cases of dog rabies reported in California during the 11-year period 1959–1969 occurred in San Diego and Imperial Counties in association with California/Baja California, Mexico outbreak 1959–1969.

Source: State of California, Department of Public Health, Morbidity Records.

Fig. 11. Canine Rabies, California, 1954–1969

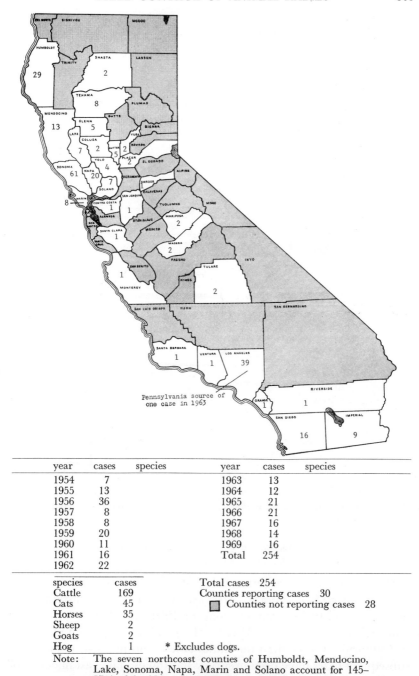


| year | cases | species | year | cases | species |
|---|---|---|---|---|---|
| 1954 | 7 | | 1963 | 13 | |
| 1955 | 13 | | 1964 | 12 | |
| 1956 | 36 | | 1965 | 21 | |
| 1957 | 8 | | 1966 | 21 | |
| 1958 | 8 | | 1967 | 16 | |
| 1959 | 20 | | 1968 | 14 | |
| 1960 | 11 | | 1969 | 16 | |
| 1961 | 16 | | Total | 254 | |
| 1962 | 22 | | | | |

| species | cases |
|---|---|
| Cattle | 169 |
| Cats | 45 |
| Horses | 35 |
| Sheep | 2 |
| Goats | 2 |
| Hog | 1 |

Total cases 254
Counties reporting cases 30
▨ Counties not reporting cases 28

* Excludes dogs.

Note: The seven northcoast counties of Humboldt, Mendocino, Lake, Sonoma, Napa, Marin and Solano account for 145–57% of the 254 cases reported.

Source: State of California, Department of Public Health, Morbidity Records.

Fig. 12. Rabies in Domestic Animals*, California, 1954–1969

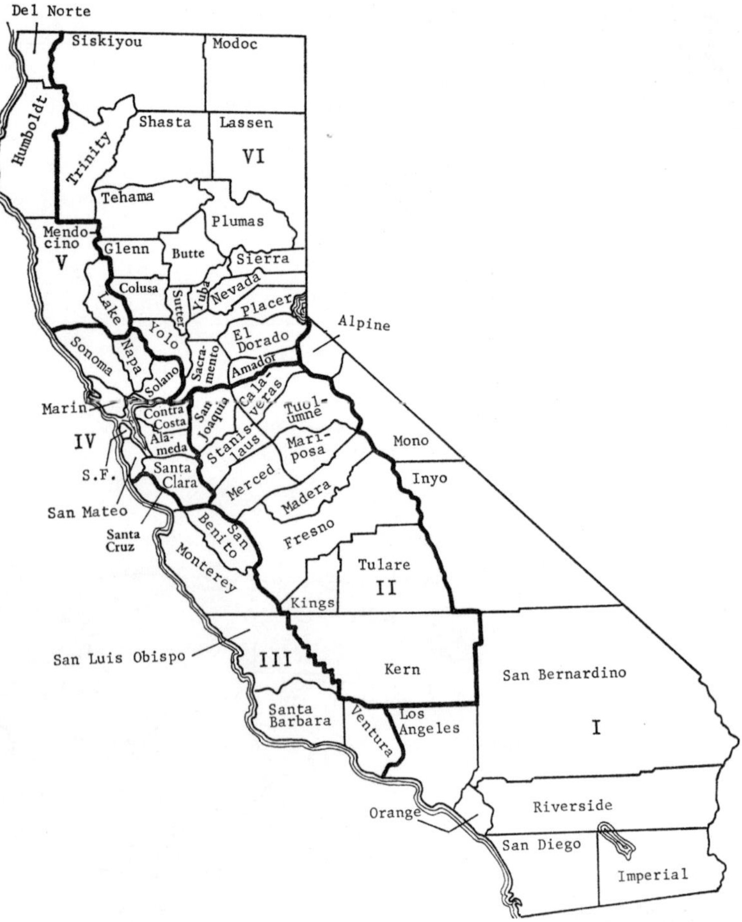


*a* Established by the State of California, Department of Public Health under provisions of Section 1901.2 of the California Health and Safety Code.

Fig. 13. California's Rabies Regions I–VI*a*

Rabies in bats in California was first identified in a Mexican free-tail bat *Tadarida brasiliensis* (*Mexicana*) collected by Constantine in Sonoma County in a survey done in 1954 (Enright *et al.*, 1955). Through 1969, a total of 484 cases of bat rabies have been identified in California. Other than the initial case found in 1954, none of the subsequent cases have been in survey specimens. The vast majority of cases in bats have been in individuals found ill (partially paralyzed) or dead. Only one instance of frank unprovoked attack on man and two probable instances of similar behavior, one involving man and one a dog, have occurred among the 484 confirmed cases of bat rabies in California. Most human exposures to rabies in bats can be avoided if persons would refrain from handling ill appearing or partially paralyzed bats. This is considered more a matter of public education than control and is particularly important with respect to young children who are apt to come in contact with infected ill bats in the course of play. Where infected bats are picked up by children, multiple exposures commonly occur.

Where bats inhabit buildings, effort should be undertaken to correct construction defects so as to preclude occupancy and use by bats. Since bats are migratory in habit, cases have been discovered in sporadic fashion throughout most (53 of 58) counties in the state and constitute the most widely distributed source of infection in California (Fig. 6).

Fox rabies has occurred in a generally sporadic fashion over a large area of California (Fig. 7). A concentration of cases has occurred in the north coastal counties of Marin, Sonoma, Napa, Mendocino, and Humboldt Counties (37.5 percent of the total of 152 cases during the period 1954–1969). During 1966–1968 a total of 48 cases of fox rabies occurred in San Diego County in connection with an epizootic of wildlife rabies which also involved Baja California, Mexico (Table 6).

Bobcat rabies has occurred primarily on a sporadic basis in areas affected by rabies in skunks. However, 23 or 61 percent of the total of 38 cases reported during the 16-year period 1954–1969, occurred during the four years 1966–1969 in San Diego County in connection with the above mentioned wildlife epizootic involving Baja California, Mexico, and San Diego County (Fig. 8). The wildlife outbreak in San Diego County, which began in March 1966, provided the highest recorded incidence of rabies in foxes and bobcats in the history of the disease in California. The 23 cases of bobcat rabies recorded in San Diego County during 1966–1969 constitutes the largest outbreak in that species in the United States. To our knowledge, the bobcat problem in San Diego County constitutes the first evidence to date of bobcat to bobcat transmission of rabies in the United States. The three bobcat cases reported from San Diego County in 1969 occurred as part of a sharply circumscribed focus which developed in the Lakeside area starting in September 1968.

Nineteen cases of rabies in coyotes were recognized during the

Table 4. Examinations for Rabies by Animal Species: 1950–1963 (14 years)

| Species[a] | Total Examined | Positive for Rabies[b] | |
|---|---|---|---|
| | | Number | Percent |
| Totals | 22,369 | 1,652 | 7.4 |
| Skunk | 1,988 | 1,028 | 51.7 |
| Bovine | 373 | 101 | 27.1 |
| Badger | 10 | 2 | 20.0 |
| Bobcat | 62 | 12 | 19.4 |
| Equine | 96 | 14 | 14.6 |
| Fox | 598 | 83 | 13.9 |
| Bat | 1,071 | 138 | 12.9 |
| Goat | 9 | 1 | 11.1 |
| Coyote | 93 | 7 | 7.5 |
| Sheep | 19 | 1 | 5.3 |
| Dog | 6,054 | 232 | 3.8 |
| Racoon | 285 | 7 | 2.5 |
| Monkey | 153 | 2 | 1.3 |
| Cat[c] | 4,730 | 24 | 0.5 |
| Gopher | 1,412 | – | – |
| Squirrel[d] | 1,358 | – | – |
| Rat[e] | 1,090 | – | – |
| Mouse[f] | 942 | – | – |
| Hamster | 639 | – | – |
| Rabbit[g] | 319 | – | – |
| Chipmunk | 262 | – | – |
| Muskrat | 129 | – | – |
| Opossum | 128 | – | – |
| Guinea Pig | 113 | – | – |
| Mole | 92 | – | – |
| Weasel | 89 | – | – |
| Deer | 26 | – | – |
| Chinchilla | 13 | – | – |
| Mink | 12 | – | – |
| Vole | 9 | – | – |
| Pig | 8 | – | – |
| Ocelot | 8 | – | – |
| Bear | 7 | – | – |
| Porcupine | 5 | – | – |
| Mountain Lion | 3 | – | – |
| Gibbon Ape | 3 | – | – |
| Prairie Dog | 3 | – | – |
| Beaver | 2 | – | – |
| Coatimundi | 2 | – | – |
| Ferret | 1 | – | – |
| Wolf | 1 | – | – |
| Nutria | 1 | – | – |
| Tapir | 1 | – | – |
| Kinkajou | 1 | – | – |
| Others and Unknown | 149 | – | – |

period 1959–1969 in California. None were reported in the preceding 5-year period 1954–1958. Eleven of the 19 coyote cases were reported from San Diego County (Fig. 9), eight in connection with the wildlife rabies outbreak during 1966–1969. All of the 11 cases in coyotes in San Diego County relate directly to the wildlife epizootic in Northern Baja California, Mexico, beginning about 1958 or to a second wave in 1965–1966. Cases in coyotes in the balance of the state have occurred as single sporadic cases, with the possible exception of the 1961 case in Yosemite National Park (Mariposa County); here epidemiologic evidence strongly suggests that a number of cases occurred in coyotes during the same time period. However, no specimens were submitted for laboratory examination from other suspect animals in the area. While the exact role of the coyote in the ecology of rabies is unknown, infected coyotes could easily serve to move rabies infection from one locality to another, since the species is capable of moving over long distances.

Rabies in racoons, badgers, and opossums in California are not common, 14 cases only (racoons-9, badgers-3, opossums-2) being reported in the 16-year period 1954–1969 (Fig. 10). The cases in the foregoing species are spread over nine years of the 16-year period and have occurred as single sporadic cases. Cases in the foregoing three species are considered a reflection of the disease in such vector species such as skunks and foxes.

The distribution of cases of rabies in dogs and other domestic animals such as cattle, cats, horses, sheep, goats, and swine, since 1958, with the exception of those in the immediate area of the Mexican border, are also a reflection of the distribution of infection in wildlife (Table 2 and Figs. 11, 12).

---

⇦

*a* Species underlined represent those in which rabies have been confirmed in California.
*b* Positive for rabies by microscopic examination for Negri bodies, mouse inoculation or fluorescent rabies antibody (FRA).
*c* Includes both owned and feral domestic cats.
*d* Includes both tree and ground squirrels..
*e* Includes both wild and pet white rats.
*f* Includes field and house mice and pet white mice.
*g* Includes both domestic and wild rabbits.
Source: State of California, Department of Public Health, Laboratory Records.

## RABIES SURVEILLANCE LEVELS AND FREQUENCY OF POSITIVE LABORATORY FINDINGS BY SPECIES

The 58 counties and over 400 cities in California are served by 56 county health departments (two of which provide bi-county service) and two city health departments. Thirty-eight of the local health departments have public health laboratory facilities, all of which are capable of performing rabies examinations. The California Department of Public Health provides laboratory services to those local health departments without laboratory facilities as well as providing reference diagnostic service to all local health department laboratories in the state. Five of the 38 local health department laboratories doing rabies examinations use Seller's stain with microscopic examination for Negri bodies and 33 use the fluorescent rabies antibody (FRA) test (as of December 31, 1969). Several local laboratories are also capable of performing mouse inoculation for rabies.

The State Department of Public Health laboratory is capable of carrying out rabies examinations using the FRA, Seller's stain, mouse inoculation, and serum neutralization tests. Between October 1959 and September 1962, over 4,230 specimens routinely submitted for rabies examination to the department were comparatively examined using the FRA test, microscopic examination for Negri bodies, and mouse inoculation test (Magoffin, 1964; Lennette *et al.*, 1965). The FRA test was adopted as the routine procedure for rabies examination in January 1963 (Calif. Dept. of Pub. Hlth., 1963). To date, the department has accumulated over 11 years of experience in use of the FRA procedure (See Lennette, E. H. Diagnosis of Rabies-Classical and Modern Methods, this meeting).

Since January 1, 1964, statewide data on animals examined for rabies by local health departments and by the California Department of Public Health have been accumulated on an annual basis. These annual tabulations provide valuable information on the number of animals examined annually for rabies in California by county and species and the number which have been found positive. Statewide figures for the 5-year period 1964–1968 show that a total of 46,039 animals were examined for rabies, 1,515 or 3.3% of which were positive (Table 5). The frequency of positive examinations by species vary from nearly 31% for skunks to 0.2% for domestic cats.

Similar figures are available for rabies examinations performed by

Table 5. Examinations for Rabies by Animal Species Examined in California, 1964–1968

| Species[a] | Total Examined | Positive for Rabies[b] | |
|---|---|---|---|
| | | Number | Percent |
| Total | 46,039 | 1,515 | 3.3 |
| Skunk | 3,003 | 927 | 30.9 |
| Bovine | 223 | 52 | 23.4 |
| Bobcat | 126 | 24 | 19.1 |
| Equine | 102 | 17 | 16.7 |
| Fox | 787 | 76 | 9.7 |
| Bat | 2,958 | 268 | 9.1 |
| Coyote | 193 | 10 | 5.2 |
| Badger | 20 | 1 | 5.0 |
| Ocelot | 22 | 1 | 4.5 |
| Dog | 7,949 | 118 | 1.5 |
| Opossum | 308 | 1 | 0.3 |
| Racoon | 326 | 1 | 0.3 |
| Cat[c] | 10,407 | 19 | 0.2 |
| Gopher | 4,298 | – | – |
| Hamster | 3,906 | – | – |
| Mouse[d] | 3,677 | – | – |
| Squirrel, Ground | 1,227 | – | – |
| Squirrel, Tree | 212 | – | – |
| Squirrel, N.S. | 850 | – | – |
| Rat[e] | 2,266 | – | – |
| Rabbit[f] | 1,026 | – | – |
| Guinea Pig | 588 | – | – |
| Chipmunk | 438 | – | – |
| Monkey | 370 | – | – |
| Weasel | 229 | – | – |
| Muskrat | 159 | – | – |
| Mole | 147 | – | – |
| Rodent, N.S. | 26 | – | – |
| Mink | 23 | – | – |
| Deer | 21 | – | – |
| Sheep | 17 | – | – |
| Goat | 14 | – | – |
| Pig | 11 | – | – |
| Other and Unknown | 110 | – | – |

*a* Species underlined represent the 18 in which rabies have been confirmed in California.
*b* Positive for rabies by microscopic examination for Negri bodies, mouse inoculation or fluorescent rabies antibody (FRA).
*c* Includes both owned and feral domestic cats.
*d* Includes both field and house mice and pet white mice.
*e* Includes wild rats and pet white rats.
*f* Includes both wild and domestic rabbits.
NS Not Specified.
Source: State of California, Department of Public Health, Laboratory Records; local health department laboratory reports.

the California Department of Public Health laboratory for the 14-year period 1950–1963 (Table 4). Of a total of 22,369 animals examined, 1,652 or 7.4% were reported positive for rabies.

Availability of the FRA test plus a policy of encouraging examinations for rabies by local health departments, since 1963, has increased the number of animals examined for rabies from an estimated average of approximately 3,000 per year, during the period 1950–1963 to an average of 9,211 animals per year during the period 1964–1968, approximately a three-fold increase in the level of rabies surveillance carried out in the state. An increase of such a magnitude in rabies surveillance backed by laboratory diagnosis is of tremendous value in administration of a large scale program for control of the disease, such as that in California. The availability of the FRA test can be said to account for a large portion of the increase in surveillance level noted above.

## MEASURES FOR THE CONTROL OF RABIES IN DOGS

### *Early legislation*

As the result of the rapid spread of rabies in dogs throughout California during the 4-year period 1909–1913 (Fig. 1), the 1913 state legislature adopted a rabies control law which provided authority to the State Board of Public Health to establish rabies quarantines in areas affected by the disease, the right of entry upon private property for enforcement purposes, and the authority to impound or kill dogs found at-large in violation of the quarantine, as well as other related powers (Calif. State Board of Health, 1913). Local authorities were required to enforce the quarantine provisions. The statutory provisions adopted in 1913, augmented by later additions, remain in effect at the present time (State of Calif., 1969).

Despite the broad authority to restrict animal movement provided under the 1913 legislation, even with widespread application and vigorous enforcement, including muzzling requirements, canine rabies continued to occur as a series of local epizootics in California rarely affecting any one locality for more than a few years at any one time. An exception to the above migrating epizootic pattern was Los Angeles County where dog rabies remained a continuing problem during the 36-year period 1922–1957. During the foregoing 36-year period, a total of 13,877 cases of canine rabies were reported from

Los Angeles County, over 70% of the total of 19,643 cases of canine rabies reported in California during the same period.

*Failure to secure new state legislation*

In 1952, the California Department of Public Health drafted proposed legislation for the control of canine rabies with assistance from an advisory group consisting of representatives from 15 statewide organizations and official agencies. The proposed law was introduced into the 1953 legislature where it was bitterly opposed by dog lovers and antivivisectionists. An amended version of the proposed law died at the end of the 1953 session. The will of the antivivisectionists prevailed in opposing the legislation proposed by the department advisory group.

*Declaration of rabies endemic areas (1955–1957)*

In 1955, the California Department of Public Health, faced with the unprecedented increase in incidence of rabies in wildlife during 1954 and early 1955, added regulations supplementing the 1913 statutory provisions for rabies control which provided for the declaration of rabies affected counties as so-called *rabies endemic areas* (State of Calif., 1955). The initial declaration of 26 counties as *rabies endemic areas* was made by the department on October 10, 1955. The declaration included all counties which had reported one or more cases of animal rabies since January 1, 1955.

The new regulations made mandatory that all local health officers in declared *rabies endemic areas* establish rabies quarantines within their respective jurisdictions. The quarantines required under the above declaration would thus cover the entire area of each county declared. The regulations required that quarantines remain in effect for 365 days after the last reported case of rabies in the county.

The key to the success of the above action existed not so much in the regulations themselves but rather in a policy formulated by the department of accepting as a substitute for the required quarantine, the adoption and enforcement of an ordinance by a city or a county which provided for (1) registration of all dogs, (2) maintenance of a pound and pickup system, and (3) compulsory rabies vaccination of all dogs allowed to run-at-large. The application and enforcement of local ordinances requiring vaccination of dogs against rabies demonstrated the feasibility of such a program and proved that local governing bodies could adopt such ordinances without committing political suicide. The program made possible the promotion and securing of new state legislation in 1957.

The *rabies endemic area* program was carried out during the period October 10, 1955, through December 1, 1957. During the foregoing period, a total of 40 rabies-affected counties were declared as *rabies endemic areas*. While the program was in operation, 13 counties and 120 cities adopted ordinances requiring vaccination of dogs against rabies in order to avoid being placed under quarantine (Humphrey, 1966). Prior to the initial declaration of counties as *rabies endemic areas*, in October 1955, only nine counties and 55 cities required vaccination of dogs against rabies. The status of counties as *rabies endemic areas* was terminated on December 1, 1957, and were replaced by new declarations as *rabies areas* on December 2, 1957, under provisions of new statutes adopted by the 1957 California Legislature (State of Calif., 1969).

*New state legislation (1957)*

In 1956, the California State Chamber of Commerce organized a rabies committee consisting of representatives of some 17 statewide organizations and official agencies. This committee drafted proposed legislation for the control of rabies in dogs which was introduced into the 1957 state legislature. Those supporting the proposed legislation were successful in securing passage. The new law, which as implemented on December 2, 1957, added Sections 1901.2, 1920 and 1921 to the California Health and Safety Code, as follows:

Section 1901.2. *Rabies area* shall mean any area not less than a county as determined by the director within a region where the existence of rabies constitutes a public health hazard, as found and declared by the director, after consultation with, and the approval of, the regional advisory committee. A region shall be composed of two or more counties as determined by the director. For each such region there shall be an advisory committee. The regional advisory committee shall consist of nine persons which shall include a health officer, a representative of the medical profession, a veterinarian, the mayor of the city having the largest population in the area, the chairman of the board of supervisors of the county having the largest population in the area, and such representatives of the livestock industry, civic, dog owning, and humane groups as may be appointed by the director to serve without compensation, but shall be reimbursed for actual and necessary expenses incurred during service on the committee. The status of an area as a rabies area shall terminate at the end of one year from the date of the declaration unless, not earlier than two months prior to the end of such year, it is again declared to be a rabies area in the manner provided in this section. If, however, the director at any time finds and declares that an area has ceased to be a rabies area its status as such shall terminate upon the date of such declaration.

Section 1920. In rabies areas:

(a) Every dog owner, after his dog attains the age of four months, shall annually secure a license for said dog. License fees shall be fixed by the responsible city, city and county, or county, at an amount not to exceed limitations otherwise prescribed by state law or city, city or county, or county charter.

(b) Every dog owner, after his dog attains the age of four months, shall at such intervals of time not more often than once a year as may be prescribed by the department procure its vaccination by a licensed veterinarian with a canine antirabies vaccine approved by and in a manner prescribed by the state department.

(c) All dogs under four months of age shall be confined to the premises of, or kept under physical restraint by, the owner, keeper or harborer. Nothing in this chapter shall be construed to prevent the sale or transportation of a puppy four months old or younger.

(d) Any dog in violation of the provisions of this article, and such additional provisions as may be prescribed by any local governing body, shall be impounded as provided by local ordinance.

(e) It shall be the duty of the governing body of each city, city and county, or county to maintain or provide for the maintenance of a pound system and a rabies control program for the purpose of carrying out and enforcing the provisions of this section.

(f) It shall be the responsibility of each city, county, or city and county to provide dog vaccination clinics, or to arrange for dog vaccination at clinics operated by veterinary groups or associations, held at strategic locations throughout each city, city and county, or county. The vaccination and licensing procedures may be combined as a single operation in such clinics. No charge in excess of actual cost shall be made for any one vaccination at such clinic. No owner of a dog shall be required to have his dog vaccinated at a public clinic if the owner elects to have the dog vaccinated by a licensed veterinarian of the owner's choice. All public clinics shall be required to operate under antiseptic immunization conditions comparable to those used in the vaccination of human beings.

Section 1921. Nothing in this chapter is intended or shall be construed to limit the power of any city, city and county, or county in its authority in the exercise of its police power or in the exercise of its power under any other provisions of law to enact more stringent requirements, to regulate and control dogs within the boundaries of its jurisdiction.

The major problem with regard to the control of rabies in dogs in California for many years was the lack of adequate continuing or permanent local control programs. While some cities and counties enforced adequate control measures within their respective jurisdictions, many neighboring cities and counties did not. Many jurisdictions enforced control measures during periods when rabies was an acute problem locally, only to drop enforcement as the problem decreased and the state established quarantines were removed. The result was a lack of continuing application of control measures which weakened and nullified rabies control throughout the state.

Legislation, adopted in 1957, has provided adequate local control and enforcement by establishing minimum standards for local control programs as well as providing a mechanism whereby the provisions of the law can be applied to rabies affected areas of the state.

*Implementation and administration of the 1957 law*

In implementing the new law, the California Department of Public Health divided the state into six rabies regions (Fig. 13) and appointed a 9-member advisory committee for each region in accordance with provisions of Section 1901.2. An initial combined orientation meeting of the members of all six regional advisory committees was held followed by meetings with each individual advisory committee within their respective regions. In the course of the latter six meetings, the advisory committees formally approved the declaration of 31 rabies affected counties as *rabies areas*, effective December 2, 1957.

To assist implementation and administration of the new law, the California State Board of Public Health adopted additions and changes in rabies regulations on December 13, 1957, which became effective on January 18, 1958 (State of Calif., 1957). Those portions of the revised regulations, pertaining to the administration of local control programs in declared *rabies areas*, are still in effect and are included under Section 2606.4, Title 17, California Administrative Code, as follows:

Section 2606.4. Officially Declared Areas.

(a) Administration and Enforcement. For purposes of administration and enforcement of Section 1920, California Health and Safety Code, in officially declared rabies areas, the following shall apply:

(1) Licensing and Vaccination Procedure. The vaccination of dogs four months of age or older as required by subdivision (b), Section 1920, California Health and Safety Code, shall be held a requisite to licensing as required under subdivision (a) therein. Completion of the licensing procedure consists of issuance of license and vaccination tags or vaccination tag bearing the license data and shall be carried out only after presentation of a valid official vaccination certificate indicating that the period of time elapsing from the date of vaccination to the date of expiration of the license being issued does not exceed 30 months in the case of vaccination with chick-embryo rabies vaccine or 18 months in the case of vaccination with nerve-tissue rabies vaccine.

(2) Interval Permitted for Procurement of Vaccination and Licensing. The vaccination of dogs four months of age against rabies as required under subdivision (b), Section 1920, California Health and Safety Code, and the license required by subdivision (a) of said section shall be procured not later than 30 days after the dog attains the age of four months. The annual renewal of licensing as required under subdivision (a) of said section and revaccination as may be required under subdivision (b) of said section shall be procured not later than 60 days after expiration of the previously issued license.

(3) Rabies Control Activities Reporting. During such time as a county is under official declaration as a rabies area, each local official responsible for the various phases of local dog or rabies control within each city, county and city or cities, or county shall make quarterly rabies control activities reports to and on forms furnished by the department. Such reports shall be submitted to the department by the local officials responsible for the various phases of local dog or rabies control through the local health officer so as to reach the department not later than 30 days following each quarter.

(b) Vaccination of Dogs Against Rabies. Dogs shall be considered to be properly vaccinated for the purposes of Section 1920, California Health and Safety Code, when injected at four months of age or older with canine chick-embryo origin modified live-virus rabies vaccine or canine nerve-tissue killed-virus rabies vaccine in a manner prescribed by the department.

Dogs receiving INITIAL injection of rabies vaccine shall be confined to the premises of, or kept under physical restraint by, the owner, keeper or harborer until 30 days have elapsed following vaccination.

Certain provisions of the law and regulations are of particular import and should be emphasized: (1) the law places direct responsibility for maintaining or providing for a pound system and a rabies control program for the purpose of carrying out and enforcing the law, upon the boards of supervisors and the city councils, (2) regulations adopted by the State Board of Public Health require that local enforcement authorities hold vaccination requisite to licensing and (3) regulations require the reporting of local rabies control activity by each control jurisdiction within declared *rabies areas* (Table 1, Fig. 15).

The vaccination requirements of the 1957 law do not constitute a hardship for the dog owner. The law requires the holding of low-cost public vaccination clinics. The common fee for immunization in the public clinics is $1.50 to $2.00. Chick-embryo origin (CEO), low-egg-passage (LEP), Flury strain, which is accepted for a maximum period of 30 months under regulations, constitutes the vast majority (over 95 percent) of the rabies vaccine used in the state. With use of public clinics, the average cost to the dog owner for rabies immunization is thus only $0.75 to $1.00 annually.

From implementation of the new law on December 2, 1957, through December 31, 1969, a total of 52 of the 58 counties in the state have been declared as *rabies areas* one or more times. Some counties have been under declaration as *rabies areas* continually since the initial declaration made on December 2, 1957, due to the constant presence of rabies within the state, primarily in wildlife. As of December 31, 1969, 49 or nearly 85% of the state's 58 counties and over 300, 76%, of the nearly 400 incorporated cities in California require compulsory rabies vaccination of dogs by local ordinance—a 5.5 fold increase in the number of such local ordinances since 1955.

The implementation and administration of a rabies control program at the state level in an area such as California is complicated by a multiplicity of local government jurisdictions varying from concentrated urban (over 7.5 million population in the Los Angeles metropolitan area) to sparsely populated rural areas (less than 500 population). The program is further complicated by a wide variety and number of local government agencies and officials having responsibility for dog control and licensing. City and county tax collectors and city and county clerks are involved in many areas with the collection of dog license fees. City and county pounds are administratively responsible to city councils or boards of supervisors or to local health departments, police departments, the county sheriff, city and county administrators, county agricultural commissioners and county veterinarians. In addition, many county pounds are serving cities through contract; counties are contracting with cities for use of city-owned pound facilities, and humane societies are serving cities and counties via contract. All the foregoing are concerned with dog license sales, stray dog control, and animal bite investigation, dependent upon the varying pattern which may exist in a particular jurisdiction. Local health departments, veterinary practitioners as individuals or as organizations or groups, together with various enforcement agencies and in some cases volunteer organizations, are concerned with the holding of low-cost public rabies vaccination clinics. Last, but not least, city councils and county boards of supervisors are concerned with the adoption of local ordinances, the setting of policy, and the appropriation of necessary funds for local program operation.

The role of the state is that of administration of the law but not enforcement which is the responsibility of local authorities. In addition to such administration, the California Department of Public Health carries out various rabies related activities not associated with the administration of control statutes. At the present time, approximately 0.6 time of one veterinarian and 0.4 time of one clerk is spent on rabies-related activities of the department, including administration of the control law.

Two forms are used which greatly reduce the amount of time spent in administering the law. The first of these is the so-called "Statement of Enforcement" form (262-110) which is utilized to secure acknowledgment from the governing bodies affected by the declarations of *rabies areas* of the fact of declaration and to assure that they are complying with the provisions of the law (Fig. 14). The second form is the "Quarterly Report of Local Rabies Control Activities" (262-109) used to ascertain that enforcement is being carried out during the period under declaration as a *rabies area* (Fig. 15). Annual local control statistics collected under the program are included in Table 1.

## EFFECTIVENESS OF CANINE RABIES CONTROL PROGRAM (1955–1969)

The primary objective of the California rabies control program is prevention of canine rabies. With any program of control or prevention, there comes a time of appraisal as to how effective the program has been in achieving its objective. An easily available means of evaluation in a continuing program of rabies control is to compare what occurred before and after implementation of the program in question. The figures included in Table 2 provide some insight into the question of the effectiveness of the California program.

From 1922 through 1953, the rabies problem in California consisted of rabies in dogs, primarily urban in distribution. During the 32-year period 1922–1953, a total of 20,801 cases of animal rabies was reported in California, 19,173 or 92% of which were in dogs. Only 150 or 0.7% was reported in wildlife during the same period. Sixty-four of the above 150 cases in wildlife occurred in the last four years (1950–1953) of the 1922–1953 period. Forty-four cases were reported in wild animals during 1954 (Table 2).

By 1958, canine rabies as a major problem in California was largely resolved and has continued to remain so through the present time with the exception of the area of the state immediately adjacent to the Mexico border. However, the annual incidence of the disease in wildlife increased tremendously and has remained high since 1955 (Table 2).

From 1954 through 1969, a total of 4,156 cases of animal rabies was reported, 784 or nearly 19% were in dogs and 3,111 or nearly 75% in wildlife. In considering the effectiveness of the California program for prevention of rabies in dogs, it is of interest to examine the 784 cases in dogs which have been reported in the past 16 years and to determine when, where and why they occurred.

Of the total of 784 cases (excluding two from out of state) reported in dogs during the 16-year period 1954–1969, 470 were reported during the four years 1954–1957 (Table 2). Of the latter, a total of 470, 414 cases occurred in connection with an outbreak in Los Angeles and Orange Counties during the 3-year period 1954–1957. The balance of 314 cases in dogs that have been reported during the 12-year period 1958–1969 has not been considered a major problem in California. The statement that canine rabies has not been a major problem in the state during a period when 314 cases of rabies in dogs were reported may appear to be in conflict. Nevertheless, the above statement is factual.

Of the 314 cases of canine rabies reported in California during the 12-year period 1958–1969, 278 or nearly 90% occurred in the immediate area of the California-Mexico border as compared to only 36 cases (excluding two from out-of-state) in the balance of the state. Of the latter 36 cases, one case occurred in a California dog which developed rabies five days after return from a 7-week stay in Mexico; and 35 or an average of 2.9 cases annually are considered to have incurred infection as the result of exposure to infected wildlife in the areas of the state where they occurred (Fig. 11 and Table 2).

There is little question but what ample opportunity exists in California for dogs to be exposed to rabies. The disease in wildlife has been widespread in the state since 1954. Of the total of 4,156 cases of animal rabies reported during the past 16 years, (1954–1969), 3,111 or nearly 75 percent have been in wildlife species. Rabies infection in wildlife has been reported from all of the 53 counties reporting cases of rabies in California since 1950. Rabid skunks have been found in 43 counties since 1950; and rabid bats have been found in 53 counties since 1954. The reduction and prevention of canine rabies infection in all but two California counties (San Diego and Imperial) has, thus, occurred in the presence of an exceedingly large reservoir of rabies in wildlife. This fact raises the question of why dog rabies in Imperial and San Diego counties has continued to persist (147 cases since 1959 and 128 cases since 1962, respectively) if California can so successfully prevent the canine disease in the other 56 counties of the state.

The reason for the continued persistence of dog rabies in Imperial and San Diego counties was a reservoir in Mexico. Imperial County (since 1959) and San Diego County (since 1962) have both continuously enforced outstanding programs of rabies control. The rabies programs carried out by these two counties have included unprecedented enforcement of stray dog control, licensing and vaccination of dogs against the disease. Both have included measures aimed at reducing the hazard of transmission of rabies from wildlife to dogs. Both have continued to find rabid dogs within their respective areas due to repeated crossing of rabid dogs from northern Baja California, Mexico.

There is ample evidence that the continuing rabies problem in Imperial and San Diego counties has had its source in the uncontrolled occurrence of rabies in dogs in the adjoining areas of Mexico (cities of Tijuana and Mexicali and the Mexicali Valley). Of the total of 275 cases of dog rabies reported from Imperial and San Diego Counties, since 1959 and 1962, respectively, through 1969, 232 cases were found less than five miles from the Mexican border, 37 cases between 5–10 miles, and only six cases at distances over 10 miles.

The distribution of dog rabies cases in Imperial and San Diego counties is not consistent with the distribution of the human and dog populations in either county. Numerous rabid dogs have been shot in California after crossing the border from Mexico. Figures emphasizing this point are available from the Port of Entry, Calexico, Imperial County, where a 24-hour dog guard was maintained for the 65-month period January 22, 1964, through June 30, 1969, to prevent the entry of stray dogs from the city of Mexicali, Mexico. During the approximately 65-month period the dog guard was in operation, a total of 547 dogs were apprehended. Of these 547 apprehended dogs, 12 were returned to owners in Mexico, 528 were examined for rabies in the laboratory, and four were not examined due to freezer failure. Of the 528 on which examination was completed, 33 were found positive, approximately 6.3% of those examined. During 1964, positive examinations ran nearly 30%. Under the conditions which exist along the border, it is remarkable that the two counties have succeeded in containing the rabies problem to areas so closely adjacent to the Mexican border.

## CONTROL OF RABIES IN WILDLIFE

### *Problems of control*

The present situation with regard to rabies in wildlife in California is not good. Rabies in wildlife has been justification for the state to require institution of adequate canine rabies control programs by city and county government including the mandatory immunization of dogs against the disease. As a result, an efficient and effective program for prevention of canine rabies is maintained in California; and, rabies in dogs has not constituted a problem in the state, with the exception of the areas of San Diego and Imperial Counties immediately adjacent to the Mexico border. On the other hand, the incidence of rabies in wildlife has ranged unchecked throughout most of the state since 1955.

Rabies in wildlife is not well understood. As a result, effective means of control of the disease in wild animal populations are not easily implemented. There are, for example, no methods available 1) to determine the actual incidence of rabies infection in wildlife of an affected area, 2) to ascertain the wild animal population in an area, nor 3) to determine the number of animals which must be removed from a wildlife population in order to reduce transmission to below the threshold population density necessary for maintenance of the disease.

From an epidemiologic standpoint, a disease outbreak can be stopped if a critical proportion of susceptible hosts can be removed from an affected population. In the case of rabies in dogs, susceptible animals are removed by 1) rabies immunization and identification (licensing) of immunized animals, 2) pickup and elimination of stray, unowned nonvaccinated animals, and 3) restriction of dog movement (quarantine) to reduce dog-to-dog contact.

In any disease control program, it is not necessary to eliminate all susceptibles in a population to prevent an outbreak. Not all dogs in California have been immunized against rabies. With new introductions into the dog populations (estimated at 20–25% turnover annually) coupled with noncompliance, only about 50–60% of the dog population can be considered immune to rabies at any one time. Despite the foregoing immune status of the dog population, rabies does not constitute a problem in dogs in California even with the presence of an extensive reservoir of the disease in wildlife.

With rabies in wildlife, however, the only available technique for control of the disease is population reduction of the affected species. The objective of reduction work is the same as that in the prevention of rabies in dogs—reduction of contact between infected and susceptibles to a point where transmission of the disease cannot be maintained. In doing reduction work on rabies affected wildlife species in an area, it is true that we cannot differentiate between infected and noninfected or between exposed and nonexposed individuals. However, simple removal or reduction in numbers serves the same end point that is reduction of contact and thus reduction in transmission of rabies infection in the control area.

Population reduction measures have proved effective in controlling rabies in wild animals despite the many difficulties involved. Wildlife rabies control is usually most effective when the work can be applied in an area circumscribed by physical barriers, for example, San Diego County.

*San Diego County wildlife rabies control project*

San Diego County is bounded on the west by the Pacific Ocean and on the east by an arid desert barrier not conducive to support of any sizable population of animals of the species affected in the wildlife rabies outbreak. The outbreak can be considered to be a northward extension of a recognized wildlife rabies outbreak in adjacent Baja California, Mexico. There was no evidence of involvement to the north of the affected areas of San Diego County.

An accelerated control project was implemented using a total of eight trappers on December 15, 1966. The project was an effort to reduce the wildlife vectors of rabies (fox, bobcats, coyotes, and skunks) in an area extending 50 miles beyond the recognized affected portions of San Diego County (Table 6). The program was continued through June 30, 1968, when it was terminated somewhat prematurely by the San Diego County Board of Supervisors. There is every evidence that the program was effective during the period it was carried out. That termination of control work was premature, was borne out by subsequent events in the Lakeside area of the county.

On September 28, 1968, a rabid fox was identified in the Lakeside area. The September case was followed by a series of cases in animals and one in man, all in the Lakeside area as follows:

Rabies Cases, Lakeside Area, San Diego County, California, September 28, 1968-June 30, 1970

| *Date Found* | *Species* | *Comments* |
|---|---|---|
| September 28, 1968 | Fox | - |
| October 21, 1968 | Skunk | - |
| December 17, 1968 | Cat (stray) | - |
| March 21, 1969 | Bobcat | Child bitten |
| April 1, 1969 | Bobcat | Source of April 18 human case |
| April 18, 1969 | Human | Onset April 18 |
| May 6, 1969 | Calf | - |
| June 16, 1969 | Horse | - |
| December 20, 1969 | Bobcat | Man bitten |
| February 26, 1970 | Fox | - |

Table 6. Wildlife Rabies Outbreak, San Diego County, California
March, 14, 1966–June 30, 1970

| Year | Total | Cases Associated with the Wildlife Rabies Foci | | | | | |
|---|---|---|---|---|---|---|---|
| | | Wildlife Species | | | | | Domestic Species[1] |
| | | Fox | Bobcat | Coyote | Skunk | Bat | |
| Total | 105 | 49 | 23 | 8 | 9 | 4 | 12 |
| 1966 | 57 | 39 | 10 | 3 | 4 | – | 1 |
| January | – | – | – | – | – | – | – |
| February | – | – | – | – | – | – | – |
| March | 3 | 1 | 2 | – | – | – | – |
| April | 4 | 1 | 2 | – | – | – | 1 dog[a] |
| May | 3 | 2 | 1 | – | – | – | – |
| June | 3 | 3 | – | – | – | – | – |
| July | 4 | 3 | 1 | – | – | – | – |
| August | 11 | 10 | – | – | 1 | – | – |
| September | 5 | 4 | 1 | – | – | – | – |
| October | 6 | 3 | – | – | 3 | – | – |
| November | 7 | 4 | 2 | 1 | – | – | – |
| December | 11 | 8 | 1 | 2 | – | – | – |
| 1967 | 28 | 7 | 8 | 3 | 4 | 2 | 4 |
| January | 7 | 2 | 2 | 1 | 2 | – | – |
| February | 8 | 1 | 2 | 2 | 1 | 1 | 1 cat[a] |
| March | 5 | 3 | 1 | – | – | – | 1 dog[a] |
| April | 2 | 1 | – | – | – | – | 1 dog[a] |
| May | 1 | – | 1 | – | – | – | – |
| June | – | – | – | – | – | – | – |
| July | – | – | – | – | – | – | – |
| August | – | – | – | – | – | – | – |
| September | – | – | – | – | – | – | – |
| October | 3 | – | 2 | – | – | 1 | – |
| November | – | – | – | – | – | – | – |
| December | 2 | – | – | – | 1 | – | 1 horse |
| 1968 | 8 | 2 | 2 | – | 1 | – | 3 |
| January | 1 | – | – | – | – | – | 1 dog |
| February | 1 | – | 1 | – | – | – | – |
| March | – | – | – | – | – | – | – |
| April | – | – | – | – | – | – | – |
| May | 2 | – | 1 | – | – | – | 1 bovine |
| June | – | – | – | – | – | – | – |
| July | – | – | – | – | – | – | – |
| August | – | – | – | – | – | – | – |
| September | 1 | 1[b] | – | – | – | – | – |
| October | 1 | – | – | – | 1[b] | – | – |
| November | 1 | 1 | – | – | – | – | – |
| December | 1 | – | – | – | – | – | 1 cat[a,b] |

| Wildlife Rabies Control | | | | | Remarks |
|---|---|---|---|---|---|
| | Animals Trapped | | | | |
| Trappers | Coyote | Bobcat | Fox | Skunk | |
| | 5,827 | 1,297 | 778 | 1,089 | |
| – | 1,385 | 220 | 294 | 340 | |
| 3 | 168 | 23 | 21 | 57 | |
| 3 | 101 | 9 | 14 | 46 | First case in outbreak appeared on March 14, 1966. |
| 3 | 66 | 14 | – | 23 | |
| 3 | 50 | 7 | 3 | 15 | One additional trapper added; supported by county funds. |
| 4 | 63 | 20 | 28 | 16 | |
| 4 | 72 | 18 | 53 | 23 | |
| 4 | 77 | 21 | 27 | 30 | |
| 4 | 123 | 15 | 36 | 26 | |
| 4 | 103 | 22 | 22 | 26 | |
| 4 | 128 | 23 | 14 | 19 | |
| 5 | 118 | 20 | 42 | 34 | An accelerated wildlife rabies control project initiated December 15, 1966, using county funds supplemented by $17,164 from the California Department of Agriculture. |
| 8 | 148 | 28 | 34 | 25 | |
| – | 2,090 | 622 | 380 | 323 | |
| 8 | 220 | 34 | 31 | 27 | |
| 8 | 249 | 58 | 25 | 14 | County wide quarantine restricting movement of all dogs and cats affected January 1, 1967. |
| 8 | 230 | 83 | 25 | 17 | |
| 8 | 133 | 48 | 26 | 12 | |
| 8 | 196 | 71 | 30 | 27 | |
| 7 | 133 | 75 | 21 | 45 | |
| 7 | 129 | 27 | 20 | 13 | During the period July 1, 1967–June 30, 1968, program supplemented by $17,520 in border rabies control funds from N.C.D.C., P.H.S., U.S.D.H.E.W. |
| 7 | 151 | 37 | 32 | 32 | |
| 7 | 127 | 35 | 43 | 39 | |
| 5 | 189 | 72 | 72 | 41 | |
| 7 | 161 | 49 | 37 | 20 | |
| 6 | 172 | 33 | 18 | 36 | |
| – | 975 | 229 | 72 | 192 | |
| 6 | 214 | 55 | 19 | 56 | |
| 6 | 172 | 40 | 11 | 22 | |
| 6 | 126 | 42 | 20 | 10 | Trapper force reduced to 3 men during part of May, 1968. Wildlife rabies control projects terminated by the San Diego County Board of Supervisors effective June 30, 1968. Control work done only during one week in June. |
| 6 | 126 | 44 | 9 | 17 | |
| 5 | 72 | 23 | 9 | 9 | |
| 2 | 35 | 5 | – | 3 | |
| 2 | 33 | 2 | 3 | 21 | |
| 2 | 48 | 7 | – | 23 | |
| 2 | 35 | 5 | – | 15 | Two man crew retained during July 1968 through June 1969 constitutes level of work normally maintained by county to control livestock predation. |
| 2 | 30 | 2 | – | 6 | |
| 2 | 44 | 2 | 1 | 9 | |
| 2 | 40 | 2 | – | 1 | |

| | | | | | | | |
|---|---|---|---|---|---|---|---|
| 1969 | 10 | – | 3 | 2 | – | 1 | 4 |
| January | – | – | – | – | – | – | – |
| February | – | – | – | – | – | – | – |
| March | 1 | – | 1[b] | – | – | – | – |
| April | 3 | – | 1[b] | 1[b] | – | – | 1 human[b] |
| May | 2 | – | – | – | – | – | (2 calf[b]) |
| | | | | | | | horse[b]) |
| June | 1 | – | – | – | – | – | 1 dog |
| July | 1 | – | – | – | – | 1 | – |
| August | – | – | – | – | – | – | – |
| September | – | – | – | – | – | – | – |
| October | 1 | – | – | 1 | – | – | – |
| November | – | – | – | – | – | – | – |
| December | 1 | – | 1[b] | – | – | – | – |
| 1970 | 2 | 1 | – | – | – | 1 | – |
| January | – | – | – | – | – | – | – |
| February | 1 | 1[b] | – | – | – | – | – |
| March | – | – | – | – | – | – | – |
| April | – | – | – | – | – | – | – |
| May | 1 | – | – | – | – | 1 | – |
| June | – | – | – | – | – | – | – |

1 Cases in domestic species represent those associated with the foci of wildlife rabies in south central San Diego County. Cases associated with the foci of canine rabies in the South Bay San Diego-Tijuana, Mexico, are not shown in this table.

*a* Stray animals without owner.

Four of the six cases recognized in the Lakeside area during the six month period December 17, 1968, through June 16, 1969, constitute spillover of rabies infection into domestic animals (cat, calf, horse) and man from wildlife. The April 1, 1969, bobcat case was the source of infection for a $2\frac{1}{2}$ year old boy bitten in his own backyard during daytime. This is the first instance of human rabies being incurred from a bobcat in California and possibly in the United States.

Lakeside is a small rural community located near the northeastern edge of the metropolitan San Diego area. Due to its somewhat semi-urban nature, Lakeside was essentially by-passed during the course of the wildlife rabies control work conducted from December 15, 1966, through June 30, 1968. It is unfortunate that the wildlife rabies control work was terminated. Had the staff of six trappers been maintained, it is possible that effective reduction work could have been initiated in the Lakeside area in early 1969, perhaps with an outcome differing from that which occurred.

Control work was re-implemented in the Lakeside area using a total of four trappers starting July 1, 1969. The total force was increased to six trappers during January 1–June 30, 1970, following which all trapping was terminated by the Board of Supervisors. It

| | | | | | |
|---|---|---|---|---|---|
| 2 | 862 | 105 | 14 | 129 | |
| 2 | 60 | 1 | – | 12 | |
| 2 | 42 | – | – | 3 | |
| 2 | 65 | – | – | 4 | |
| 2 | 42 | 4 | – | 10 | April bobcat case source of infection for human case of rabies. |
| 2 | 25 | 2 | 1 | 2 | |
| 2 | 38 | 7 | 2 | 16 | |
| 4 | 69 | 15 | – | 7 | Two trappers added July 1, 1969, by county for wildlife rabies control work. |
| 4 | 82 | 11 | 3 | 10 | |
| 4 | 92 | 10 | – | 19 | |
| 4 | 107 | 26 | 1 | 23 | |
| 4 | 122 | 18 | 4 | 13 | |
| 4 | 118 | 11 | 3 | 10 | |
| 6 | 515 | 121 | 18 | 105 | Two additional trappers added using border rabies control funds from the N.C.D.C., P.H.S., U.S.D.H.E.W. |
| 6 | 108 | 23 | – | 20 | |
| 6 | 113 | 25 | 3 | 17 | |
| 6 | 95 | 18 | 2 | 10 | |
| 6 | 90 | 24 | 7 | 8 | Total control program terminated June 30, 1970, by the San Diego County Board of Supervisors. |
| 6 | 57 | 16 | 1 | 25 | |
| 6 | 52 | 15 | 5 | 25 | |

*b* Cases involved in the circumscribed wildlife outbreak in the Lakeside area, September 28, 1968–February 26, 1970.

Source: State of California, Department of Public Health, Morbidity Records and Fish and Wildlife Service, U.S. Department of Interior, Sacramento, California.

should be noted that the on-off again nature of wildlife rabies control work done in San Diego County was due to public opposition to the control program. Notwithstanding the opposition and obstacles to conducting wildlife rabies control work in San Diego County, there is evidence that what has been done may be effective (Table 6).

*Limitations of wildlife rabies control in California*

In general, it has not been possible to implement organized wildlife control work in other areas of California on a scale comparable to that done in San Diego County. Control work, where done, has been aimed at localized areas of peak incidence supported by funds made available by county boards of supervisors. The widespread, diffuse nature of wildlife rabies in California defies attempts to promote an organized program for its control. The simple problem of manpower and funds for any serious attempt at control on a statewide basis are considered prohibitive at the present time.

There is serious need for organized government support of basic research on the ecology of rabies in wildlife and to develop more adequate methods for control of rabies in wildlife populations. There is little such work being carried out in the United States today.

## CONCLUSION

Legislation adopted in 1913 to control rabies in dogs, based upon the establishment of area quarantines requiring confinement of animals to owner premises, restriction of movement on leash, muzzling, licensing, pickup and destruction of dogs at-large, was never successful in controlling or preventing the disease, despite extensive application and enforcement during the epizootic-enzootic occurrence of canine rabies in California from 1914–1953.

Changes in state rabies control regulations, adopted in October 1955, which provided for the declaration of rabies affected counties as so-called *rabies endemic areas* for the first time gave official state recognition of local ordinances requiring rabies vaccination of dogs. The *rabies endemic area* program was instrumental in promoting the adoption of local ordinances requiring rabies vaccination by 13 counties and 120 cities between October 10, 1955, and December 1, 1957.

New state legislation, adopted by the 1957 state legislature which made rabies vaccination of all dogs four months of age or older mandatory in rabies affected counties declared as so-called *rabies areas* further enhanced rabies vaccination as a rabies control measure in California when implemented on December 2, 1957. The application of mandatory rabies vaccination coupled with other control measures have proved their worth in California over the past 14-year period, despite the continual presence of an extensive reservoir of rabies in wildlife throughout California and in dogs in adjacent Baja California, Mexico.

Rabies control legislation adopted in 1957 basically prescribes minimum standards for local control programs enforced by the counties and cities in so-called *rabies areas* declared by the California Department of Public Health. Declaration of *rabies areas* effected during 1969 encompassed 48 of the 58 counties in the state. Declarations are primarily effected through six regional block declarations of *rabies areas* made annually on December 2nd, the anniversary date of the first declarations made in implementing the law in 1957. Individual declarations of counties as *rabies areas*, however, can be made at any time of the year with approval of the regional rabies advisory committee, should the need arise.

Beyond necessary state legislation, the key to good rabies control is good dog control. The mere imposition of rabies vaccination and licensing requirements will not control canine rabies. The legal responsibility for program enforcement is placed upon the local governing bodies.

In California, as in other parts of the United States, dog and rabies control programs are becoming increasingly more sophisticated. Coordinated countywide pound systems, operated by county government contracting with the various incorporated cities within the county to provide program enforcement service to the cities, are becoming more and more commonplace. Under these coordinated countywide control programs, county dog licenses are usually sold within the cities.

IBM record-keeping on dog license and rabies vaccination data together with input and feedback on enforcement time and cost analysis, level of service provided to contracting cities, and so on are being used more and more in rabies control program administration, as well as in other local government operations.

Other measures include: (1) the holding of low-cost public rabies vaccination clinics (over 1,400 annually in California) during the annual grace periods when dog licenses become due (Table 1), (2) the holding of rabies vaccination as a requisite to licensing, (3) house-to-house canvass for license and rabies vaccination enforcement, and (4) the issuance of citations for violations in the same manner as for traffic violations, all greatly increase the efficiency of enforcement and thus compliance.

Where control programs operate on a complaint basis only, it is seldom that 20% compliance with licensing and vaccination requirements is achieved. House-to-house canvassers more than pay their way and license and rabies vaccination compliance can be greatly increased. Program revenue can be significantly increased by house-to-house canvass, making control programs more self-supporting.

The issuance of citations for violations greatly increases program efficiency. The impoundment of animals is reduced by a citation system relieving pressure on pound facilities and field enforcement personnel. The natural reluctance of city and county attorneys to prosecute minor violations is avoided; and the time spent by field enforcement personnel in attending court sessions is greatly reduced.

The annual billing of dog owners for payment of license renewal fees is accomplished in many areas by routine mailing of license card files at the end of the license year. Rabies vaccination notice reminders are included on license notice cards where revaccination against rabies is due. The dog owner completes the card, a license renewal application, encloses a valid rabies vaccination certificate where re-immunization is due, together with a check or money order covering the license fee, and mails them to license collection authorities. A new license tag is sent to the dog owner by return mail. The foregoing procedure is simple, is greatly appreciated by the dog owner, and the expense of license collection is reduced. In some jurisdictions, self-addressed envelopes are used by control agencies.

Two-year licensing on either a mandatory or an optional basis in connection with the use of CEO, MLV, LEP rabies vaccine is provided for by local ordinance in several jurisdictions in California. Where optional two-year licenses are provided, the dog owner may purchase the two-year license at a saving over the cost of buying an annual license, for example, a two-year license for $5.00 or an annual license for $3.00.

Late license penalty fees are commonly charged in most areas. An alternative to the late license penalty fee which gains public goodwill and encourages license compliance during the annual grace period for license renewal is to require a basic license fee (equal to that which would normally be charged plus the added delinquent penalty fee) which if paid during the annual grace period for license renewal can be purchased for a reduced amount. Public resentment at being charged the penalty fee for late licensing is no longer a factor where the reduced fee scheme is in effect during the annual license renewal period.

In urban areas, the holding of rabies vaccination as a requisite to licensing, house-to-house canvass for license and vaccination enforcement, the use of a citation system for violations are the important program tools for enforcement work.

The holding of training sessions at the state level for city and county dog and rabies control personnel on a regular basis provides an effective means of educating local field enforcement personnel regarding rabies and its control, particularly supervisory staff and program heads. The development of adequate printed training material for use and distribution at training sessions will be rewarded by long-term reference use at the local program level. An example of such training material are the *Rabies Control Manuals* prepared by the California Department of Public Health for distribution at the series of four two-day Rabies Institutes held bi-annually by the California Department of Public Health in various areas of the state.

The above phases of program enforcement coupled with state legislation requiring minimum standards for local control programs and mandatory rabies vaccination of dogs in counties declared as *rabies areas* has prevented canine rabies in California. While statewide compulsory rabies vaccination of dogs would seem less cumbersome than the existent method of declaring rabies affected counties as *rabies areas* with the necessary holding of regional rabies advisory meetings, present legislation provides an effective program basis which has enabled local governing bodies to implement efficient programs of rabies control without having to face the protests of a vocal antivivisection-antivaccination minority.

The program has proved its worth over the past 12 years of application from 1958–1969. The present wildlife rabies situation in California warrants continued application and enforcement of current control measures. More adequate control of canine rabies in the adjoining areas of Mexico which were initiated under a cooperative agreement with the federal Mexican and United States governments in September 1966 is greatly enhancing the effectiveness of canine rabies control work being done in Imperial and San Diego Counties—adjacent to the Mexican border. The increasing control work being done in the border cities in Baja California, since 1966, is being reflected in fewer cases of dog rabies crossing from Mexico into California.

Fig. 14

State of California
Department of Puclic Health
VETERINARY SECTION

## STATEMENT OF ENFORCEMENT

*Completed Form to be Sent to the County Health Officer*

Statement of Enforcement of Rabies Control Requirements for Rabies Areas Applying to

____________________ Effective ____________________
(County) (Date)

________________________________________
Area or Jurisdiction for Which Statement is Made

| Statement Completed By: | Endorsement by Local Health Officer or Authorized Representative: |
|---|---|
| Date | Date |
| ▶ Signature | ▶ Signature |
| Name (print) | Name (print) |
| Title | Title |
| Address | Local Health Department–Address endorsed form to the VETERINARY SECTION, California State Department of Public Health, 2151 Berkeley Way, Berkeley, California 94704 |

1. Licensing required? Yes☐ No☐ AGE at which licensing required ________

2. Vaccination required? Yes☐ No☐ If yes, answer a and b below.

   a. As a requisite to licensing? Yes☐ No☐

   b. By local ordinance? Yes☐ No☐

3. Dog pound maintained? Yes☐ No☐ If yes, answer a and b below.

   a. Government owned? Yes☐ No☐

   b. Contract with ________

4. Dogs under four months required to be kept confined to the premises of owner, keeper or harborer? Yes☐ No☐

5. Impound stray unowned dogs and those in violation of provisions of Section 1920, California Health and Safety Code, and 2606.4, California Administrative Code. Yes☐ No☐

   a. Government employed enforcement personnel? Yes☐ No☐

   b. Contract with ________

6. Provide or arrange for low cost rabies vaccination clinics? Yes☐ No☐ If yes, answer a and b below

   a. Number of clinics held per year ________

   b. Vaccination fee charged at clinics ________

(See Reverse for Instructions)

# INSTRUCTIONS FOR COMPLETING "STATEMENT" FORM

A. This statement should be completed in its entirety by the appropriate official designated by the local governing body (city council, county board of supervisors) having responsibility for enforcement of State rabies control provisions applying to declared rabies areas (Sections 1901.2, 1921 and 1921, California Health and Safety Code and Section 2606.4 of Title 17, California Administrative Code).

B. Upon completion of the "Statement" form, it should be sent to the Local Health Officer for endorsement. The Local Health Officer will forward the endorsed form to the Veterinary Section, California State Department of Public Health.

C. The "Statement" form deals with local enforcement of State required rabies control provisions applying to declared rabies areas. A short summary of requirements follows:

Item 1: Section 1920(a), Health and Safety Code requires licensing of all dogs beginning at four months of age.

Item 2: Section 1920(b), Health and Safety Code requires vaccination of all dogs against rabies beginning at four months of age.

Item 2a: Section 2606.4(a) of Title 17, Administrative Code requires that rabies vaccination be held requisite to the licensing requirement. This Section permits the collection of the license fee and issuance of an interim receipt prior to vaccination. However, the license certificate or receipt and license/vaccination tag(s) cannot be issued until a valid vaccination certificate is presented. A reasonable length of time may be permitted the dog owner, e.g., 10–15 days, to submit the vaccination certificate following issuance of the interim license receipt. Enforcement agencies are obligated, however, to follow up instances where the vaccination certificate is not submitted within the allotted time.

Item 3: Section 1920(e), Health and Safety Code requires that the governing bodies (board of supervisors and city councils) in declared rabies areas to maintain or provide for the maintenance (e.g., contract) of a pound system and a rabies control program for the purpose of carrying out and enforcing the provisions of Section 1920.

Item 4: Section 1920(c), Health and Safety Code requires that all dogs under four months of age be confined to the premises, or kept under physical restraint by the owner, keeper or harborer, Section 2606.4(b) of Title 17. Administrative Code additionally requires that dogs receiving initial injections of rabies vaccine be similarly confined until 30 days have elapsed following vaccination (the period of time necessary for full immunity to develop).

Item 5: Section 1920(d), Health and Safety Code requires the impounding of dogs in violation of the provisions of Article of said Code.

Item 6: Section 1920(f), Health and Safety Code makes it a responsibility of the counties and cities in declared rabies areas to provide or arrange for low cost public rabies vaccination clinics. The charge at such clinics cannot be in excess of actual cost.

Fig. 14 (revarse side)

Fig. 15

# QUARTERLY REPORT OF LOCAL RABIES CONTROL ACTIVITIES

*Completed Reports to be Forwarded to the County Health Officer*

| AREA FOR WHICH REPORT IS MADE: (On county reports, indicate if report covers only unincorporated area. If cities are served by contract or other arrangement, please list.) | REPORT FOR QUARTER: (Check one)<br>☐Jan–March Due Date Apr 30<br>☐Apr–June Due Date Jul 30<br>☐Jul–Sept Due Date Oct 30<br>☐Oct–Dec Due Date Jan 30<br>YEAR______ |
|---|---|

| NOTE: Please add numbers to subtotals and totals as indicated; if report for any items is "none" or "zero", so indicate. | | | NUMBER THIS QUARTER |
|---|---|---|---|
| RABIES VACCINATION | | A. Dogs vaccinated in low cost public vaccination clinics | |
| | | B. Number of low cost public vaccination clinics held during quarter | |
| | | C. Individual vaccination fee charged in above low cost public vaccination clinics $______ | |
| CANINE RABIES CONTROL | Licensing | D. Total number of dogs licensed (include those shown under 1 and 2 below) | |
| | | 1. Dogs licensed for which valid vaccination certificates were submitted | |
| | | 2. Dogs licensed with vaccination exemption certificate approved by the local health department (for acute illnesses only) | |
| | Stray Dog Control | E. Dogs impounded | |
| | | F. Dogs redeemed | |
| | | G. Dogs sold or given away | |
| | | H. Dogs destroyed | |

| | | |
|---|---|---|
| Enforcement | I. Warnings issued for violations, vaccination and/or license requirements of State law or local ordinance provisions | |
| | J. Number prosecuted | |
| | K. Convictions obtained | |
| ANIMAL BITES REPORTED | L. Animal bites reported, TOTAL: | |
| | 1. Dog bites reported, Total: | |
| | a. Licensed and vaccinated | |
| | b. Licensed only | |
| | c. Vaccinated only | |
| | d. Neither licensed nor vaccinated (but owned) | |
| | e. Neither licensed nor vaccinated (strays) | |
| | 2. Other animal bites reported, Total: | |
| | a. Domestic | |
| | b. Wild | |
| ADMINISTRATION | Name of agency or organization responsible for administration of dog control in above jurisdiction | |
| | Address | |

COMPLETED BY:

Signature ______________________

Name (print) ______________________

Title ______________________

Agency ______________________

Endorsement by Local Health Officer or authorized representative:

Signature ______________________

Name (print) ______________________

Title ______________________

## REFERENCES


Black, S. P. and Powers, L. M. (1910). History of Rabies in Southern California. *Calif. State J. Med.*, **8**, 369–372.

California Dept. of Public Health (1963). Change in California State Laboratory Test Procedure for Rabies Examination. California Surveillance Report, Rabies Report No. 1, Jan.

California State Board of Health (1910). Twenty-first Biennial Report for the Fiscal Years from July 1, 1908 to June 30, 1910, 228–230.

California State Board of Health (1915). Rabies in Coyotes in California. Monthly Bulletin, **11**, 215–216.

California State Board of Health (1916). Rabies Campaign (Modoc and Lassen Counties). Monthly Bulletin, **12**, 59.

California State Board of Health (1916). Report on Rabies Conference. Monthly Bulletin, **11**, 400.

California State Board of Health (1913). Special Bulletin No. 3. Regulations for Enforcement of an Act to Prevent the Introduction and Spread of Rabies (14 pages).

California State Dept. of Public Health (1932). Rabies. Thirty-Second Biennial Report for the Fiscal Years July 1, 1930 to June 30, 1932, 20–22.

Enright, J. B., Sadler, W. M., Moulton, J. E. and Constantine, D. (1955). Isolation of Rabies Virus from an Insectivorous Bat (*Tadarida mexicana*), in California. *Proc. Soc. Exp. Biol. Med.*, **89**, 94–96.

Gieger, J. C. (1913). The Work of the Pasteur Division of the State Hygienic Laboratory. Special Report to the California State Board of Health, August 4.

Hebert, H. J. and Humphrey, G. L. (1961). Rabies Outbreak in Imperial County. *Pub. Hlth. Repts.*, **76**, 391–397.

Hovey, H. G. (1874). Rabies Mephitica. *Amer. J. Sci. and Art.*, **7**, 477–783; reprinted in *Fur Bearing Animals*. Washington, D.C., U.S. Government Printing Office, 1877, 223–235.

Humphrey, G. L. and Hebert, H. J. (1960). The California (U.S.A.) -Baja California del Norte (Mexico) Rabies Outbreak of 1959–1960. California Surveillance Report, Rabies Report No. 3, California Dept. of Public Health, Berkeley, Calif., 94704.

Humphrey, G. L. (1966). California State Rabies Control Program. Proc. National Rabies Symposium, N.C.D.C., P.H.S., U.S.D.H.E.W., Atlanta, Georgia.

Lennette, E. H., Woodie, J. D., Nakamura, K. and Magoffin, R. L. (1965). The Diagnosis of Rabies by Fluorescent Antibody Method (FRA) Employing Immune Hamster Serum. *Hlth. Lab. Sci.*, **2**, 24–34.

Lyman, G. D. (1930). *John Marsh, Pioneer*, New York, N.Y., Scribner.

Magoffin, R. L. (1964). Fluorescent Antibody Test for Diagnosis of Rabies Proves Fast and Reliable. California's Health, **22**, 79.

Mallory, L. B. (1915). Campaign Against Rabies in Modoc and Lassen Counties. Calif. State Board of Health, Monthly Bulletin, **11**, 273–277.

Nelson, E. W. (1918). *Wild Animals of North America.* Washington, D.C., National Georgraphic Society.

Rand McNally (1962). California Pocket Reference Map. San Francisco, Rand McNally and Co.

Rand McNally (1967). Standard Reference Map and Guide of California. San Francisco, Rand McNally and Co.

Records, Edwards (1932). Rabies-Its History in Nevada. *Calif. and West. Med.*, **37**, 90–94.

Sawyer, W. A. (1912). Rabies in California for the Year Ending March 31, 1912. Special Report to the California State Board of Health, July, 3.

Sawyer, W. A. (1912). Rabies in Its Present Status in California. *Calif. State J. Med.*, **10**, 318–329.

Sikes, Keith (1968). Need for Developing Uniform Rabies Control Practices in the United States. *J.A.V.M.A.*, **153**, 1793–1797.

State of California Health and Safety Code (1969). Sections 1900–1901, and 1902–1918.

State of California (1955). Title 17, Administrative Code (1955), Section 2606(d) and (e).

State of California (1957). Title 17, Administrative Code (1957), Section 2606.4(a) and (b).

State of California (1969). Health and Safety Code (1969), Sections 1901.2, 1920 and 1921.

World Health Organization Expert Committee on Rabies (1950). Report on the First Session. Wld. Hlth. Org. Techn. Report Ser., 28.

World Health Organization Expert Committee on Rabies (1954). Second Report, Wld. Hlth. Org. Techn., Report Ser., 82.

World Health Organization Expert Committee on Rabies (1957). Third Report. Wld. Hlth. Org. Techn. Report Ser., 121.

World Health Organization Expert Committee on Rabies (1960). Fourth Report. Wld. Hlth. Org. Techn. Report Ser., 201.

For Discussion, see page 335.

# Discussion*

DAVENPORT: The outlook for eradication of rabies from these areas with dog control would be greatly enhanced if it were known there were not reservoirs in species other than dogs.

It is often stated in the recommendations that the physician has the option of not instituting post-bite prophylaxis—I am not talking about postexposure but post-bite prophylaxis— if rabies has not occurred in that specific area for a sufficient period of time. What are your views on the "sufficient" length of time that canine rabies has been absent to make it safe to withhold treatment in the case of the unapprehended or unidentified dog? I am speaking about this one particular instance where the recommendations say that if you cannot find the dog or if the dog cannot be identified, you should treat, but then there is the loophole that at the discretion of the physician, if there has been no dog rabies in the area, donot treat.

HUMPHREY: This is always a difficult situation. We do not have any hard and fixed rule. We look at each case on its individual merit. There are many factors which we consider, such as the recognition of wildlife rabies in the area where the dog is, the past history of where the dog has been, and whether the dog has been vaccinated or not. We do not have any set period of time for the absence of dog rabies in an area for saying that we will or will not recommend treatment. In the five-year period, 1964–1968, we examined nearly 8,000 dogs for rabies in California, of which 118 were positive. These figures include dogs from the Mexican border areas as well. This is about 1.5%. If it were in the area of the Mexican border, at the present time I probably would recommend treatment. In other areas of the state, particularly an area like San Francisco or other urban areas, somewhat removed from where we have found cases of rabies in wildlife, I would probably recommend against treatment. But I think it is important that you look at each case individually. Cat rabies is a similar problem. We probably have more cat bites than we do dog bites. For ex-

* This Discussion refers to the report by Humphrey.

ample, during the time period 1964–1968 in California, we examined over 10,000 cats, only 19 of which were positive, less than 0.2% but you still have the problem of decision regarding treatment if the animal is not available for observation or laboratory examination.

LENNETTE: This is really what was behind my remarks yesterday when I talked about the need for complete epidemiologic information, and the data that Dr. Humphrey is talking about are always referred to whenever there is a reported bite, or suspected rabies. We go through these various records and make an evaluation according to where the animal is, where the individual resides, how much rabies has been there, when the last case of rabies was reported, and so on. Is this a fair statement, Dr. Humphrey? Each one of these cases thus takes a tremendous amount of time on the part of the epidemiologic staff as well as the laboratory staff, and yet the files are quite complete. They have to be, if one is going to make the kind of judgments you are talking about, Dr. Davenport.

HUMPHREY: I think really the biggest factor to help us has been the use of the FRA test. We have enough confidence in our laboratory that if an animal is negative, we recommend against treatment. I won't go so far as to make this recommendation based on a local laboratory exam. In that sort of a situation I usually try to get material sent in to the state lab for confirmation. We have confidence in the FRA procedure, and this has been the biggest factor, as far as I am concerned, in a long, long time in making these kind of decisions.

LENNETTE: It is also helpful because, as I say, you don't have to wait for the animal to show signs of infection. You kill the animal promptly, examine the brain by the FRA technique, and you have got an answer, yes or no. This is also a big time-saver from the standpoint of initiating treatment. Any other comments or questions?

HADDOCK: The proper treatment of animal bite patients has been a thorny and persistent problem on Guam and the prospects are that it will continue to be so even after Guam is declared rabies-free. We have not been able to obtain any practical assistance on what changes, if any, we should make in our treatment recommendations at that time. At present we are using the U.S. Public Health Service recommendations for rabies prophylaxis in rabies endemic areas (which all areas of the continental United States are considered to be at the present time).

I would like to ask the delegates from Japan under what circumstances, if any, humans exposed to animal bites in Japan are given rabies vaccine or other specific anti-rabies treatment.

If you have any information on rabies prophylaxis regimens of other areas assumed to be rabies-free, that would be helpful also.

SHIMADA: Before we became rabies-free in Tokyo, I would carry out examinations and report the results of these examinations to Dr. Otani (laboratory of Prof. Kitamoto, the Institute for Infectious Diseases, the University of Tokyo) and he would treat if the results were positive and would not treat if the results were negative. What is being done now, I do not know accurately because I am no longer engaged in this work, but I think no vaccinations are being carried out now.

OKUNO: To the question of Dr. Haddock, I would like to comment on the current rabies situation in rabies-free Taiwan. Taiwan has been free from reported incidence of rabies 1960 and that makes almost ten years now. Last year, it was declared by WHO that this country is free from rabies. Even before that declaration, most of the people, including myself, were getting too optimistic about the situation. Even though the doctor recommends the vaccination, people would not receive any. Especially after the declaration, I do not think any doctor recommends the vaccination to people bitten by the suspicious dog. Regarding the examination the national laboratory is carrying out the routine checks for stamp specimens from these dogs for Negri body by Seller's stain. In conclusion, I am confident about that not even a single case of bitten humans has received immunization since 1967.

HAMMON: We have been talking about California and I am wondering about some of the legal aspects there. If a doctor fails to give prophylaxis following a bite and he has been advised that it is probably not necessary by somebody in the health department, perhaps somebody who is not a physician, and the patient develops rabies, legally where does the responsibility lie? Is the doctor only sued for not having used good judgment or are his advise sued?

HUMPHREY: The only thing I can say is that we have not had any suits. My recommendations to treat or not to treat are based on the veterinary aspects of the exposure. There is very close collaboration when it comes to the medical aspects of such recommendations. It is not uncommon to have a physician and a veterinarian both consulting on the same telephone with the physician. We had an instance like this involving a cat bite in Davis on a very small child, 2 and one-half years old. Obviously bitten, she said it was a cat but no adult observed the bite incident, there was no animal available, and on this instance both a physician and myself were on the telephone and both of us recommended treatment.

LENNETTE: There is a little bit more to this too. If you notice Dr. Humphrey's paper, at the bottom it shows that he is on the staff of the Consumer Research Program in Environmental Health. Under our re-organization, he was divorced from the communicable disease and laboratory group but we are still fighting to keep him in the same location because we do have this very close consultation between the physician and the veterinarian. It is true that if there is a problem it always involves Dr. Humphrey or Dr. Emmons or myself as administrative officials of the State of California. If Dr. Harald Johnson, being a staff member of the Foundation, gave us some advice, I do not know where he would stand legally. This has never come up, but of course it does not mean it might not. I think this points up the sort of thing I was talking about yesterday and which Dr. Humphrey has mentioned today, i.e., the close collaboration which is needed between the two groups, so that the epidemiological and laboratory data are available in one place. You can not have the whole series of records scattered about a bureau or department on different floors or even in different cities (as you know, we are divided between Sacramento Berkeley, which are some 65 or 70 miles apart)—the records have to be in one place and readily available for consultation.

I think that is an important point. This has troubled us too in the past. Dr. Hammon?

HAMMON: I was simply curious and I still am somewhat curious whether our attorney friend Mr. Melvin Belli has not brought up some cases in which some one has made a mistake involving complications from the Pasteur or Semple vaccine, central nervous system accidents where the vaccine was used when some might judge that it was not necessary, or somebody died from rabies and the vaccine was not used; or perhaps the serum was not used according to recommendations. What is the legal position of the person who gives advice, whether it be the health department or the individual? Since you have so many more law suits against physicians in California and liability insurance is so difficult to get for this reason, I am just wondering what the history has been.

LENNETTE: Dr. Humphrey can answer that but I think all the questions you have been asking plus some of these others are the reasons for the title of a paper some years back called "Rabies: The Physician's Dilemma."

HUMPHREY: To my knowledge, Dr. Hammon, there have been no suits. There have been some threats of suits, one involved a rabid ocelot in the city of Berkeley. This was an imported animal from Peru and very shortly after it was brought in it became sick. There were five people bitten. One of them was a mighty sick man and spent 3 or 4 weeks in the hospital as a result of delayed serum sickness. I have not heard what the outcome is or whether it is even gone to suit. As far as people working for the state health department, mal-practice protection is a question which has been discussed many times. Dr. Lennette is aware of the fact that physicians within the department have asked for the state to pay for malpractice suit. We have been uniformly turned down, with the assurance, however, that the state attorney general will defend us.

DAVENPORT: I would like to approach the question in another way. In one of his papers I think Dr. Habel gave a statistic that over 30,000 dog bites per annum in the United States were treated recently with the post-exposure program. I wonder if you have the figures for California. You are entitled to one-tenth of the total population of the United States and that should give you 3,000 if you are treating at the same rate as other people are.

HUMPHREY: We do not have any figures on number of anti-rabies treatments administered in California; it is not a reportable item. Our only source of information is the epidemiologic report card we receive from the local health department on each case of rabies which contains space for inserting the number of persons exposed, whether there were saliva contacts or bites together with space for indicating the type of treatment given. Oftentimes, however, the space is left blank and if I went through and tabulated them I would not have any confidence that I had all of the information. It used to be possible to make some guesses as to how many people were being treated; for example, in prior years we have collected figures on the number of doses of human antirabies vaccine distributed by the various manufacturing firms to California. But this does not help us much any more because of the widespread use of duck embryo vaccine for pre-exposure immunization. You can not separate amounts used for pre-exposure from that being given for post-exposure treatment. I really do not have any good figures.

DAVENPORT: Well—at 30,000 level, do you think there is over-use or under-use in the United State?

HUMPHREY: I think, if anything, that there is gross over-treatment. The factor that Dr. Hammon brought up regarding suits influences many physicians strongly and if they did not fear a malpractice suit for not administering, treatment, I am sure that there would not be nearly as much human vaccine sold in the United States. The only consolation that a physician can take, if he does make a decision not to treat in a particular instance is that he does have company, in other words quite often he will have somebody in the local health department and it is not unusual to have two or three people in our department involved in making a decision. We have recourse to records on cases and with a consensus on recommending a decision, to treat or not to treat, on a particular case, I believe the attending physician's ultimate decision is greatly strengthened. We also have state health department recommendations or guidelines for treatment which have been published in "California Medicine", and in "A manual for the Control of Communicable Disease in California" which is put out by the state health department. I think that within these guidelines and with uniformity in making a recommendation, even though you may err sometimes, and it is very possible that you could err, it might be difficult to collect in a mal-practice suit, although I am only guessing.

LENNETTE: Dr. Davenport might be interested to know that the recently issued copy of our Statistical Summary on Communicable Disease has a picture of the structure of an adenovirus on the front cover, which is a new departure, I think, for a communicable disease manual.

SOEKAWA: I would like to add to Dr. Shimada's statement on the treatment of persons bitten by dogs. When the dog cannot be captured, it is another matter, but when the dog can be found, we act on the premise that the dog will show signs of rabies within ten days if it is rabid. With the vaccine, we inject intradermally 0.2 m*l* of vaccine for 7 days as preliminary treatment, or we inject hyperimmune serum, and observe the dog. And complete vaccination will be conducted when the positive diagnosis is made on the animal. I would like to ask the doctors here whether this observation period of ten days is sufficient.

SIKES: It seems to me that to answer this question about what they should do in this case with treatment of an individual, the key point seems to me the question is this an indigenous dog? And if this dog is an indigenous animal and shows absolutely no abnormal behavior at the time of the bite, I think you would not be expected to treat, but simply detain the dog for ten days. Legally this would certainly prove your point. If the dog started showing signs during the ten days, then you would start treatment, but the indigenous factor is the key here.

The key point here is: was the animal emitting virus in his saliva? The evidence that we have is that a dog does not emit virus more than five days before he shows clinical signs, and if you double this length of time, then you are covered; that if these dogs later become sick the person that was bitten at this particular incident is not at risk. In other words, if you hold an animal ten days, if he dies within that ten days, you start treatment. If he does not die within ten days and he waits three months to die, the people that are bitten henceforth at that situation, that is another matter, but the first person bitten is not at risk.

HUMPHREY: In California, under regulations we will release a dog five days after bite with veterinary observation and examination. This means a complete physical examination with the veterinarian certifying that he can find no signs or symptoms of any infection.

ISHII: I would like to explain Dr. Soekawa's statement in detail, so that there is no misunderstanding. Dogs suspected of being rabid are immediately killed and we carry out a laboratory examination. Dogs that are not obviously rabid or are not suspected of being rabid are observed for ten days and a decision is made.

DAVENPORT: It is still not clear to me what is done in Japan when the dog cannot be found.

LENNETTE: I gathered from what was said here that if the dog cannot be found, treatment is initiated.

# Evaluation of Canine Rabies Vaccines

R. K. Sikes

*Viral Zoonoses Section, Center for Disease Control, Atlanta, Georgia 30333*

## INTRODUCTION

The first practical vaccine for dogs was developed in the early 1920s by Umeno and Doi (1921). This phenolized rabbit brain vaccine was used to control dog rabies successfully in Japan and its success stimulated interest in dog vaccination in the United States. It was not until 1940, however, when Habel developed a standard potency test for Semple type vaccines that real improvement in vaccines occurred (Habel, 1940). Johnson (1945) provided the first significant experimental contribution to our knowledge of the duration of immunity in dogs following rabies vaccination. His results indicated excellent protection in dogs for one year after a single dose of phenolized vaccine.

Koprowski and Cox (1948) developed a modified, live virus rabies vaccine of chick embryo origin (CEO-MLV). This CEO vaccine, low egg passage (LEP) type was proven by Tierkel *et al.* (1953) to have a 39-month duration of immunity in adult dogs. This vaccine was the primary type of vaccine used in the United States between 1953 and 1965 when dog rabies was reduced from 5,688 confirmed cases to only 412 (Center for Disease Control, 1969). Similar results with the CEO-LEP type were obtained in other countries also.

Following Kissling's successful adaptation of fixed rabies virus to primary hamster kidney tissue culture cells (Kissling, 1958), several vaccine producers in the United States and Canada developed various types of tissue culture rabies vaccines for use in domestic animals (Ott & Heyke, 1962; Kucera *et al.*, 1969; Abelseth, 1964; Brown *et al.*, 1967; Cabasso *et al.*, 1965; Emery *et al.*, 1968). Also two suckling mouse brain origin vaccines were developed for possible use in animals and in humans (Fuenzalida *et al.*, 1964; Sikes & Larghi, 1967).

I shall now review three years of data from a study comparing these eight different vaccines in dogs. The purpose of this study was to determine the relative immunogenicity of these vaccines and ultimately to determine if the newer types of vaccines provided as long a duration of immunity in dogs as the LEP-CEO type.

(The final observation period of challenged dogs will be completed in February 1971.)

## PROCEDURES AND RESULTS

*Vaccines—potency tests*

The tissue culture and CEO-LEP vaccines were prepared by the manufacturer licensed for their production. Suckling mouse brain vaccine (SMBV) was obtained from the Pan American Health Organization (PAHO) and the purified rabies vaccine (PRV) was prepared at the Center for Disease Control (CDC). Potency and infectivity tests were conducted at CDC where the complete duration-of-immunity study was carried out. Results of the virus potency tests on all vaccines supplied to CDC by the USDA are shown in Table 1.*

*First year results—vaccination, bleeding, challenge of dogs*

A total of 320 dogs were vaccinated with a single dose of vaccine administered in the biceps femoris muscle. Forty dogs were vaccinated with each of the eight vaccines and 100 additional dogs were maintained in the same kennels as unvaccinated controls. At the time of vaccination, all dogs were young adults 9 to 12 months of age. The total 420 purebred beagles had been purchased from a single breeder 6 months earlier and had never received any rabies vaccine. They were bled prior to vaccination and their serum tested for rabies SN antibody; none had detectable antibody at a 1:2 dilution.

All vaccinated dogs were bled at 7 intervals the first year—after 1, 2, 3 and 4 weeks, as well as at 2, 6 and 12 months; each serum was tested separately for rabies SN antibody. These individual results will be published in a more detailed paper. The median antibody titers of each group of 40 vaccinated dogs are presented in Figs. 1–8.

One year after vaccination, 10 dogs from each group were selected at random for challenge with the NYC-Ga. dog salivary gland strain of rabies virus. Those dogs vaccinated with tissue culture and CEO, LEP-Flury vaccines were challenged with 20,000 mouse $I.C.LD_{50}$

* The SMBV arrived 3 months later than the others, so the potency tests in mice and vaccination of dogs were conducted 3 months later.

Table 1. Results of Potency and Infectivity Tests on Rabies Vaccines Considered for Use in Canine Duration-of-Immunity Study

| Type of vaccine | Infectivity titer in mice | Guinea pig potency test-dog dose dilutions 1/80 | 1/20 | 1/10 |
|---|---|---|---|---|
| 1. Chick Embyo Origin (LEP-FLURY) | | | | |
| [a]Company A | $10^{4.3}$ | 0/10[b] | | |
| 〃 B | $10^{4.6}$ | 0/10[b] | | |
| 〃 C | $10^{4.4}$ | 0/0[b] | | |
| 〃 D | $10^{5.0}$ | | | |
| 2. Chick Fibroblast T.C. (LEP-FLURY) | | | | |
| Company E, Lot 1 | $10^{2.0}$ | | | |
| 〃 , Lot 2 | $10^{3.6}$ | 3/11[c] | | 0/10[b] |
| 〃 , Lot 3 | $10^{3.6}$ | 7/12[c] | | |
| [a]Company F | $10^{3.5}$ | 2/10[b] | | 0/9[b] |
| 3. Hamster Kidney T.C. (LEP-FLURY) | | | | |
| Company G, Lot 1 | $10^{3.3}$ | 5/10[b] | | 1/10[b] |
| 〃 Lot 2 | $10^{2.9}$ | | | |
| [a]Company H | $10^{4.0}$ | 2/10[b] | | 0/8[b] |
| 4. Hamster Kidney T.C. (CVS) (INACTIVATED+ADJ.) | | | | |
| [a]Company I Lot 1 | | | 0/12[c] | |
| 〃 , Lot 2 | | | 1/12[c] | |
| 〃 , Lot 3 | | | 1/12[c] | |
| 5. Porcine Kidney T.C. (ERA) | | | | |
| [a]Company J | $10^{4.1}$ | 2/10[b] | | 0/10[b] |
| 6. Canine Kidney T.C.[d] (HEP-FLURY) | | | | |
| [a]Company K, Lot 1 | $10^{4.3}$ | 0/11[c] | | |
| 〃 , Lot 2 | $10^{4.3}$ | 1/12[c] | | |
| 〃 , Lot 3 | $10^{4.4}$ | 0/12[c] | | |
| 7. Suckling Mouse Brain *VACC.*[e] (INACTIVATED) | | NIH Potency test A.V.=1.5 | | |
| 8. Purified Rabies Vaccine (*PPV*)[e] (INACTIVATED) | | NIH Potency test A.V.=4.0 | | |

*a* Vaccine selected for study

*b* Control mortality—8/10—Rabies deaths/Inoculated

*c* Control mortality—9/9—Rabies deaths/Inoculated

*d* Titrated suckling mice, 0.02 ml I.C. Adult mouse potency test also done, values of $10^{3.2}$, $10^{3.3}$ obtained.

*e* NIH Test control data: $ED_{50}$ of NIH ref. vacc. lot 173+0.25 mg (challenge=10 MIC $LD_{50}$, CVS-27).

three months prior to those vaccinated with the SMBV and PRV which were challenged with 8,500 mouse I.C. $LD_{50}$ (Tables 2 and 3).

Group I LEP-CEO

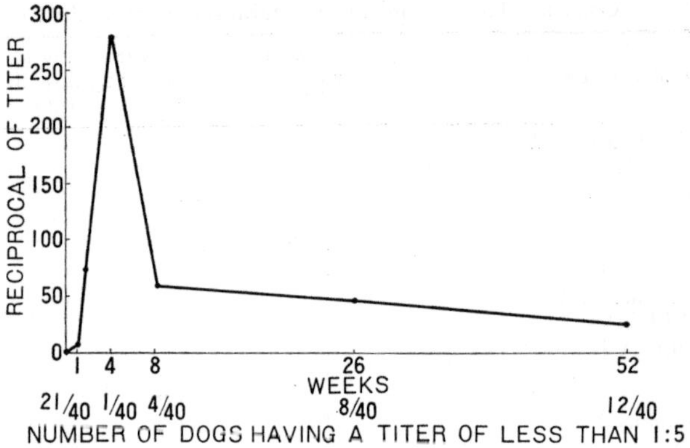


**Fig. 1.** Rabies Duration of Immunity Study Median SN Antibody Profile

Group II LEP-CFTC

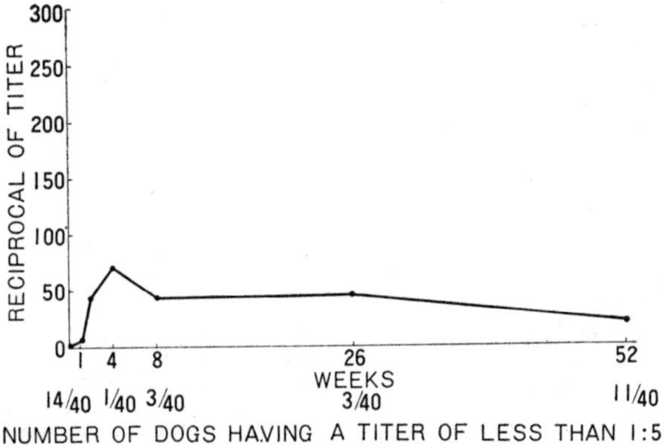


**Fig. 2.** Rabies Duration of Immunity Study Median SN Antibody Profile

Group III LEP-HKTC

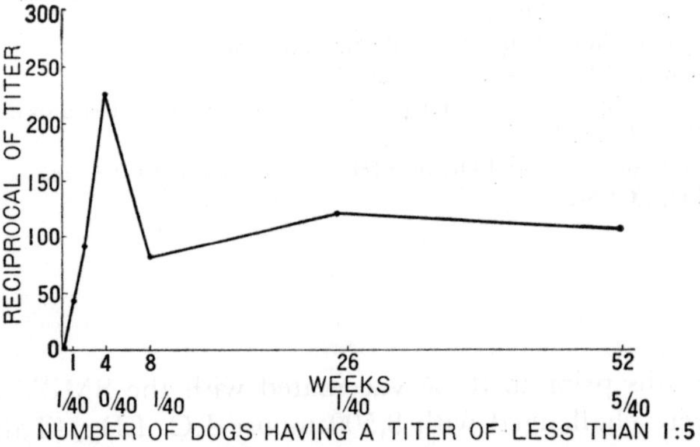


**Fig. 3.** Rabies Duration of Immunity Study Median SN Antibody Profile

Group IV CVS-HKTC (ADJUVANT)

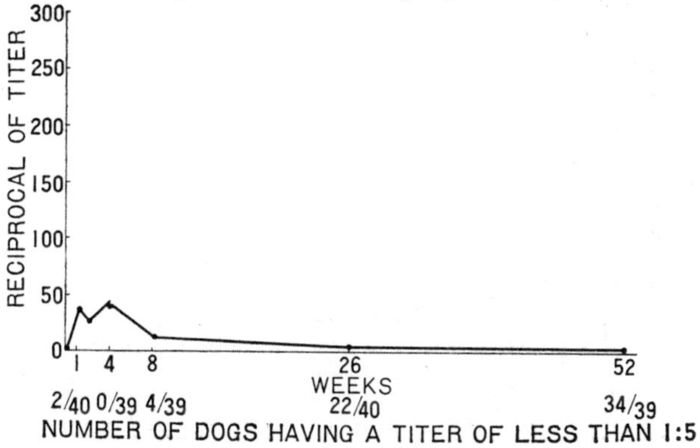


Fig. 4. Rabies Duration of Immunity Study Median SN Antibody Profile

Group V HEP-CKTC

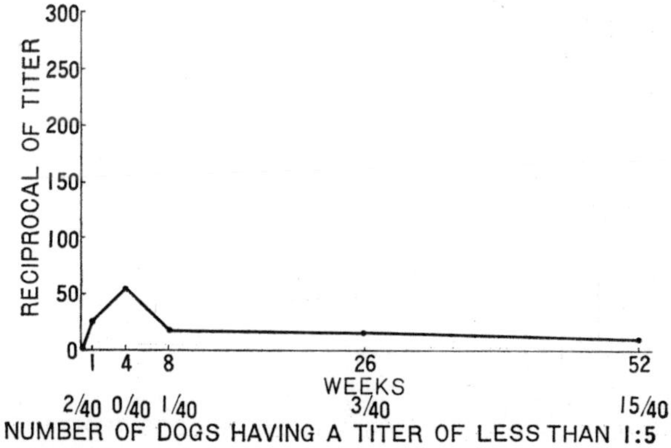


Fig. 5. Rabies Duration of Immunity Study Median SN Antibody Profile

Group VI ERA-PKTC

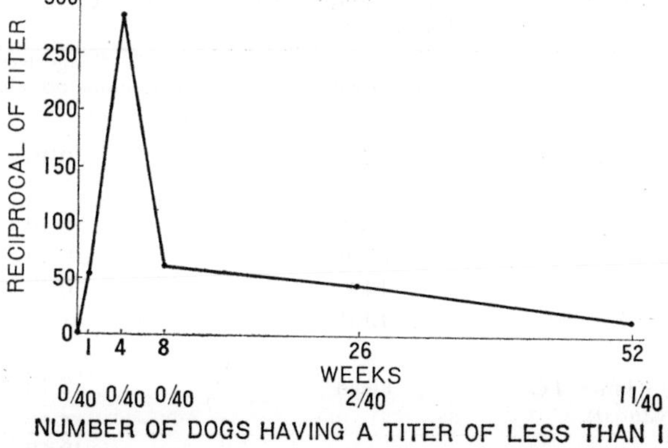


Fig. 6. Rabies Duration of Immunity Study Median SN Antibody Profile

Group VII SMV

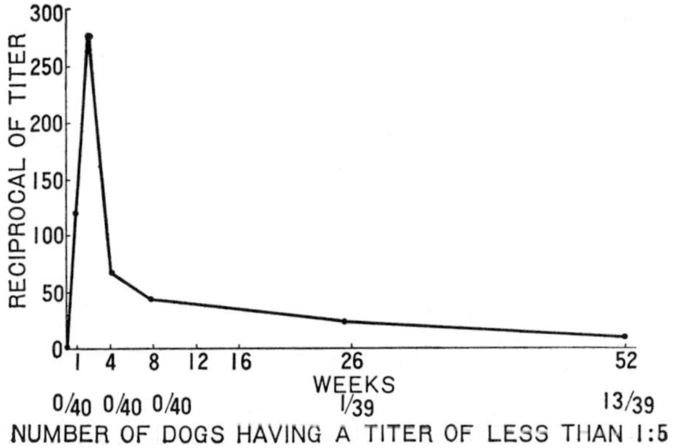


Fig. 7. Rabies Duration of Immunity Study Median SN Antibody Profile

Group VIII PRV

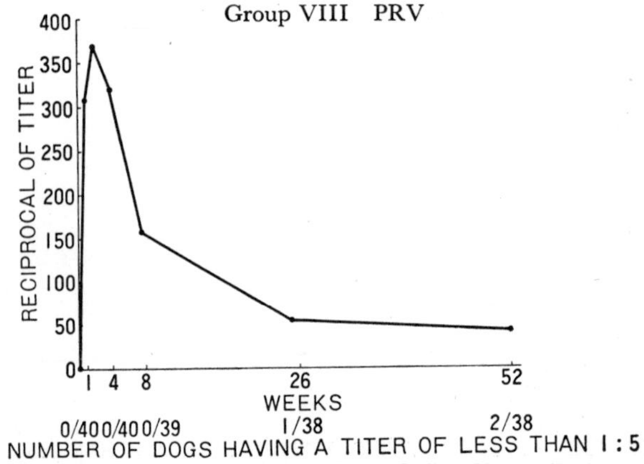


Fig. 8. Rabies Duration of Immunity Study Median SN Antibody Profile

Table 2. Rabies Duration of Immunity Study; Results of Challenge 12 Months after Vaccination

| Type of Vaccine | Virus Strain | Challenge Results* (rabies deaths/no. challenged) |
|---|---|---|
| Love: | | |
| Chick Embryo Origin | LEP | 0/10 |
| Tissue Culture: | | |
| Porcine Kidney | ERA | 0/10 |
| Canine Kidney | HEP | 0/10 |
| Chick Fibroblast | LEP | 0/10 |
| Hamster Kidney | LEP | 1/10 |
| Inactivated: | | |
| Hamster Kidney TC (Adjuvanted) | Fixed | 3/10 |
| Nonvaccinated Controls | | 10/10 |

* Challenge dose of 20,000 Mouse I.C. $LD_{50}$ contained in the 0.6 m*l* volume used in each dog.

Table 3. Rabies Duration of Immunity Study; Results of Challenge 12 Months after Vaccination with SMBV and PRV

| Type of Vaccine | Virus Strain | Challenge Results* (rabies deaths/no. challenged) |
|---|---|---|
| Inactivated: | | |
| Suckling Mouse Brain (SMBV), PAHO | Fixed | 0/10 |
| Purified (PRV), CDC | Fixed | 0/10 |
| Nonvaccinated Controls | | 4/10 |

* Challenge dose of 8,500 Mouse I.C. $LD_{50}$ contained in the 0.6 m*l* volume used in each dog.

Group I LEP-CEO

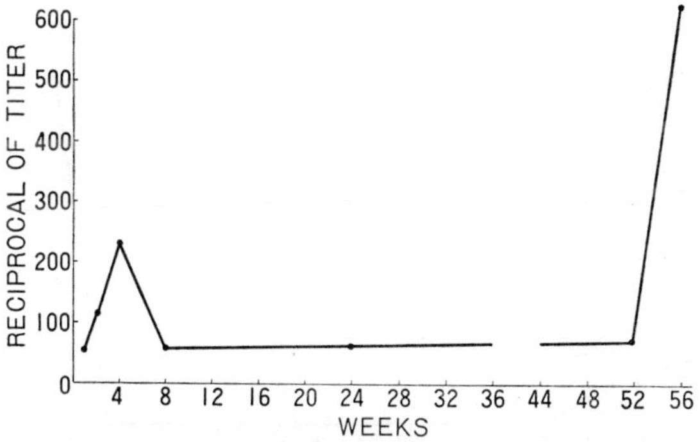


Fig. 9. Rabies Duration of Immunity Study Effect of Challenge on Titer One Year after Vaccination Median SN Antibody Profile

Group II LEP-CFTC

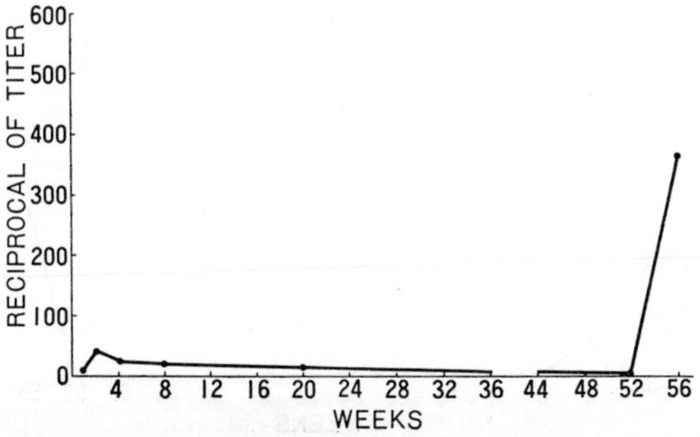


Fig. 10. Rabies Duration of Immunity Study Effect of Challenge on Titer One Year after Vaccination Median SN Antibody Profile

Group III LEP-HKTC

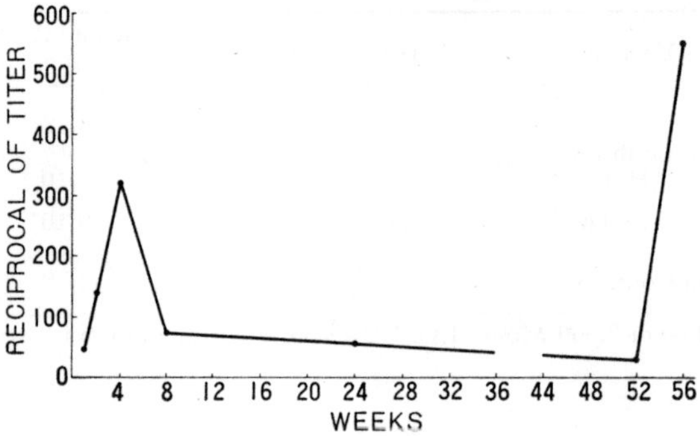


Fig. 11. Rabies Duration of Immunity Study Effect of Challenge on Titer One Year after Vaccination Median SN Antibody Profile

Group IV CVS-HKTC

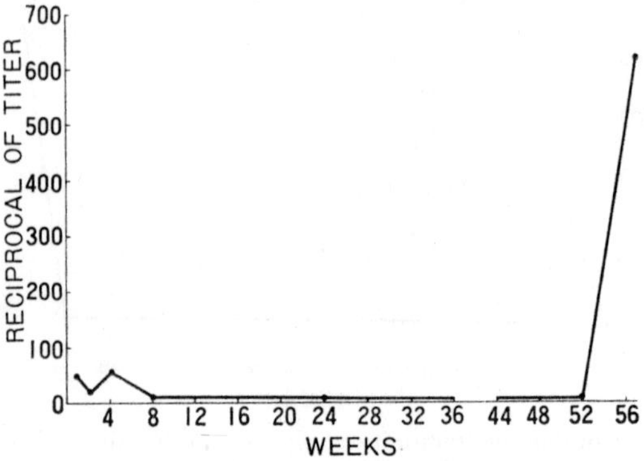


Fig. 12. Rabies Duration of Immunity Study Effect of Challenge on Titer One Year after Vaccination Median SN Antibody Profile

Group V HEP-CKTC

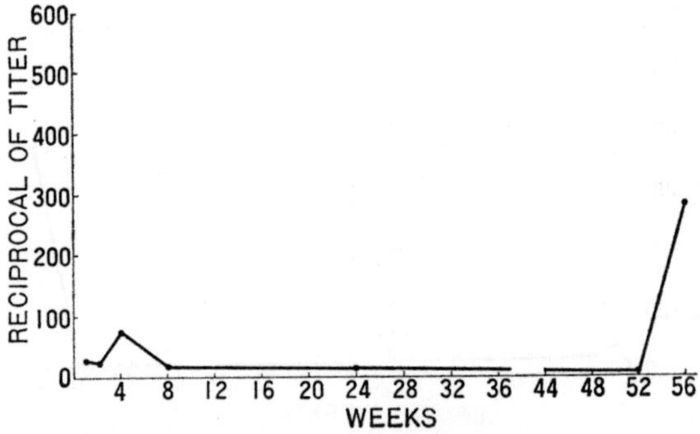


Fig. 13. Rabies Duration of Immunity Study Effect of Challenge on Titer One Year after Vaccination Median SN Antibody Profile

Group VI ERA-PKTC

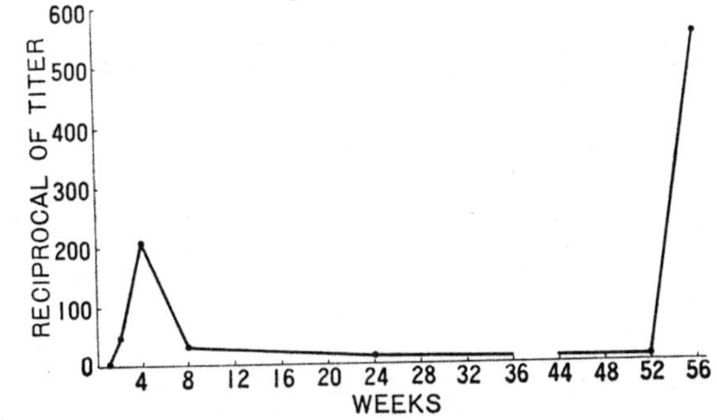


Fig. 14. Rabies Duration of Immunity Study Effect of Challenge on Titer One Year after Vaccination Median SN Antibody Profile

Group VIII PRV

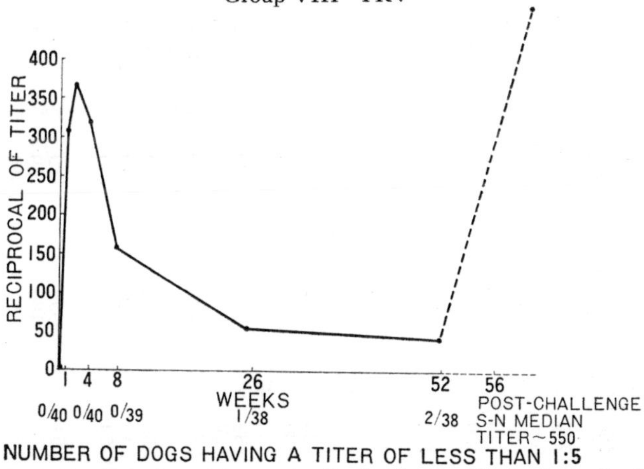


Fig. 15. Rabies Duration of Immunity Study Median SN Antibody Profile

Group VII SMV

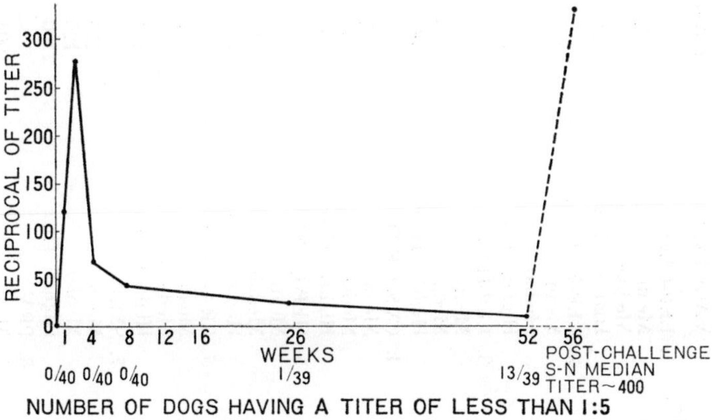


Fig. 16. Rabies Duration of Immunity Study Median SN Antibody Profile

Table 4. Canine Immunity Duration Study
Mean, Median and Highest Rabies Serum Neutralization Titers at Various Times after Vaccination

| VACCINE | 1 WK. | 2 WKS. | 3 WKS. | 1 MO. | 2 MOS. | 6 MOS. | 1 YR. | 2 YRS. |
|---|---|---|---|---|---|---|---|---|
| 1. LEP-CEO | | | | | | | | |
| Mean | 11 | 186 | 341 | 325 | 93 | 89 | 45 | 67 |
| Median | <5 | 75 | 230 | 280 | 56 | 56 | 25 | 33 |
| Highest Titer | 95 | 1750 | 1400 | 1400 | 350 | 480 | 282 | 350 |
| 2. LEP-CETC | | | | | | | | |
| Mean | 18 | 76 | 203 | 118 | 44 | 71 | 35 | 86 |
| Median | 5 | 46 | 96 | 70 | 45 | 45 | 14 | 39 |
| Highest Titer | 125 | 400 | 625 | 350 | 230 | 280 | 280 | 800 |
| 3. LEP-HKTC | | | | | | | | |
| Mean | 102 | 128 | 540 | 280 | 106 | 199 | 139 | 207 |
| Median | 46 | 95 | 280 | 230 | 70 | 230 | 84 | 143 |
| Highest Titer | 480 | 800 | 1400 | 1160 | 350 | 800 | 480 | 480 |
| 4. CVS-HKTC | | | | | | | | |
| Mean | 58 | 45 | 144 | 56 | 14 | <5 | <5 | <5 |
| Median | 40 | 25 | 80 | 46 | 11 | <5 | <5 | <5 |
| Highest Titer | 480 | 280 | 480 | 280 | 45 | 56 | 18 | 9 |
| 5. HEP-CKTC | | | | | | | | |
| Mean | 35 | 32 | 138 | 130 | 80 | 79 | 20 | 23 |
| Median | 18 | 18 | 70 | 56 | 19 | 18 | 8 | 11 |
| Highest Titer | 125 | 330 | 625 | 1400 | 1750 | 1750 | 350 | 160 |
| 6. ERA-TKTC | | | | | | | | |
| Mean | 82 | 358 | 490 | 310 | 165 | 87 | 32 | 55 |
| Median | 56 | 230 | 300 | 280 | 60 | 46 | 14 | 19 |
| Highest Titer | 232 | 1750 | 1400 | 1150 | 1150 | 800 | 160 | 480 |
| 7. SMBV | | | | | | | | |
| Mean | 275 | 294 | 339 | 125 | 62 | 49 | 37 | 11 |
| Median | 125 | 280 | 180 | 69 | 46 | 25 | 10 | 6 |
| Highest Titer | 2400 | 1150 | >625 | 350 | 280 | 232 | 480 | 56 |
| 8. PRV | | | | | | | | |
| Mean | 1004 | 1003 | 724 | 565 | 173 | 91 | 35 | 24 |
| Median | 350 | 480 | 625 | 365 | 160 | 56 | 33 | 18 |
| Highest Titer | 12000 | 5900 | >3125 | 1800 | 480 | 625 | 125 | 95 |

The calculated dose of virus was injected bilaterally into the masseter muscle. The dogs that survived the challenge were bled 30 days after challenge to determine the effect of challenge on antibody titer. These results are shown in Figs. 9–16. The dogs were observed for 6 months after challenge but no deaths occurred more than 20 days after challenge.

*Second year results*

The mean and median SN antibody titers, as well as the individual with the highest titer of each group of dogs for all bleedings through the second year, are presented in Table 4.

*Third year results*

See p. 308

## CONCLUSIONS

*Potency*

Although a difference in potency was noted among various vaccines, each type used in this study passed the required test set by the USDA-VBD.

*Immunogenicity—general*

Each vaccine was sufficiently immunogenic to stimulate detectable antibody. A titer of at least 1:5 was detected in all except one of 320 vaccinated dogs.

*Comparative immunogenicity*

1. Speed of Antibody Development: Three vaccines stimulated development of antibody faster than the other five. All 40 dogs of each group vaccinated with ERA-PKTC, SMBV and PRV had detectable antibody one week after vaccination. Three other vaccines stimulated antibody almost as rapidly. The LEP-HKTC vaccine stimulated antibody in 39 of 40 dogs after one week.

The LEP-CEO and LEP-CFTC vaccines stimulated antibody at a slower rate than the other six vaccines. Twenty-one of 40 (55%) dogs vaccinated with LEP-CEO and 14 of 40 (35%) with the LEP-CFTC type failed to develop a detectable titer one week after vaccination.

2. Highest Titers (Median): The PRV vaccine produced the highest median titer (1:625) of all vaccines tested. Four vaccines, LEP-CEO,

LEP-HKTC, ERA-PKTC and the SMBV, produced peak median titers of 1:200 to 300.

3. Duration of Antibody Titer: After one year, 36 of 38 dogs vaccinated with PRV retained a titer of 1:5 or greater. The other vaccines ranked in the following order for stimulating antibody that lasted one year:

| | |
|---|---|
| LEP-HKTC | (35/40) |
| LEP-CFTC | 29/40 |
| ERA-PKTC | |
| LEP-CEO | (28/40) |
| HEP-CKTC | (25/40) |
| SMBV | (13/39) |
| CVS-HKTC | (5/39) |

Thus, as regards the duration of antibody:

(1) The CVS-HKTC inactivated vaccine is significantly worse ($p < .01$) than any other vaccine or any combination of the other vaccines.

(2) PRV is significantly better ($p < .01$) than the other vaccines, taken as a group.

4. First Year Challenge: There was no statistically significant difference (at .05 level) between the inactivated CVS-HKTC vaccine and the other types. There did appear to be a biologically significant difference, however.

5. Second Year Results: No dogs were challenged after 2 years but all were bled and their serum antibody titers determined. Antibody not only persisted in most instances of dogs vaccinated with live rabies vaccines but there was frequently an increase in titer. This is evidence that live virus vaccines do multiply and it appears that when antibody declines to a certain low threshold that an anamnestic response occurs.

6. Third Year Results: Antibody titers (Table 5)

A. Rabies SN antibody persisted for 3 years in 15x of 233 (68%) of the vaccinated dogs.

B. Dogs vaccinated with live rabies vaccines licensed for use in the U.S.A. had significantly longer lasting antibody than those vaccinated with licensed, inactivated vaccines, 77% to 31% ($p < .01$).

Challenge results (Table 6)

A. The only vaccine which protected 100% of the dogs was the experimentally-produced PRV type made at CDC. This proves that an inactivated vaccine can be as immunogenic as

Table 5. Persistence of Rabies SN Antibody in Dogs Vaccinated; 3 Years Prior with Live or Inactivated Vaccines

| Type Vaccine | Number of Dogs Vaccinated | | |
|---|---|---|---|
| | with antibody after 3 years | without antibody after 3 years | Total No. with antibody/No. vaccinated |
| Licensed | | | |
| live, attenuated | 115 | 32 | 115/147 (77%) |
| inactivated | 18 | 41 | 18/59 (31%) |
| Non-licensed | | | |
| purified, inactivated | 24 | 3 | 24/27 (90%) |
| TOTAL | 157 | 76 | 157/233 (68%) |

the live vaccines presently in use for dogs. The PRV had a high value of antigenic mass—approximately 10 to 100 times greater than most vaccines of nervous tissue origin.

B. Two inactivated vaccines, the CVS-HKTC and SMBV, protected the least number of dogs in this study.

C. There was a statistically significant difference in mortality between the group of dogs vaccinated with the CVS-HKTC vaccine and all other vaccinated groups.

Table 6. Results of Dogs Challenged with Street Rabies Virus 36–39 Months after Vaccination

| Vaccine Type | Rabies deaths/No. Challenged | % Mortality |
|---|---|---|
| Inactivated: | | |
| CVS-HKTC with adjuvant | 12/29 | 41.3 |
| SMBV | 6/30 | 20.0 |
| PRV | 0/27 | 0.0 |
| Live: | | |
| ERA-PKTC | 3/29 | 10.3 |
| LEP-CFTC | 3/29 | 10.3 |
| HEP-CKTC | 2/29 | 6.8 |
| LEP-CEO | 2/30 | 6.6 |
| LEP-HKTC | 1/30 | 3.3 |
| Nonvaccinated controls | 27/30 | 90.0 |

Table 7. Relationship of SN Rabies Antibody to Protection of Dogs Challenged 3 Years after Vaccination

| | Number of Dogs Vaccinated | | |
|---|---|---|---|
| | With antibody after 3 years | Without antibody after 3 years | Total |
| Died | 2 | 28 | 30 |
| Survived | 158 | 45 | 203 |
| Total deaths/ No. challenged | 2/160 (1.3%) | 28/73 (38.4%) | 30/233 (13.0%) |

## Relationship of Antibody to Protection in Dogs (Table 7)

In this study, as in many others, presence of rabies SN antibody at the time of challenge did not indicate protection for all of the animals. Likewise, absence of antibody at the time of challenge did not mean the animals were unprotected. However, there was strong statistical significance ($p<.01$) that animals with SN antibody at the time of challenge were better protected than those with no detectable SN antibody. Only 2 of 160 (1.3%) animals with antibody at the time of challenge died while 28 of 73 (38.4%) of those without antibody at the time of challenge died. (The 2 animals with antibody which died had titers of 1:3 and 1:5.)

## FINAL CONCLUSION

Since there was no significant difference in the duration of immunity between the groups of dogs vaccinated with any type of the modified live virus rabies vaccines of either chick embryo or tissue culture origin, it may be assumed that any of these types provide equal immunity in adult dogs for 39 months.

On the basis of this study, the inactivated rabies vaccine of tissue culture origin does not provide protection of dogs for 39 months. At best, that type vaccine might be considered for providing one-year duration of immunity.

There was an indication that the SMBV (another inactivated vaccine) does not provide as solid an immunity as any of the live vaccines but it was better than the inactivated vaccine or HKTC origin. On the basis of this study, it appears to be capable of providing solid immunity for at least one to two years.

## ACKNOWLEDGMENT

This work was done in cooperation with the U.S. Department of Agriculture, Veterinary Biologics Division, and the Pan American Health Organization.

## REFERENCES

Abelseth, M. K. (1964). An attenuated rabies vaccine for domestic animals produced in tissue culture. *Canad. Vet. J.*, **5**, 279–286.

Brown, A. L., Davis, E. V., Merry, D. L., Jr. and Beckenhauer, W. H. (1967). Comparative potency tests on modified live-virus rabies vaccine produced from Flury high egg-passage virus grown on permanent dog kidney cell line. *Am. J. Vet. Res.*, **28**, 751–759.

Cabasso, V. J., Stebbins, M. R., Douglas, A. and Sharpless, G. R. (1965). Tissue-culture rabies vaccine (Flury LEP) in dogs. *Am. J. Vet. Res.*, **26**, 24–32.

Center for Disease Control (1969). Public Health Service, USDHEW, Zoonoses Surveillance, Annual Summary, Rabies.

Emery, J. B., Elliott, A. Y., Bordt, D. E., Burch, G. R. and Kugel, E. E. (1968). A tissue-culture, modified live-virus rabies vaccine for dogs: Report on development and clinical trial. *J.A.V.M.A.*, **152**, 476–482.

Fuenzalida, E., Palacios, R. and Borgono, J. M. (1964). Antirabies antibody response in man to vaccine made from infected suckling-mouse brains. *Bull. WHO*, **30**, 431–436.

Habel, K. (1940). Evaluation of a mouse test for the standardization of the immunizing power of antirabies vaccines. *Public Health Rep.*, **55**, 1473–1487.

Johnson, H. N. (1945). Experimental and field studies of canine rabies vaccination. Proceedings of the 49th Annual Meeting of the U.S. Livestock Sanitary Association, Chicago, Dec. 5–7, pp. 99–107.

Kissling, R. E. (1958). Growth of rabies virus in non-nervous tissue culture. *Proc. Soc. Exp. Biol. & Med.*, **98**, 223–225.

Koprowski, H. and Cox, H. R. (1948). Studies on chick-embryo adapted rabies virus. I. Cultural characteristics and pathogenicity. *J. Immun.*, **60**, 533–554.

Kucera, C. J., Sandvig, D. C. and Johnson, A. F. (1969). A formalinized and adjuvanted rabies vaccine of tissue culture origin. I. Preparation and evaluation of the vaccine. *Biochem. Rev.*, **33**, 3–9 (No. 2).

Ott, G. L. and Heyke, B. (1962). Preliminary trials of a new tissue culture rabies vaccine. *Vet. Med.*, **57**, 158–159.

Sikes, R. K. and Larghi, O. P. (1967). Purified rabies vaccine. Development and comparison of potency and safety with two human rabies vaccines. *J. Immun.*, **99**, 545–553.

Tierkel, E. S., Kissling, R. E., Eidson, M. and Habel, K. (1953). A brief survey and progress report of controlled comparative experiments in canine rabies immunization. Proceeding of the 90th Annual Meeting of the American Veterinary Medical Association, Toronto, July 20–23.

Umeno, S. and Doi, Y. (1921). A study in the antirabic inoculation of dogs. *Kitasato Arch. Exp. Med.*, **4**, 89–108.

For Discussion, see page 359.

# Discussion*

NOMURA: Dr. Sikes, you said that when you examined the groups 36 and 39 months afterwards, the immunity of the group inoculated with live virus lasted for a considerably long time. The immunity rate was about 90% and the mortality rate about 10% in the 36-month-challenge group. Is this immunity based on the replication of the virus?

SIKES: We have indirect evidence in this study that there was virus replication, namely the antibody titers first were increased slightly between the one-and two-year bleedings. We have seen it with one vaccine between six months and one year. So there was evidence based on antibody titer that the virus was still present at least enough to stimulate antibody in these groups of dogs. But regardless of whether there is replication or not, I think this data on the duration of immunity and the earlier data with the live vaccines, compared with the conventional inactivated vaccines, show that they are superior for providing longer duration of immunity in adult dogs.

NOMURA: In that case, do you think that the virus was replicating extraneurally, and if not, where do you think the virus was still present?

SIKES: It apparently occurs extraneurally, according to evidence seen by a pathologist at the University of Missouri. He vaccinated dogs with the usual dose and then ten times the dose of the live vaccine, sacrificed the animals at periodic intervals within the first month and was never able to show any virus present in the neural tissue of the brain. Circumstantial evidence indicates, therefore, that the virus certainly is present extraneurally. There is no indication by the FA of these dogs so vaccinated that there is any virus detectable by the FA or the mouse inoculation method in the neural tissue.

* This Discussion refers to the report by Sikes.

JOHNSON, R. T.: There was some discussion of the challenge dose. What was the final total amount of virus given in the challenge dose?

SIKES: That is a good point. Dr. Johnson knows the slight problem we were having at this 39-month time when we were ready to challenge. To answer your question, we used the same dose. It came out within 2/10 of a log of the exact same dose we used at one year. It was not the identical same stock, however, it was NYC—Georgia type of rabies salivary gland virus. We had to go back to an earlier stock, passage it in some dogs, and then use this fresh stock, meaning that the original stock virus suspension that was planned to be used for challenge somehow lost its effectiveness for the dogs of this age group that we were pre-challenging. So we did end up using NYC-Georgia, roughly 20,000 mouse intracerebral $LD_{50}$. We gave this intramuscularly.

TAGAYA: Are the differences in the immunogenicity between the inactivated tissue culture vaccine and the suckling mose brain vaccine based on the virus concentration of starting materials used for preparation of the vaccine or on some factors derived from the host cells in which the virus multiplied. Which do you think is more important for these differences in immunogenicity?

SIKES: Comparing the suckling mouse brain vaccine and the hamster kidney tissue culture-CVS inactivated vaccine, I think the differences noted were due to the antigenic mass based on the previous titrations done before inactivation. The suckling mouse brain vaccine has roughly $10^8$ log of virus, then it is reduced to a 2% concentration. The reduction down to about $10^{6.5}$ would be a little over a million mouse $LD_{50}$, whereas with the hamster kidney, this is around $10^{4.5}$ so that there is that much difference in antigen.

HAMMON: To those who might be philosophically or otherwise opposed to the use of live virus vaccine and would want to use the inactivated vaccine, what about the comparative cost of purified, concentrated inactivated vaccine as opposed to the ordinary type? You say it has been concentrated 100 times. Have you any idea as to the difference in cost of the final product if it were commercially made?

SIKES: If it were commercially made, I would think that this could be done for approximately 10 times more than the cost of the tissue culture inactivated vaccines. We did make this particular purified vaccine using the suckling mouse to grow the virus. We have rather easy methods for harvesting the brain infected tissues and then making large lots, centrifuging them, running them through the column and so forth. As I would see it, the cost would be roughly 10 times more than the usual tissue type, because it must be concentrated back.

# Epidemiological Studies and Control Projects on Rabies in the Philippines

George W. Beran

*Silliman University, Dumaguete City, Negros Oriental, Philippines*

## INTRODUCTION

Rabies is an endemic zoonotic infectious disease throughout the Philippines (Beran & de Mira, 1966). The incidence is highest on the coastal and central plains of inhabited islands and lowest in the central mountain areas, whether densely populated or not. Dogs, most of which are owned but permitted much independence by their owners, are the primary hosts of the virus. Sporadic cases of rabies in other pet and domesticated animals usually follow exposure by rabid dogs. The wildlife population of the Philippines is low, due to extensive hunting and destruction of natural habitats. Remaining monkeys (*Macaque cynomolgous*) and wild felidae (*Viviera tangalunga* and *Paradoxorus philippinensis*) are principally found in mountain forests away from human habitation (Taylor, 1934). Mongooses (*Herpestes brachyurus*) are present in small numbers on Palawan and adjacent islands (Sanborn, 1946–1947). Rats of at least 12 species and bats of about 67 species are present in especially large numbers (Carter *et al.*, 1946), but there is as yet no evidence that rabies is present in either.

The annual incidence of rabies in dogs in the Philippines can only be estimated, perhaps at about 25,000 cases. A mean of 253 human cases has been reported to the Department of Health annually over the past decade (Desease, 1969). Animal bites are routinely handled as possible exposures to rabies throughout the nation. Approximately 100,000 people receive a partial or complete series of antirabies vaccine each year (Desease, 1969). Phenol inactivated 2% goat brain tissue origin vaccine is produced and distributed by the Department of Health; administration is in 25 daily doses of 1 m*l* each. Duck embryo propagated inactivated rabies vaccines are imported.

# EPIDEMIOLOGICAL STUDIES ON RABIES IN NEGROS ORIENTAL

Negros Oriental Province comprises the eastern half of Negros Island and the island of Siquijor in the central Philippines. The present population is about 700,000 people (Office of Gov., 1970). Before rabies control was instituted in the province, about 1500–2000 series of human antirabies vaccinations were begun annually and the annual incidence of human rabies was about 5 cases. An analysis of medical records on 21 human rabies deaths in 2 hospitals during the past 10 years revealed that 11 had completed full courses of prophylactic vaccine, 2 were receiving vaccine and only 5 definitely received no vaccine between exposure and onset of rabies (data collect., 1965–1969).

Rabies diagnostic service, using direct light and fluorescent antibody microscopic techniques as well as mouse inoculation tests (WHO, 1966), is offered as a public service by this laboratory. In a small surveillance study during 1967–1968, carcasses of dogs which died of any cause were purchased for examination for rabies. An effort was made to exclude from the study any animals submitted because of possible exposure of human beings to rabies and which would not have been obtained otherwise for the study. Among 93 carcasses included in this study, 25 were positive for rabies. Twenty-seven of the dogs had manifested symptoms suggestive of rabies; 21 of these were found to be positive. Twenty-eight of the dogs had shown illness not suggestive of rabies. Only 1 of these, a dog which had shown clinical and gross pathological manifestations of pneumonia was also found to be rabid. Among 38 dogs which were found dead or were killed for disposal, only 2 were rabid. Both were found along roads, one having been run over by a vehicle, the other showing no evidence of trauma.

Clinical and epidemiological data have been collected on 61 laboratory confirmed cases of rabies in dogs. Of these, 49 showed a furious form of the disease; 12 showed a dumb form. The average clinical period in the 18 of these which were not euthanized was 4.1 days (range 1–8). Fifty-two of the rabid dogs had bitten an average of 1.8 persons each (range 1–6). Fifty of the dogs were owned; 11 were strays (Beran *et al.*, 1968).

Among other animals submitted for examination as rabies suspects, 1 of 20 cats, 2 of 5 pigs, 2 of 2 cattle, but none of 2 horses, 1 sheep,

7 *Rattus rattus*, 2 *Suncus occultidens*, 4 bats of three species, 3 *Macaque cynomolgous*, or 3 *Paradoxorus philippinensis* were found to be rabid. A total of 812 bats of 13 identified species which were netted live has been negative for rabies on laboratory examination using direct microscopic examination of Seller's stained smears on all, with 447 also examined by fluorescent antibody (F.A.) microscopy (Gregorio *et al.*, 1969). These negative findings in 816 bats examined in this laboratory corroborate results reported in other Philippine studies which included negative findings in 980 bats of 2 or more species examined by direct light microscopy (Tacal & Boad, 1966) and 133 bats of 10 species examined by F.A. microscopy for rabies (Westerlund, 1966). The composite of these Philippine studies in bats represent species with a variety of food habits, habitats and gregariousness.

A total of 236 rats of 4 *Rattus spp.* and 11 *Suncus occultidens* shrews were live trapped and examined in this laboratory, all but 58 by both direct light and F.A. microscopy; all yielded negative findings. An additional 115 *R. norvegicus* examined by light microscopy (Tacal & Geronimo, 1965) and 123 rats of 3 *Rattus spp.* examined by F.A. microscopy (Westerlund, 1966) have been reported as negative in 2 other Philippine studies. These Philippine studies which comprise a total 1929 bats and 492 rats and small mammals collected in widely scattered areas of the country provide evidence that rabies is not endemic in these Philippine mammals, an important asset for rabies eradication programs based on dog vaccination.

## RABIES CONTROL PROGRAMS

Extensive rabies control programs have been promulgated in the city of Manila by the Veterinary Inspection Board, in the cities of Angeles and Olongapo with the assistance of the U.S. Department of Defense, and in Negros Oriental in a joint project of the Provincial and Duamguete City governments and this laboratory. The Negros Oriental program has combined research with community dog vaccination campaigns. Accurate dog censuses are prerequisites to organization of community campaigns. In urban Dumaguete City, the number of dogs was found to be 9.0% of the number of human residents or 61.2% of the number of households. In rural Negros Oriental, the number of dogs has been calculated as equal to 10.7 to 12.2% of the human population or 67.4–86.9% of the number of households.

Community dog vaccination campaigns have been conducted in

house to house visits by vaccinators working in teams of 3 men each. Vaccinators have been assigned to the teams from this laboratory as on-the-job trainers, working with personnel from the provincial and municipal governments. Locally recruited personnel have been essential in the vaccination teams as they are well acquainted with the campaign areas and are well accepted by the residents. Vaccinating teams have averaged 80 dogs each per working day and the number of teams organized in a community has been based on the period during which the campaign was to be conducted, practically not less than 2 weeks or more than 2 months. Vaccination teams have been provided with kits containing syringes and needles, alcohol pledgets, vaccine, certificates, identification collars, and rope dog snares with bamboo handles. Economy has been paramount in all aspects of the campaigns. Two milliliter (m*l*) disposal syringes with 22 guage, $1\frac{1}{2}$ inch needles have been rewashed and reautoclaved for use until warped beyond function, usually about 20 cycles. Identification collars have been made of plastic tubing threaded with wire and twisted together about the dogs' necks; different color tubing has been used in each community. Vaccinators have been given pre-exposure rabies immunization to afford protection in case of exposure to rabies during performance of duty (Fox, 1958).

Flury strain attenuated live rabies virus vaccines of embryonating hens' egg or cell culture origin have been used in all Negros Oriental campaigns; those since 1969 have been using vaccine produced in this laboratory. All campaigns have been based on the vaccination of a minimum of 80% of the dogs 3 months and older in each community (Tierkel *et al.*, 1950); usually 85% to 94% was achieved. Depending upon the peripheral re-entry pressure on a vaccinated community from unvaccinated areas, rabies has reappeared in 19–33 months, by which time only 20–40% of the dogs in the vaccinated community remained effectively immunized (Tierkel *et al.*, 1953). On the island of Siquijor, a subprovince of Negros Oriental, 85% of the 6650 dogs enumerated in the 6 communities were vaccinated during 1968–1969. Vaccination of incoming dogs has been instituted at the ports and it is hoped that the present rabies free status may be maintained.

Studies on age distribution of dogs in Negros Oriental has indicated that 25% of all puppies die by 6 months of age and 90% of all dogs die by 4 years of age. Rabies has not been detected in this laboratory in any of nearly 20,000 dogs which have been vaccinated in campaigns conducted since 1964.

## SOCIOLOGICAL ASPECTS OF RABIES CONTROL

The sociological aspects of planning and carrying out community rabies control programs have posed greater problems than the technical procedures involved. Philippine society is highly individualistic and is family rather than community oriented. Middle and upper class families which understand and respond readily to community programs comprise less than 10% of the population of this area. Extensive education campaigns preceding actual vaccination campaigns have been based on public seminars, movies and slide shows, posters in public places and coloring book-brochures distributed through elementary schools, and have been highly effective.

The role of the dog in the community social structure is quite different in rural areas from that of pet animals kept by middle class families. In areas of subsistence agriculture, most dogs are of nondescript breeding, very strong and quite independent. They live a partially self-sufficient existence and depend on the owners for only part of their subsistence. Surplus dogs, though usually traceable to an original owner, wander through communities searching for anything edible and congregate in packs, especially at mating season. People do not commonly play with dogs and most dogs are extremely apprehensive of anyone who attempts to handle them in any way. Dogs serve as valuable guards where houses are open and property lines have few demarcations, thus affording a degree of privacy and protection to the residents. The fear of dog bites with the attendant discomfort of antirabies prophylactic vaccination enhances the effectivity of dogs as guards.

Community acceptance of the semi-independent status of dogs and of the right of initial owners to reclaim even essentially stray dogs any time they wish to care for the animals again has mitigated against widespread destruction of unkept dogs.

Rabies has been part of the social milieu of Philippine communities as long as residents can remember and people have become somewhat adjusted to living with it. It has been generally considered that exposure to rabies can be avoided by care not to molest dogs, and unprovoked animal bites have been attributed to fate as frequently as to a diseased condition of the biting animals. Since antirabies vaccination has traditionally been administered to all persons bitten by dogs, there has been little internal community motivation to ensure that biting dogs shall be rabies free. Since few people die of rabies who received a full course of postexposure vaccination, some plausible explanations of rabies fatalities have usually been possible without recognition of the fact that such deaths could be completely prevented by community eradication of rabies. Persons who seek change from the highly stabilized pattern of life in rural communities characteristically find it by emigration rather than by affecting internal changes within the social structures. Only when educational programs reach into the community structure and residents begin to comprehend the benefits of rabies eradication will they give the wholehearted participation essential to the success of such programs (Beran & Gregorio, 1966).

## PROJECTION OF SUCCESS IN RABIES ERADICATION

Rabies vaccination campaigns conducted at the grass roots level in 13 communities in Negros Oriental have been very well received. As realization of the benefits of rabies control has affected the relationships of community residents toward dogs and of physicians toward dog bite patients, popular acceptance of rabies control has been gratifying. Communities not so protected, have clamored for campaigns upon hearing about these benefits and have cooperated well in vaccination programs conducted there.

It is sincerely hoped that upon completion of rabies control in all of Negros Oriental, that public support of a nationwide rabies eradication program will be realized. The Philippines has a number of favorable factors in achievement of this goal. On the basis of laboratory and epidemiological studies the dog appears to be the significant, if not the sole, reservoir host of the disease; disappearance of the disease in dogs has led to its disappearance in other animals and man. The natural division of the nation into islands or distinct geographical regions facilitates a step by step eradication program. The separation of the Philippines by water from the large land masses of Asia would afford protection from re-entry of rabies following eradication. We need not continue to die of rabies in the Philippines (Nat. Rabies Com., 1967).

## SUMMARY

Rabies is a serious public health problem in the Philippines, but one which may be solved by eradication of the disease from dogs. Rabies has not been found in Philippine bats or rats. Occasional findings of rabies in domesticated animals have been traced to exposure by rabid dogs. Rabies control based on vaccination of 80–94% of dogs in 13 communities have been effective in elimination of the disease. The sociological aspects of community control programs have required more attention than technical problems. The need for rabies eradication in the entire Philippines is imminent.

## REFERENCES

Beran, G. W. and Gregorio, S. B. (1966). Sociological problems in a rabies control program in a community in the Philippines. Proc. Nat. Rabies Symposium, Atlanta, Georgia, pp. 144–145.

Beran, G. W. and de Mira, O. (1966). Community wide campaign of rabies in Duamguete City, Phillippines. *Publ. Hlth. Rep.*, **81**, 169–173.

Beran, G. W., Gregorio, S. B. and Elviña, O. (1968). Epidemiology of rabies in Dumaguete City and Negros Oriental. *Silliman Jour.*, **15**, 357–364.

Carter, T. D., Hill, J. E. and Tate, G. H. (1946). Mammals of the Pacific World. MacMillan, New York. pp. 40–49.

Data collected from the Negros Oriental provincial and Municipal Health Offices and by medical surveys (1965–1969).

Disease Intelligence Center (1969). Philippines Health Statistics. Dept. of Health, Manila, pp. 261.

Fox, J. P. (1958). Prophylaxis against rabies in humans. *Ann. N.Y. Acad. Sci.*, **70**, 480–494.

Gregorio, S. B., Beran, G. W. and Elviña, C. (1969). Rabies in animals other than dogs with emphasis on Negros Oriental. *Phil. J. Anim. Sci.*, **6**, 97–106.

National Rabies Eradication Committee (1967). A plan for rabies eradication in the philippines. Dept. of Health, Manila, pp. 23.

Office of the Governor (1970). Province of Negros Oriental, Dumaguete City.

Sanborn, C. C. (1946–1947). Mammals. Philipine Zoological Expedition. Chicago Natural History Museum, Chicago. pp. 104–141.

Tacal, J. R., Jr. and Boado, P. A. (1966). Examination for Negri bodies of the brains of a species of Philippine bat (*Scotophilus temmenckii*). *Acta Med. Phil.*, **3**, 103–106.

Tacal, J. V., Jr. and Geronimo, P. A. (1965). Examination of rat brains for the presence of Negri bodies. *Nat. & Appl. Sci. Biol.*, **19**, 161–164.

Taylor, E. A. (1934). Philippine Land Mammals. Bureau of Printing, Manila. p. 543.

Tierkel, E. S., Graves, L. M., Tuggle, H. G. and Wadley, S. L. (1950). Effective control of an outbreak of rabies in Memphis and Shelby Country, *Tenn. Am. J. Publ. Hlth.*, **40**, 1084–1089.

Tierkel, E. S., Kissling, R. E., Edison, M. and Habel, K. (1953). A brief survey and progress report of controlled comparative experiments in canine rabies immunization. *Proc. Amer. Vet. Med. Assn. Convention*, Toronto, Canada, pp. 443–445.

Westerlund, N. C. (1966). Survey of rat and bat brains for the presence of rabies antigen using fluorescent antibody techniques. U.S.A.F. Technical Report., p. 5.

World Health Organization (1966). Laboratory Techniques on Rabies. Second Edition Monograph series No. 23, Geneva. p. 178.

For Discussion, see page 391.

# Progress towards Rabies-Free Status for the Territory of Guam

ROBERT L. HADDOCK

*Teritorial Public Health Veterinarian and Chief, Zoonosis Control Section, Department of Public Health and Social Services Government of Guam, Agana, Guam 96910*

## SUMMARY

The island communities of the Pacific remained free of rabies throughout recorded history until March 1967, when an outbreak occurred in the Territory of Guam, largest and most populous of the Mariana Islands. During the subsequent eight month period, 89 animal rabies cases were reported by one or more laboratories; no human cases were reported. By 1969 rabies had apparently been eliminated from the island through a combination of intensive application of classical rabies control measures and fortuitous circumstance.

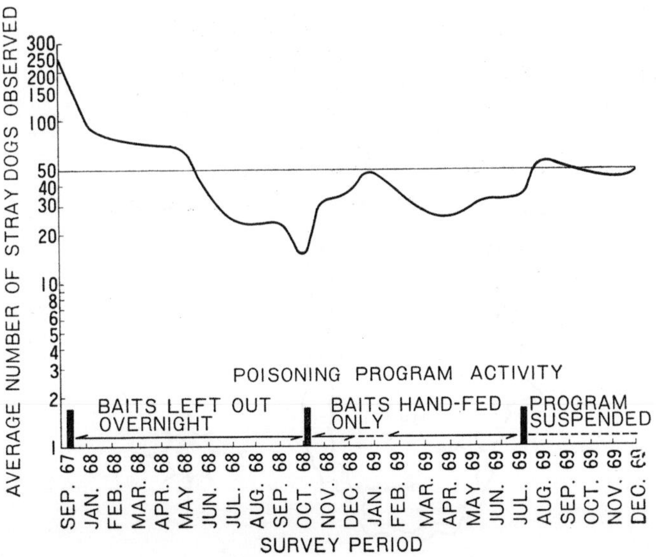


Fig. 1. Summary of Stray Dog Surveys

## THE ENVIRONMENT

The Territory of Guam is the largest and southernmost of the island chain comprising the Marianas district of Micronesia. Located in the western Pacific approximately 1,600 miles due east of Manila, the island enjoys a tropical climate with monthly average median temperatures ranging from a low of 79.3°F in February to a high of 81.8°F in June. Seasons are determined primarily by rainfall which is heaviest in July, August and September (averaging about 13 inches per month) and lightest in February, March and April (averaging about 3 inches per month). The island flora, dominated by tangan-tangan (a woody shrub) and coconut palm, forms a dense jungle along the coastline, river valleys and other scattered areas. Much of the interior, a coral plateau to the north, rolling to mountainous

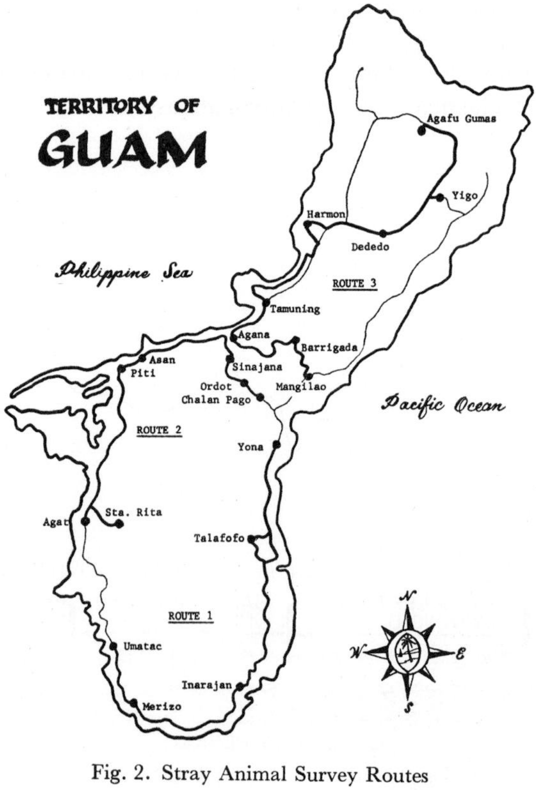


Fig. 2. Stray Animal Survey Routes

terrain of volcanic origin to the south, is grass-covered as a result of frequent brush fires during the dry season.

Total population (1969) is estimated to be 105,000 of which 45,000 are military personnel or their dependents. Civilians reside in 19 villages distributed along the coasts and central waist of the island; military personnel reside primarily on the four principal navy and air force installations. Principal occupations of civilians are, in order: public administration, construction, service industries and retail sales. Local agriculture plays an insignificant part in the economy accounting for, in 1969, approximately 0.3% of the work force and 0.4% of gross sales. Eight hundred-twenty acres or 0.6% of Guam's 225 square mile land mass were devoted to crop lands in 1969.

Guam had for many years been plagued by a large stray animal population. Estimates of the total dog and cat population in 1967 ranged from 20 to 60 thousand and may have exceeded the total civilian population; perhaps 50% of these were strays. A number of reasons have been proposed for this unusually large population including the salubrious climate, abundant shelter, permissive attitude of the islanders and the absence of a control program. Another factor that may have been important is the large percentage of transients (nearly 50%) in the island population. Rotating military

Table 1(a). Animals Disposed (Includes animals shot, poisoned, unclaimed strays, pet turned in for disposal and animals found dead)

| | Dogs | Cats | Others | Total |
|---|---|---|---|---|
| 1967 | 13,406 | 3,393 | Not Available | 16,799 |
| 1968 | 1,641 | 916 | 133 | 2,690 |
| 1969 | 563 | 690 | 208 | 1,461 |
| Totals | 15,610 | 4,999 | 341 | 20,950 |

Table 1(b). Biting Animals Impounded

| | Dogs | Cats | Others | Total |
|---|---|---|---|---|
| 1967 (6 mos.) | 241 | 101 | Not Available | 342 |
| 1968 | 313 | 64 | Not Available | 377 |
| 1969 | 380 | 71 | 17 | 468 |

Table 1(c). Biting Animals Not Caught for Impoundment

| | Dogs | Cats | Others | Total |
|---|---|---|---|---|
| 1967 (6 mos.) | 44 | 32 | 20 | 96 |
| 1968 | 21 | 17 | 22 | 60 |
| 1969 | 36 | 15 | 16 | 67 |

and civil service personnel are known to have abandoned many animals when they left for other duty stations.

Table 2

ZCS-21
10-69

## GOVERNMENT OF GUAM
## DEPARTMENT OF PUBLIC HEALTH AND SOCIAL SERVICES

To: Chief, Zoonosis Control Section
From: Officer-In-Charge, Animal Control Unit
Subject: Monthly Animal Control Report

ANNUAL SUMMARY

| Month: January–December, 1969 | Dogs | Cats | Others |
|---|---|---|---|
| Biting Animals | | | |
| 1. Impounded at Dog Pound | 311 | 54 | 5 |
| 2. Impounded at owner's property | 69 | 17 | 12 |
| 3. Not located | 36 | 15 | 16 |
| 4. Released from observation | 378 | 62 | 13 |
| 5. Died during observation | 2 | 9 | 4 |
| Other Animals Impounded | | | |
| 6. Stray animals | 39 | 32 | 6 |
| 7. Others | 19 | 28 | 0 |
| Animals Released to Owner | | | |
| 8. Biting animals | 160 | 9 | 14 |
| 9. Stray animals | 2 | 1 | 5 |
| 10. Others | 2 | 0 | 0 |
| Animals Destroyed | | | |
| 11. Owner request | 87 | 41 | 1 |
| 12. Stray unclaimed | 113 | 80 | 7 |
| Dead Animals Picked-Up | | | |
| 13. Poisoned | 71 | 17 | 0 |
| 14. Dead-on-road | 290 | 543 | 196 |
| 15. Other | 0 | 0 | 1 |
| Dog Pound Census (Average Daily) | | | |
| 16. Bite cases | 9 | 1 | <1 |
| 17. Strays | <1 | <1 | <1 |
| 18. Other | <1 | <1 | <1 |
| 19. Total Citations Issued for Months January to December. | 41 | 0 | 0 |
| 20. Rabies Vaccinations for Months January to December. | 43 | × | × |
| 21. Total Fees Collected for Months January to December. | $ 2,788.00 | | |

Guam is fortunate in apparently not having an efficient rabies reservoir present in its wildlife population. Feral species currently inhabiting the island are a variety of deer (*Cervus mariannus*); 3 species of rats, *R. exulans*, *R. rattus* and *R. norvegicus*; *Suncus murinus*, the house shrew; fruit bats (*Pteropus mariana*); wild pigs; and several species of reptiles and amphibians. Fortunately, amateur ecologists who have suggested controlling the rodent population by introducing the mongoose or Japanese weasel have not gained a sympathetic ear on Guam.

## HUB OF THE WESTERN PACIFIC

Although traffic to Guam from nearby rabies-enzootic areas such as the Philippines and the Asian mainland is known to have taken place sporadically for the past several hundred years, the advent of rapid transportation during the modern era has significantly increased the danger of introducing the disease. Not only have planes and modern ships eliminated the "natural" quarantine imposed by the relatively slow sea traffic of earlier eras, but traffic volume has also increased many-fold, particularly in the 25 years since World War II. Guam is becoming increasingly popular as a vacation spot for affluent Asians, particularly Japanese and Filipinos. In 1968, for instance, there were 35,000 visitor arrivals on Guam (exclusive of military) and approximately 50% of these were traveling from points in Asia. In addition, Guam serves as a trans-shipping port for the Trust Territory of the Pacific Islands.

## THE EPIZOOTIC

Guam's index rabies case, a stray dog which died during observation as a biting animal, was apprehended in a residential area near the main commercial and military harbor centrally located on the western coast. The second case, detected one month later, was from the same area and was known to have had contact with the first case. A third case occurred during May in the same general area. In June cases were detected with increasing frequency (total of 5) and a spreading of the epizootic in a northerly direction was apparent. Thirteen cases were reported in July, 9 of these occurring in the northern half of the island. In August 36 cases were reported, again the majority (22) occurred in the northern half of the island. The 18 cases reported in September and the 14 cases reported in October ended the epizootic. Other statistics concerning the epizootic are summarized in Table 7.

## HUMAN EXPOSURES

Animal bite or scratch cases reported during the epizootic totaled 995. Of these, 131 (13%) received at least one dose of specific antirabies therapy and the balance received only tetanus antitoxin and local wound treatment. No deaths due to rabies or antirabies therapy were recorded.

Records for the calendar year 1968 are incomplete. During 1969, 252 bite treatment cases were reported; of these 65 (26%) received specific antirabies therapy. Other data on animal bites are presented in Table 3.

Table 3. Data on Animal Bite Patients Reported to the Dog Pound-1969

| Age | Male | Female | Total |
|---|---|---|---|
| <1 | 3 | 1 | 4 |
| 1–5 | 46 | 29 | 75 |
| 6–9 | 38 | 30 | 68 |
| 10–14 | 26 | 13 | 39 |
| 15–19 | 6 | 8 | 14 |
| 20–24 | 1 | 3 | 4 |
| 25–29 | 8 | 3 | 11 |
| 30–39 | 12 | 6 | 18 |
| 40–49 | 6 | 1 | 7 |
| 50–59 | 5 | 1 | 6 |
| 60–69 | 1 | 2 | 3 |
| 70 and above | 1 | 2 | 3 |
| Grand Total | 153 | 99 | 252 |

| | | |
|---|---|---|
| Mode (Age group most frequently bitten) | Male | 1–5 |
| | Female | 6–9 |
| Average age of bite victims | Male | 14 |
| | Female | 13 |

| | |
|---|---|
| Treatment | |
| Tetanus prophylaxis and/or local cleansing only | 131 |
| Antirabies vaccine | 62 |
| Antirabies serum | 3 |
| No treatment indicated | 56 |
| Total | 252 |

NOTE: Specific antirabies treatment may have been discontinued if biting animal was apprehended for observation.

## INITIAL CONTROL MEASURES

As early as January 1966, the air force veterinarian stationed at Andersen Air Force Base had recognized the escalating danger of importing rabies due to increased traffic from the Asian mainland as a result of the Viet Nam conflict. Impoundment facilities were established on the base and the recommendation that an island-wide embargo or 120-day quarantine be established was forwarded to the civilian Department of Public Health and Social Services (November 1966). Unfortunately the first rabies case occurred before these recommendations had been put into effect.

Table 4(a). Vaccination Status of Biting Dogs Examined For Rabies (1969)

| | Vaccinated | Unvaccinated | Unknown |
|---|---|---|---|
| January | 2 | 5 | 0 |
| February | 0 | 0 | 0 |
| March | 2 | 3 | 0 |
| April | 0 | 1 | 2 |
| May | 2 | 2 | 0 |
| June | 3 | 4 | 0 |
| July | 2 | 7 | 0 |
| August | 0 | 13 | 0 |
| September | 2 | 2 | 0 |
| October | 0 | 9 | 1 |
| November | 2 | 8 | 2 |
| December | 0 | 12 | 0 |
| Total | 15 | 66 | 5 |

Table 4(b). Unvaccinated+Unknown/Vaccinated Ratio*

| | |
|---|---|
| 1969 | 4.7/1 |
| 1968 | 2.9/1 |
| 1967 | 6.5/1 |

* This ratio has a bias in favor of unvaccinated dogs as most vaccinated dogs are reclaimed by their owners from the dog pound.

Table 4(c). Estimate of Total Dog Population (Unvaccinated+Unknown/Vaccinated Ratio×Number Vaccinated)+Number Vaccinated

| | |
|---|---|
| 1969 | (4.7×2,783)+2,783=15,863 |
| 1968 | (2.9×2,070)+2,970= 8,073 |
| 1967 | (6.5×3,258)+3,258=24,435 |

Table 5. Rabies Vaccination Clinics in 1969; Summary by Village

| Day | Date | Village | Dogs, Vacc. & License | License only* | Cats | Total |
|---|---|---|---|---|---|---|
| Monday | 3–31 | Umatac | 26 | 0 | 3 | 29 |
| Tuesday | 4–1 | Merizo | 37 | 0 | 7 | 44 |
| Wednesday | 4–2 | Inarajan | 34 | 0 | 0 | 34 |
| Thursday | 4–3 | Talofofo | 54 | 0 | 11 | 65 |
| Saturday | 4–5 | Mangilao | 52 | 0 | 6 | 58 |
| Monday | 4–7 | Yona | 71 | 0 | 15 | 86 |
| Tuesday | 4–8 | Santa Rita | 74 | 3 | 6 | 83 |
| Wednesday | 4–9 | Asan | 42 | 5 | 7 | 54 |
| Thursday | 4–10 | Piti | 49 | 0 | 16 | 65 |
| Monday | 4–14 | Barrigada | 106 | 2 | 7 | 115 |
| Tuesday | 4–15 | Yigo | 61 | 6 | 8 | 75 |
| Wednesday | 4–16 | Yigo | 59 | 0 | 5 | 64 |
| Thursday | 4–17 | Mongmong-T-M | 51 | 0 | 10 | 61 |
| Friday | 4–18 | Tamuning | 62 | 0 | 22 | 84 |
| Saturday | 4–19 | Tamuning | 74 | 0 | 14 | 88 |
| Tuesday | 4–22 | Chalan Pago-Ordot | 93 | 0 | 12 | 105 |
| Wednesday | 4–23 | Sinajana | 72 | 0 | 12 | 84 |
| Thursday | 4–24 | Sinajana | 58 | 0 | 11 | 69 |
| Friday | 4–25 | Agana Heights | 66 | 0 | 20 | 86 |
| Saturday | 4–26 | Agana Heights | 49 | 3 | 3 | 55 |
| Tuesday | 4–29 | Barrigada | 119 | 0 | 22 | 141 |
| Wednesday | 4–30 | Agat | 80 | 0 | 16 | 96 |
| Thursday | 5–1 | Agat | 59 | 0 | 16 | 75 |
| Friday | 5–2 | Dededo | 94 | 0 | 30 | 124 |
| Saturday | 5–3 | Dededo | 109 | 2 | 37 | 146 |
| Monday | 5–5 | Agana | 88 | 1 | 11 | 100 |
| Tuesday | 5–6 | Barrigada | 35 | 5 | 7 | 47 |
| Total | | | 1,774 | 27 | 334 | 2,133 |

* Includes animals which were vaccinated at private or military veterinary clinics.

| | |
|---|---|
| Village clinics | 1,774 |
| Andersen Air Force Base | 451 |
| ComNavMar (navy) | 90 |
| Private clinics | 468 |
| Total | 2,783 |

Early efforts at stray dog reduction were limited to live-capture but were only productive for several weeks after which strays learned to avoid the control crews. Many dogs were turned in for disposal by the owners and portable cages were placed at village commissioners' offices to serve as collecting points.

Two weeks after confirmation of the first case, rabies vaccination teams began a campaign that took them to each of the 19 villages at least once. In response to a call for assistance in May, the U. S. Public Health Service sent a team of experts to Guam to review the situation and offer recommendations. Their suggestions included placing an embargo on cats and dogs entering Guam for at least six months or until the situation had stabilized; instituting a 120-day quarantine after the embargo had been lifted; eliminating, as nearly as practicable, all wild-stray dogs; developing a local capability for laboratory rabies testing, starting a zoonoses control program to be coordinated by a public health veterinarian; and providing anti-rabies serum and vaccine for persons severely exposed to rabies.

## STRAY DOG CONTROL

Beginning in June 1967, police department sharpshooters shot strays at night with .22 calibre rifles. Although the marksmanship and discretion of the officers assigned this task prevented any known property damage or human injuries, this phase of the control program was soon abandoned as being too dangerous in relation to its effectiveness.

Initial attempts to use poison (meat baits of several pounds each impregnated with 1080 and staked out at village dump sites) were not effective. The baits spoiled rapidly and they did not succeed in

Table 6. Comparison of Rabies Control Statistics during (January–June 1969) and after (July–December 1969) a Stray Dog Control Program Using Poison Baits

(a) Biting Animals Impounded

| | Dogs | Cats | Others | Total |
|---|---|---|---|---|
| January–June | 162 | 26 | 7 | 195 |
| July–December | 218 | 45 | 10 | 273 |
| Total for 1969 | 380 | 71 | 17 | 468 |

(b) Biting Animals Not Located

| | Dogs | Cats | Others | Total |
|---|---|---|---|---|
| January–June | 11 | 8 | 6 | 25 |
| July–December | 25 | 7 | 10 | 42 |
| Total for 1969 | 36 | 15 | 16 | 67 |

(c) Bite Patient Treatment Reports: Species of Biting Animal

| | Dogs | Cats | Others | Not Specified | Total |
|---|---|---|---|---|---|
| January–June | 54 | 10 | 8 | 0 | 72 |
| July–December | 121 | 14 | 16 | 29 | 180 |
| Total for 1969 | 175 | 24 | 24 | 29 | 252 |

Table 7. Animal Rabies Case Data

| Species | Owned | Stray or wild | History of vaccination | | Humans exposed | Humans treated | No history available | Total cases |
|---|---|---|---|---|---|---|---|---|
| | | | yes | no | | | | |
| Cats | 33 | 14 | 20 | 27 | 57 | 26 | 2 | 49 |
| Dogs | 15 | 7 | 6 | 15 | 36 | 25 | 0 | 21 |
| Shrews | 0 | 9 | 0 | 9 | 3 | 3 | 0 | 9 |
| Deer | 0 | 7 | 0 | 7 | 0 | 0 | 0 | 7 |
| Rats | 0 | 2 | 0 | 2 | 0 | 0 | 0 | 2 |
| Pig | 0 | 1 | 0 | 1 | 0 | 0 | 0 | 1 |
| Totals | 48 | 40 | 27 | 61 | 96 | 51 | 2 | 89 |

Table 8. Rabies Testing of Guam Specimens by the National Communicable Disease Center

| NCDC No. | Species | Submission Date | FRA | Virus Isolation | Comments |
|---|---|---|---|---|---|
| 67-0579 | Canine | 3-7-67 | + | + | Initially examined at the Army Medical Laboratory, Schofield Barracks, Hawaii (A.M.L.). No. virus characterization studies recorded. |
| 67-1991 | Canine | 6-20-67 | + | + | Initially examined in Hawaii at A.M.L. and Hawaii Department of Agriculture (H.D.A.). |
| 67-1992 | Cervine | 7-27-67 | + | − | Initially examined in Hawaii (A.M.L. and H.D.A.). |
| 67-1993 | Feline | 8-3-67 | + | + | Initially examined in Hawaii (A.M.L. and H.D.A.). Chick embryo studies at NCDC suggest that their isolate was street virus. |
| 67-1994 | Feline | 8-3-67 | + | − | Initially examined in Hawaii (A.M.L. and H.D.A.). |
| 67-1995 | Feline | 8-4-67 | + | − | Initially examined in Hawaii (A.M.L. and H.D.A.). |
| 67-1996 | Cervine | 8-4-67 | + | − | Initially examined in Hawaii (A.M.L. and H.D.A.). |
| 67-1908 | Canine | 8-12-67 | + | + | Vaccinated on Guam about 1 week before being shipped to Hawaii where it died in quarantine. Chick embryo studies at NCDC suggest that their isolate was street virus. |
| 67-1997 | Feline | 8-22-67 | + | − | Initially examined in Hawaii (A.M.L. and H.D.A.). |
| 67-1998 | Canine | 8-22-67 | + | − | Initially examined in Hawaii (H.D.A.). |
| 67-1925 | Cervine | 8-25-67 | + | + | Sent directly to NCDC from Guam. Isolation of street virus confirmed by mouse neutralization tests. |
| 67-2215 | Soricine | 9-29-67 | + | − | Sent directly to NCDC from Guam. |

attracting dogs away from the village areas. Cyanide ejection cartridges, which had been used extensively for coyote control in the southwestern U. S., also did not appear to fulfill the dual requirements of both high efficiency and safety after field evaluation on Guam.

The method adopted for intensive use was the distribution of "bite-size" 1080 impregnated baits. This proved to be effective and is thought to be relatively safe and amenable to use in villages. Baits were distributed by two methods: two or three baits were left on anchored paper plates along road shoulders between the hours of 10 p.m. and 4 a.m. after which baits not consumed were retrieved, or baits were thrown individually to observed strays and retrieved if not accepted. The former method has been used only at night, the latter primarily during daylight hours. On January 1, 1969, all poisoning was stopped due to severe and protracted public criticism in the form of letters to the editor and editorial comment appearing in the local newspaper.

In an effort to gage whether these opinions were representative of the general public and to gain other information that might be useful in planning various aspects of the rabies control program, the use of a confidential opinion survey was begun during the 1969 vaccination campaign. Survey forms (Fig. 3) were made available along with license application forms at each clinic but pet owners were not required to fill them out as a condition for having their pets vaccinated and licensed.

Results of the surveys, both in 1969 and in 1970 (Tables 9 and 10) suggest that a majority of the pet owners who utilize the vaccination clinics to have their pet vaccinated are in favor of continuing the poisoning program. As it is reasonable to expect that pet owners, being those most directly affected, would be most likely to oppose the poisoning of strays, it was concluded that the public in general was solidly in favor of this aspect of the rabies control program.

Poisoning was resumed on February 10 using the "hand-feeding" method only and was continued until July 1 when the poisoning crews assumed responsibility for operation of the Animal Quarantine Station. Hand-feeding poison baits to strays was resumed on January 1, 1970, and is expected to continue indefinitely.

Fig. 3

# SURVEY

THIS IS AN ANONYMOUS SURVEY. YOU DO NOT HAVE TO SIGN YOUR NAME.

1. What village do you live in?____________________

2. How did you first learn about the rabies vaccination clinic to be held in your village?

   Commissioner ○
   Newspaper ○
   A friend ○
   Radio ○
   Television ○
   Other (please specify)_______________

3. How many stray dogs do you see in your village?

   More than last year ○
   Less than last year ○
   The same as last year ○

4. Are you in favor of continuing the poisoning program?

   Yes ○
   No ○

5. How many dogs did you own last year?_______________

6. How many cats did you own last year? _______________

7. How many dogs do you own this year? _______________

8. How many cats do you own this year? _______________

9. What suggestions do you have for improving the rabies vaccination clinics?

Table 9

# RABIES VACCINATION CLINICS—1969 PUBLIC OPINION SURVEY

2. How did you first learn about the rabies vaccination clinic to be held in your village?

| | |
|---|---|
| Commissioner | 24.5% |
| Newspaper | 49.6% |
| Radio | 15.1% |
| Television | 8.6% |
| Other | 2.2% |

3. How many stray dogs do you see in your village?

| | |
|---|---|
| More than last year | 10.9% |
| Less than last year | 76.0% |
| Same as last year | 13.1% |

4. Are you in favor of continuing the program?*

| | |
|---|---|
| Yes | 97.1% |
| No | 2.9% |

4. Are you in favor of continuing the poisoning program?*

| | |
|---|---|
| Yes | 58.2% of replies to Q. 4 |
| No | 41.8% of replies to Q. 4 |

5–8. How many dogs and cats did you own in 1968, how many do you own this year?

| | |
|---|---|
| Number of dogs per dog owner–1968 | 1.1 |
| Number of dogs per dog owner–1969 | 1.3 |
| Number of cats per dog owner–1968 | .29 |
| Number of cats per dog owner–1969 | .23 |

*The word "poisoning" was inadvertently omitted from the first survey (307 responses to question) but was included in a corrected survey (170 responses to question).

The latter survey was used in Agat, Barrigada and Dededo and probably represents a reasonably representative cross-section of the island population.

Table 10

# RABIES VACCINATION CLINICS—1970 PUBLIC OPINION SURVEY SUMMARY

Total replies to survey 371

2. "How did you first learn about the rabies vaccination clinic to be held in your village?"

| | | |
|---|---|---|
| A. | Commissioner | 31% of replies |
| B. | Newspaper | 48% of replies |
| C. | A friend | 8% of replies |
| D. | Radio | 8% of replies |
| E. | Television | 4% of replies |
| F. | Other | 1% of replies |

3. "How many stray dogs do you see in your village?"

| | | |
|---|---|---|
| A. | More than last year | 12% of replies |
| B. | Less than last year | 50% of replies |
| C. | Same as last year | 8% of replies |
| D. | Not answered | 30% of replies |

4. "Are you in favor of continuing the poisoning program?"

| | | | |
|---|---|---|---|
| A. | Yes | 51% | (59.7% of replies to Q. 4) |
| B. | No | 31% | (40.3% of replies to Q. 4) |
| C. | Not answered | 18% | |

4. "Are you in favor of continuing the poisoning program?" Response broken down on basis of answer to question number 3 above.

| Number of Stray Dogs Seen | In Favor of Poisoning Program? | | |
|---|---|---|---|
| | Yes | No | Not Answered |
| A. More than last year | 57% | 29% | 14% |
| B. Less than last year | 52% | 37% | 11% |
| C. Same as last year | 53% | 40% | 7% |
| D. Not answered | 43% | 22% | 35% |

5-8. "How many dogs and cats did you own last year, how many do you own this year?"

| | | |
|---|---|---|
| A. | Average number of dogs owned per respondent last year, | 1.2 |
| B. | Average numer of cats owned per respondent last year, | .23 |
| C. | Average number of dogs owned per respondent this year, | 1.4 |
| D. | Average number of cats owned per respondent this year, | .19 |

## EMBARGO AND QUARANTINE

By executive order of the governor, an embargo on the entrance to Guam of all dogs and cats (excepting military sentry or seeing-eye dogs) became effective August 3, 1967. It remained in effect until August 16, 1968, when dogs or cats that had undergone 120 days of quarantine in the Hawaii Department of Agriculture Animal Quarantine Station were permitted entry. Shortly thereafter, Hawaii was officially recognized as a rabies-free area.

On April 1, 1969, Hawaii found it necessary to cancel the quarantine agreement and the embargo on dogs and cats was reinstituted. Fortunately Guam's own animal quarantine facilities were nearing completion and the embargo was again lifted when the station officially opened its doors on July 2, 1969. Currently animals which have resided continuously in Australia, New Zealand, the British Isles or Hawaii for a period of not less than 120 days are permitted to enter Guam without quarantine.

## PET VACCINATION AND LICENSING

Village pet vaccination clinics at which both the annual vaccination and dog license required by law may be obtained have been held each year since 1967. As might be expected, utilization of the clinics tapered off as the dramatic events of the epizootic receded into the past. Undoubtedly efforts toward education will become increasingly important if the objective of maintaining a high level of immunity in the canine population is to be realized. Enforcement of dog vaccination and licensing requirements has, unfortunately, been sporadic due to manpower shortages. In practice, the only persons ticketed for failure to comply with leash law regulations are those whose dogs have been involved in bite incidents.

Subsequent to the 1967 clinics during which only phenol inactivated vaccine was used, the use of chick embryo origin modified live virus (CEO-MLV) vaccine for dogs and phenol inactivated vaccine for all other animals was inaugurated.

## EDUCATION

Education efforts, directed by a professional health educator, were intensive during the epizootic. An NCDC film titled "Rabies

Can Be Controlled" was shown in all elementary schools and several times on television within the first few weeks following identification of the index case. Rabies information was prepared and distributed to all island teachers. Radio, television and newspapers distributed informative articles or announcements in both English and Chamorro, the native tongue of Guam. Initial efforts were directed primarily at explaining the need for the various control measures, particularly the elimination of strays and unwanted pets. The success of these efforts are attested to by the voluntary surrender of approximately 3,000 unwanted dogs and cats for destruction during the first two months of the epizootic. The general acceptance of the drastic measures adopted to reduce the population of rabies susceptible animals (including shooting and poisoning) can also be credited, at least in part, to an effective campaign of public education.

## SURVEILLANCE

Realizing that control of the island's rabies-susceptible animal population would be a critical factor in the effort to eradicate rabies, a systematic stray dog and cat survey was initiated in September of 1967. Since then it has been our policy to conduct at least three all-island stray animal surveys per month. Data accumulated over the past three years has substantially aided in both the planning and justification aspects of the Rabies Control Program and most particularly in those areas concerned with vector control.

In addition to field or vector surveillance, laboratory surveillance for rabies cases has continued to be intensive. A technologist employed by the local health department received training at the NCDC Rabies Investigation Laboratory in Sellers staining, the fluorescent rabies antibody (FRA) technique and mouse innoculation. Only the FRA method is routinely used at the present time; questionable specimens are forwarded to the NCDC for review. An average of 15 brain specimens have been examined for rabies each month during the past three years. These have been primarily unclaimed biting animals but strays and samples of wildlife population are also examined periodically. There have been no clinically or laboratory diagnosed rabies cases reported since October of 1967.

## PROSPECTS FOR THE FUTURE

If no additional rabies case are discovered, it is anticipated that

Guam's Director of Public Health and Social Services will declare Guam to be a rabies free area on October 27, 1970, the third anniversary of the apparent end of the 1967 epizootic.

At that time all aspects of the Rabies Control Program will be subject to strenuous review. Of course any relaxation of the measures designed to prevent the reintroduction or rapid spread of rabies, e.g., quarantine and stray animal control, would seriously jeopardize this hard-won achievement and is unlikely to be adopted.

Other aspects of rabies control, particularly the handling of animal bite cases, could well be modified. Recommendations that are being considered include using home impoundment of biting dogs that have current vaccinations (at present dogs must be vaccinated with CEO vaccine within 12 months or with phenolized vaccine within 6 months), increasing the accepted duration of immunity provided by rabies vaccination to 2 years and 1 year, respectively, for CEO and phenolized types of vaccine, and recommending that human anti-rabies therapy be given only when there is substantial reason to believe that the biting animal was rabid and it is not available for laboratory examination.

On a larger scale, it is hoped that in the near future Hawaii, Guam, the Trust Territory of the Pacific Islands, American Samoa and perhaps some other communities of the Pacific as well can unite in a common rabies control and quarantine effort, thereby permitting free movement of dogs and cats between all points within the area.

## DISCUSSION

Possibly the most significant aspect of the rabies control program in the Territory of Guam was the prompt control and apparent eradication of rabies, once an effective means of eliminating stray dogs had been put into effect. Had there been an efficient rabies reservoir present in the island's wildlife population (such as the mongoose, fox, skunk, etc.), the outcome might well have been very different.

It is of interest to note that in 1967 plans for controlling the stray dog population called for a two-stage operation: 1) elimination of strays in villages (greatest priority being given to control of those vectors in close contact with humans) and 2) elimination of wild-strays (boonie dogs) in the boondocks or uninhabited areas. By the time some degree of success had been achieved in reaching the first objective, however, it was observed that the number of strays in boondocks had also dropped substantially. Apparently the strays on Guam seldom reverted to a truly wild state and when competition for food, territory, and so on, was reduced in the villages by the control program, dogs which had previously been forced to seek shelter in the boondocks reentered populated areas and were, in turn, themselves eliminated.

For Discussion, see page 391.

# Discussion*

ROSEN: Dr. Haddock commented on the large difference between the number of animals diagnosed as rabid by local laboratories in Guam and those confirmed at C.D.C. This was one of the things that led to confusion in Hawaii at the time and I wonder if he would comment further on the possible reasons for this phenomenon?

HADDOCK: First, let me say that only two animals were diagnosed as rabid by Guam laboratories; all the other "local" diagnoses were by laboratories in Hawaii. I am sure there are several possible reasons for the difference in the number of positive diagnoses reported. One that has been mentioned previously and may have been significant is the possibility of laboratory error. The FRA test, which was the one used on all of these specimens, is apparently not a test that can be conducted only once or twice a month as just one additional chore of already overworked laboratory personnel. It has to be practiced continually by the individual involved and I think that this may have been one of the problems encountered locally.

Another reason for this discrepancy is that a number of the specimens that were submitted to other labs and subsequently diagnosed as rabies positive, never did reach C.D.C. for confirmation. For this reason we can not strictly compare the number of positive cases reported by C.D.C. and the other labs. Some specimens did eventually reach C.D.C. but some were destroyed after being examined in the first laboratory.

ROSEN: Were the positive specimens that you referred to examined on Guam and if so, how many different laboratories were involved?

HADDOCK: We have records of only two specimens being tested on Guam during the epizootic. These were both shrews and both were called FRA positive by the U.S. Naval Hospital laboratory. We have no record of mouse inoculation tests being carried out on these

* This Discussion refers to the reports by Beran and Haddock.

specimens or of their being submitted to any other laboratory for further testing. The majority of the specimens from Guam were initially examined by Schofield Barracks (the U.S. Army laboratory in Hawaii). Some of these were, in turn, referred to the Hawaii Department of Agriculture or C.D.C. for confirmation. Of the specimens sent directly from Guam to C.D.C., two were FRA positive and one did yield apparent street rabies virus. Two other specimens examined first in Hawaii also contained apparent street rabies virus when subsequently examined in the C.D.C. laboratories.

DAVENPORT: I would like to ask two questions, one of each speaker. Were there special reasons why Oriental Province was selected for these studies and could you tell us a little more about the circumstances which led to selecting that area to begin this type of work? Dr. Haddock, I am a little confused by the numbers, but if you had 900 bites, as I understood, and 900 persons were treated for bites during this time interval with no human cases of rabies, and since no vaccination post-exposure treatment plan is perfect and there were no human deaths from rabies, one suspects that the true incidence of rabies in dogs on Guam must have been relatively low. I am not assuming there was no incidence, but I wonder what you consider the true incidence to be.

BERAN: Negros Oriental province is typical of the situation throughout the Philippines. The island is small enough that it is easy to work in; it has one of the best health services of any of the provinces; and it happens to be where I live.

HADDOCK: In reply to your question as to the true size of the Guam rabies epizootic, perhaps it did seem larger than it actually was. Although we would generally expect only a few of the affected animals to eventually reach the lab and be reported as rabid, there may have been conflicting factors at work. One factor which would have added to the number of animals apparently affected by the epizootic is the possibility of incorrect positive diagnoses. A conflicting factor, which would tend to lower the apparent size of the epizootic, would be those animals that may have run off into the boonies to die undetected. I do not know to which of these or other factors should be given the most weight.

BERAN: I would like to ask Dr. Haddock a question. If you had not come up with rabies in this one out of the twelve shrews, then it would have been much more difficult to evaluate the situation than it was. Is there any way that you can make some estimate as to how many animals of a species you really should examine per area or per estimated population so that there would be some kind of a working basis to go on?

HADDOCK: The problem of deciding what will constitute an adequate sample of a particular animal population from which valid epidemiologic conclusions may be drawn is a difficult one at best, and particularly so when dealing with a wild species. We have had a difficult time trying to decide how many dogs there are on Guam, let alone how many shrews. Under these circumstances it has been our policy to encourage the testing of any shrews that are seen in the daytime or otherwise behaving strangely. The same holds true for dogs; in general, we just test as many suspect animals as we can obtain.

JOHNSON, H. N.: I am still not clear as to how many and what species of animals were diagnosed as being rabid. First of all, do you do the mouse inoculation test at Guam at all? Do you use adult or infant mice for the inoculation? In the paper you mentioned 49 cats that died, and 20 of these had been vaccinated. Of the 20 that were vaccinated, how many were confirmed as having rabies by mouse inoculation? You mentioned 22 dogs that died and seven that were vaccinated; how many of those were confirmed as rabid by mouse inoculation? I think some people still are not clear as to whether one shrew was mouse inoculation test positive or negative. I understood it as being negative, so that you have yet to isolate a virus from a shrew.

HADDOCK: No mouse inoculation tests were conducted on Guam during the epizootic. Mouse inoculation was used at the Army laboratory in Hawaii and their reports indicate that the majority of their FRA positive specimens from Guam were confirmed by the mouse inoculation test. I do not know whether adult or infant mice were used in those tests.

SIKES: It is going to be difficult to get exact numbers, not knowing which to believe and which not to believe. It came out in the

Army investigation that there was a problem in Hawaii and because of this confusion about what you can or cannot believe from Hawaii labs the situation in Guam is confused because the diagnosis of most cases was done in the labs in Hawaii. The first diagnosis from Guam was confirmed. It was diagnosed in Hawaii and confirmed by Dr. John Stewart and Dr. Bob Kissling and our virus reference unit at C.D.C. A few others helped to convince us of the fact that there was at least some degree of rabies on Guam. But it is difficult to believe that all these dozens of cases, including vaccinated dogs, were truly positive. We must look at Jim Glosser's paper which was recently published in Public Health Reports, I believe, to find the ones he published as being confirmed outside Hawaii.

HUMPHREY: The 49 cat cases do not fit epidemiologically with the rest of the picture, either.

HAMMON: I think that quite a bit may be said tomorrow during the panel on pitfalls in the diagnosis of rabies, not only by Dr. Sikes but by myself, about some of the problems that occurred in the laboratories in Hawaii, where much of this material was sent. Attempting to discuss and to sort out, as Dr. Sikes has suggested, what was reliable and what was not reliable is just a waste of time, for there were many diagnoses called positive that many of us, investigating it later, were sure were not positive. But no satisfactory answers will ever be known. I think we should not discuss this further.

ROSEN: Before we leave this subject, I want to ask Dr. Haddock one question. He gave the number of cases in dogs per month and I believe that he said that these were dogs that died. Were these diagnoses based on clinical or laboratory findings?

HADDOCK: This was the composite laboratory report and was based solely on laboratory diagnoses. However, Dr. James Glosser, the U.S.P.H.S. veterinarian who was temporarily assigned to Guam while the epizootic was still in progress, reports that he observed at least one dog exhibiting classical signs of furious rabies.

SIKES: Dr. Haddock, you suggested that three of you share in some quarantine program and I am very much interested in that. I believe it was American Samoa, Guam and some other territory. Would you restate that and what you had in mind to share quarantine?

HADDOCK: At the present time, by intent rather than coincidence, Guam has rabies quarantine regulations that are almost identical to those of Hawaii. It is our hope that in the near future Hawaii will recognize Guam as a rabies-free area and extend reciprocity to us so far as rabies quarantine is concerned.

Although Dr. Willers (State Veterinarian, Hawaii) and I both believe that many of the other areas in the Pacific are indeed rabies-free (Samoa and the Trust Territory of the Pacific Islands, for instance), the problem has been that until recently they have not had rabies quarantine and control programs that could reasonably be depended on to prevent the entry of rabies or to detect and report its presence soon after it arrived. We would have been remiss in extending quarantine reciprocity to these areas in the past because of the danger of importing a rabies case from a supposedly rabies-free area. But I believe that in the near future it may be possible for all of these areas to have similar programs and to have rabies quarantine reciprocity with each other.

SIKES: Are you suggesting the operation of only the quarantine station in Hawaii, and not in Guam, or are you proposing three independent ones?

HADDOCK: I believe it will be necessary, due to political, economic and other problems, to have quarantine stations in each area.

JOHNSON, H. N.: I know it is a problem in a place like Guam to know how many dogs there are and what the normal mortality is, but I was wondering what you had done after this episode occurred to find out how many dogs were dying a day. Did you have any means to take a census, visiting homes, for example, to find out home by home what the dogs population might be. Do you have any evidence along this line?

HADDOCK: We have found conducting a population census to be very difficult and time consuming. In addition, even if you do manage to count all of the dogs in one specific area, there is no guarantee that the next day some of them would not be in a different area and counted again. Because of the difficulties and limitations inherent to the census method, we have come to depend almost exclusively on what we call the "Stray Dog Survey." Periodically counting the number of dogs seen running-large along a specified route gives us the information that we feel is most important: has the population most likely harboring and spreading the rabies virus (the stray and presumably unvaccinated dogs) undergone a relative increase or decrease. This method of population surveillance has the additional advantage of causing a minimum of disruption to normal routines and duties and we can afford to use it at frequent intervals.

One attempt that we did make at estimating the total dog population is shown on Table 4 of my report. In this case we used the unvaccinated/vaccinated ratio of those dogs actually tested for rabies to estimate the number of unvaccinated dogs on the island. This is a mathematical shortcut and is the nearest we have come to developing an accurate estimate of the total dog population.

Davenport: I would like to ask Dr. Beran another question. In Luzon there used to be two populations, the aborigines, I believe formerly called Igorot, and the Filippinos. Is it known how much trouble rabies has caused in the aboriginal population and do you anticipate that you might have greater difficulties in controlling dogs and the disease in that segment of the population?

Beran: This is no small problem. As rabies control progresses, it is going to be a real problem to get to the dogs in all of the small, isolated communities which lie at great distances from population centers. Yet these have to be reached. It is true that there is one rather large indigenous population on in Central Luzon, in the mountain area, to whom the dog is a true delicacy. These people would choose dog meat over other. Rabies is actually not a problem in that specific area, and the dog population is quite small. There are, however, other indigenous populations scattered throughout the islands; we have one in our province; and unfortunately rabies is present in many of these widely scattered areas. It is going to take a very real education program to reach these people. You get nowhere simply going in and vaccinating their dogs by force. The people must actually understand what you are doing in order to obtain their cooperation. Further it is not easy to educate these people because they speak so many different languages. There are 83 different languages and there are dialects of these languages. People are most responsive to a program if it is presented by one of the people who speak their own dialect perfectly. We have attempted to work with this problem by using vaccinating teams composed of three persons, one of whom always comes right from the specific village, one of whom is a government man who has been trained, and one more. The provincial government representative leads the team, but the local representative is the one who attempts to convince the people of the need for the vaccination campaign.

HADDOCK: Dr. Beran, you mentioned that in one instance the dog population was 9% of the human population in one area. I wonder what methods you have used and found most satisfactory to estimate the dog population?

BERAN: We have used a system of surveying the community by natural subunits of the community. Then we operate on a house-to-house basis to find out exactly how many dogs are owned by the people in the particular houses. We use these figures for estimating the dog population. Further, during our vaccination campaigns, we keep complete records so that later we can go back and see how accurate our estimates were. This has become a pretty accurate system now. In the urban communities in the provincial area, the figure of 9% of the human population is a good working figure, but the more rural the area, the sparser the population and the more numerous the dogs we find per 100 people, until we find as much as around 12.2% of the human population in these areas. If we went on a basis of 9% throughout our province, then we would be doing an inadequate job of vaccination in the rural areas.

HADDOCK: Do you feel this method adequately determines the number of stray dogs or do you feel that there are not really many stray dogs and that most of them are picked up by your house-to-house survey?

BERAN: Fortunately, when we are vaccinating dogs or when we are making dog census surveys in the more rural areas, the masters of the houses are probably out somewhere so we ask the people that are cooking in the kitchens or working on the premises. They are the ones who know exactly how many dogs there are at a particular house. In the rural areas, there really are not stray animals as you think of them in the western sense. In the urban areas, there are a few true stray dogs which live principally in the markets. After the day's work is done in the markets and the venders clean up, then the dogs come in and pick up what scraps they can find. Usually the people in the marketplace know how many stray dogs there are. In this type of community, it isn't difficult to actually count every dog.

# INDEX

**O**



**P**



**Q**



**R**

**S**